Phytochemicals in Cancer Chemoprevention and Treatment

Phytochemicals in Cancer Chemoprevention and Treatment

Guest Editors

Wojciech Trybus
Ewa Trybus
Aneta Węgierek-Ciuk

MDPI

Basel • Beijing • Wuhan • Barcelona • Belgrade • Novi Sad • Cluj • Manchester

Guest Editors
Wojciech Trybus
Department of Medical Biology
Jan Kochanowski University of Kielce
Kielce
Poland

Ewa Trybus
Department of Medical Biology
Jan Kochanowski University of Kielce
Kielce
Poland

Aneta Węgierek-Ciuk
Department of Medical Biology
Jan Kochanowski University of Kielce
Kielce
Poland

Editorial Office
MDPI AG
Grosspeteranlage 5
4052 Basel, Switzerland

This is a reprint of the Special Issue, published open access by the journal *Current Issues in Molecular Biology* (ISSN 1467-3045), freely accessible at: https://www.mdpi.com/journal/cimb/special_issues/FPTK7C396D.

For citation purposes, cite each article independently as indicated on the article page online and as indicated below:

Lastname, A.A.; Lastname, B.B. Article Title. *Journal Name* **Year**, *Volume Number*, Page Range.

ISBN 978-3-7258-5867-5 (Hbk)
ISBN 978-3-7258-5868-2 (PDF)
https://doi.org/10.3390/books978-3-7258-5868-2

Contents

About the Editors

Wojciech Trybus

Wojciech Trybus is an employee of the Department of Medical Biology at the Jan Kochanowski University in Kielce. His research focuses on assessing the potential anticancer properties of various cytostatic compounds, with a primary focus on anthraquinones (plant-derived compounds), against various cancer cell lines, primarily prostate and cervical cancer. His experiments also investigate the potential use of anthraquinones in combination therapy with inhibitors of autophagy and inhibitors of antiapoptotic protein Bcl-2. He has also co-authored articles evaluating the mechanisms of action of antihistamines for use in cancer therapy. His research includes assessing cytotoxicity and the potential ability of the tested compounds to induce various types of cell death, such as apoptosis and mitotic catastrophe. He also focuses on the effects of the phytochemicals studied on the lysosomal system, including autophagy and lysosomal cell death. To analyze changes in cancer cells, he uses various microscopic techniques, including fluorescence, confocal and transmission electron microscopy, which are additionally supplemented with biochemical and cytometric methods.

Ewa Trybus

Ewa Trybus is an employee of the Department of Medical Biology at the Jan Kochanowski University in Kielce. Her primary research focus is assessing changes in nasal mucosa cells under the influence of antiallergic drugs. Her in vitro studies identify the potential anticancer properties of antihistamines, highlighting their novel mechanisms of action and potential use in cancer therapy, in line with the strategy of repurposing old drugs. She also studies the effects of various plant compounds on cancer cells, assessing their anticancer potential. Her research focuses primarily on mechanisms related to the induction of cell death, such as apoptosis, autophagy, lysosomal cell death, and mitotic catastrophe. She utilizes a variety of research techniques, including fluorescence microscopy, confocal microscopy, and transmission electron microscopy, as well as biochemical methods and flow cytometry.

Aneta Węgierek-Ciuk

Aneta Węgierek-Ciuk is a researcher at Jan Kochanowski University in Kielce, Poland. Her scientific interests center on the biological effects of ionizing radiation, with a particular focus on natural radiosensitizers and nanomaterials in both normal and cancer cells. She focuses on protoberberine alkaloids, mainly coralyne, as potential radiosensitizing agents in cancer therapy. Dr. Węgierek-Ciuk has also conducted research on intrinsic radiosensitivity, emphasizing predictive and prognostic assays of individual patients' radiosensitivity. She has extensive expertise in in vitro cell culture, molecular biology, genotoxicity, and cytotoxicity. She specialized in flow cytometry, comet assays, micronucleus assays, chromosomal aberrations, fluorescence microscopy, and cell viability assays. Dr. Węgierek-Ciuk is also actively engaged in academic teaching and public science communication. She is the author and co-author of numerous peer-reviewed publications and is an active participant in international scientific collaborations.

current issues in molecular biology

MDPI

Editorial

Editorial for Special Issue "Phytochemicals in Cancer Chemoprevention and Treatment"

Wojciech Trybus *, Ewa Trybus * and Aneta Węgierek-Ciuk

Department of Medical Biology, Jan Kochanowski University of Kielce, Uniwersytecka 7, 25-406 Kielce, Poland; aneta.wegierek-ciuk@ujk.edu.pl

* Correspondence: wojciech.trybus@ujk.edu.pl (W.T.); ewa.trybus@ujk.edu.pl (E.T.); Tel.: +41-349-63-01 (W.T. & E.T.)

Despite significant progress in the treatment of cancer patients, modern oncological therapy faces numerous challenges that are primarily related to the lack of response to treatment caused by the resistance of cancer cells to chemotherapeutics. Another major problem is the emerging toxicity of therapy and its associated side effects. Hence, new, alternative treatments and compounds with anticancer potential are constantly sought. Phytochemicals found in plants, for example, and are currently being studied for their anticancer properties. The aim of this Special Issue was to present a range of compounds with anticancer potential in various experimental approaches to show their possible use in cancer treatments.

1. Introduction

According to statistics from the International Agency for Research on Cancer (IARC), nearly 20 million new cancer cases and 9.7 million cancer-related deaths were reported in 2022. It is estimated that about one in five people will develop cancer during their lifetime, while about one in nine men and one in 12 women will die from it. According to the forecast based on demographic data, the number of new cancer cases will reach 35 million by 2050 [1], which is a very serious social problem. The results of clinical and epidemiological studies clearly indicate that the principal factor contributing to the development and prevention of cancer is lifestyle. An incorrect diet, lack of physical activity, alcohol consumption, and smoking are the main factors inducing an increase in the incidence of various types of cancer [2].

The main methods to treat cancer are chemotherapy and radiotherapy supplemented by surgery, which, despite their constant use, also cause numerous side effects [3]. The main disadvantages of chemotherapy are possible cancer recurrences and toxic effects on non-targeted tissues, which in turn may limit the use of anticancer drugs and worsen the patient's quality of life. Another significant cause of anticancer therapy failure is the innate and acquired resistance of cancer cells regulated, among others, by genetic and epigenetic factors that allow cancer cells to survive [4]. The basic feature of cancer cells is their ability to avoid the process of apoptosis, which results from the deregulation of molecular pathways contributing to the development of multidrug resistance. This applies to Bcl-2 family proteins, the p53 tumor suppressor, the overexpression of IAP controlling the activation of caspases, and the PI3K/AKT pathway, among others [5].

Therefore, new and alternative treatments and new groups of compounds with anticancer potential are sought, an example of which are numerous phytochemicals. The attempt to draw attention to the use of plant compounds in oncological therapy results from the fact that numerous studies have highlighted their anticancer properties [3], and herbal medicine is one of the oldest forms of therapy that has developed all over the world [6,7]. An example is Traditional Chinese Medicine, the oldest field in which recognizing the use of herbs for medicinal purposes is Materia Medica, which includes over 1800 entries with over 11,000 formulas providing full information about their medicinal use [7].

Over the years, many compounds have been isolated from plants that have become extremely important to medicine. Some key examples include taxoids and taxol, discovered in the 1960s and 1970s, isolated from the bark of *Taxus brevifolia*, which remains one of the most effective methods of treating breast and ovarian cancer [8]. Another example is the alkaloid camptothecin, isolated from the bark of *Camptotheca acuminata*, whose anticancer effect is based on the inhibition of topoisomerase I [9]. Another breakthrough was the discovery of the *Vinca* alkaloids in the 1960s, i.e., vinblastine and vincristine, which have made an equally substantial contribution to oncological therapy. Vincristine is a chemotherapeutic drug used to treat acute lymphoblastic leukemia, Hodgkin's and non-Hodgkin's lymphomas, Wilms' tumor, rhabdomyosarcomas, retinoblastoma, neuroblastoma, and various brain tumors. Its analog, vinblastine, is used in chemotherapy for Hodgkin's lymphoma, Langerhans cell histiocytosis, and brain gliomas [10].

According to Choudhari et al. (2020), clinical trials on the use of phytochemicals in anticancer therapy are currently focusing on three aspects: improving the response of cancer cells to standard chemo- and radiotherapy, reducing the serious side effects of standard therapy, and looking for undesirable interactions with standard therapy [11].

2. Selected Phytochemicals with Anticancer Properties

In this summary, we focus on several groups of phytochemicals to highlight their potential anticancer properties. An example of compounds whose anticancer properties have been demonstrated in numerous literature reports are alkaloids, which are the main bioactive chemical components of the Berberis species responsible for various pharmacological effects of both the whole extract and isolated single compounds [12]. The most well-known alkaloid with anticancer effects is berberine, the mechanism of which is based on scavenging free radicals, inducing apoptosis, blocking the cell cycle, or inhibiting angiogenesis, among others [13].

In the study by Miłek et al. (2024), it was demonstrated that extracts from ornamental barberry twigs, compared to pure berberine sulfate administered in an analogous dose, present greater cytotoxicity towards HaCaT, A375, and Caco-2 cell lines. At the same time, the team showed that ornamental barberry twigs, easier to obtain with the controlled cultivation of this plant than common barberry roots, can be used as a raw material for the isolation of berberine for the pharmaceutical industry [14].

Magnolia-derived lignans, such as honokiol and magnolol, may prove to be effective compounds in treating patients with head and neck squamous cell carcinoma. A study by Klesz et al. (2024) confirmed that these compounds can limit the viability of cancer cells by regulating the cell cycle and apoptosis, which are probably related to changes in the expression level of BIRC5 and CDKN1A. It is also interesting that the tested compounds showed cytotoxicity in FaDu cisplatin persister cells, which is key to overcoming chemoresistance [15].

Statistics show that cervical cancer accounts for 70% of all cancer cases. In 2018, more than 560,000 new cases of cervical cancer were diagnosed worldwide, with more than 300,000 resulting in death. Of these, more than 80% occurred in low- and middle-income countries, such as South Africa, India, China, and Brazil, with the main contributing factor to the development of cervical cancer being infection with the sexually transmitted human papillomavirus [16].

Hence, it is important to pay attention to new methods of treatment, including the use of compounds with significant anticancer activity in relation to this type of cancer. An example is cacalol acetate, which is a derivative of cacalol, a sesquiterpene isolated from *Psacalium decompositum*. Rostro-Alonso and colleagues (2024) were the first to prove that this derivative has cytotoxic, antiproliferative, proapoptotic, and antimigratory effects in relation to the HeLa cell line studied [17].

Alaouna et al. (2024) demonstrated the efficacy of the South African plant *Tulbaghia violacea* in the treatment of metastatic triple-negative breast cancer (TNBC) [18]. This is an interesting report since TNBC is most often an invasive high-grade ductal carcinoma, which is characterized by an aggressive clinical phenotype and lack of estrogen and progesterone receptor expression and human epidermal growth factor receptor 2 (HER2) expression. It is also one of the most common subtypes of breast cancer in women with mutations in the BRCA1 gene [19,20]. It was shown that an aqueous extract containing anticancer compounds (DDMP, 1,2,4-triazine-3,5(2H,4H)-dione, vanillin, schizandrin, taurolidine and α-pinene) affected the adhesion, invasion, and migration of MCF-10A and MDA-MB-231 cell lines. Alterations in genes related to angiogenesis, metastasis, and proliferation were also demonstrated, with reduced activity in growth receptor signaling, angiogenesis, and cancer-related pathways (Wnt, Notch and PI3K pathways), which is highly relevant in the development of therapeutics targeting TNBC metastases [18].

Ashwagandha (*Withania somnifera* L. Dunal), in which withaferin A and withanolides are considered promising anticancer compounds, also shows great promise in the treatment of breast cancer, especially with estrogen receptor/progesterone receptor (ER/PR)-positive and triple-negative breast cancer [21]. Numerous studies also indicate its anti-inflammatory, antimicrobial, cardioprotective, and antidiabetic properties [22].

Anticancer therapy can also be supplemented by alternative medicinal compounds obtained from marine flora, an example of which are micro- and macroalgae containing various types of bioactive molecules, including carotenoids and various forms of polysaccharides with anticancer activity, which act by inducing apoptosis and inhibiting the cell cycle and proliferation [23]. The interest in microalgae stems from the fact that they are a component of the daily diet and a food additive, mainly in East Asian countries. Active metabolites of algae known for their anticancer and biocidal effects are also of great interest [24]. Algae are also a source of antioxidant compounds, including carotenoids, vitamins, and phenolics, used not only in medicine but also in other branches of the pharmaceutical industry [25].

Compounds with high anticancer potential also include polysaccharides, which differ from each other in both structure and toxicity profile [26]. An example is the extracellular polysaccharides (EPS) studied by Toshkova-Yotova et al. (2024) isolated from a new Bulgarian strain of the green microalga *Coelastrella* sp. BGV, which show anticancer activity in cervical and breast cancer cells based on the induction of apoptosis, inhibition of the cell cycle, and antiproliferative activity demonstrated in a wound healing test. Interestingly, the authors did not demonstrate any cytotoxic effect on normal cells (BALB/3T3 and HaCaT lines); hence, they conclude that this new microalgae strain, as a source of EPS with selective anticancer activity, should be studied in terms of its pharmacological and biotechnological potential [27].

Numerous studies have shown that polyphenols are also phytochemicals found in many plant-based diets with chemopreventive effects on various cancers. Interest in these compounds is constantly growing because studies indicate a link between a diet rich in soy and cancer avoidance, which has been linked to the presence of genistein—a phenolic component of soy [28]. Preclinical studies have shown multidirectional effects of genistein based on antioxidant, anti-inflammatory, antibacterial, and antiviral properties, and its mechanism of anticancer action has been described on many cancer cell lines [29]. However, Banyś et al. (2024) have shown that supplementation of animals with genistein in macro, micro, and nano forms increases the intensity of the neoplastic process, the level of metalloproteinase-9, and the expression of the MMP-9 gene, and significantly reduces the level of eicosanoids (HETEs, HODE, and HEPE) [30]. Also, a study by Ju et al. suggests that consuming genistein-containing products may be dangerous for postmenopausal women with estrogen-dependent breast cancer. Genistein has been shown to act in an additive manner at low levels of 17β-estradiol, stimulating estrogen-dependent tumor growth in vivo [31].

The use of an appropriate diet may also affect the activity of key multidrug resistance transporters (MRP2, BCRP, and P-gp) influencing the effects of chemotherapy. According to Brodzicka et al. (2024), such phytochemicals include catechins, flavonoids, resveratrol, curcumin, terpenoids, sterols, and alkaloids, which, by modulating the activity of MDR transporters, impact the effectiveness of chemotherapy. The authors conclude that, in the context of improving treatment results and reducing side effects, attention should be paid to the interaction between diet and the drugs used in cancer therapy [32].

Another group of biologically active compounds are ribosomally synthesized and post-translationally modified peptides (RiPP) from plants. In their review, Hwang et al. (2024) paid special attention to rubipodanin A and mallotumide A–C, which exhibit low nanomolar IC50 values against many types of cancer cells and emphasize the importance of plant RiPP in developing innovative methods of cancer treatment [33].

Rosmarinic acid, apigenin, and thymoquinone also have chemopreventive potential, inhibiting the growth of cancer cells and modulating key signaling pathways involved in cancer development [34].

Therefore, there is a constant need to study new groups of plant compounds for their anticancer properties and analyze and discover their mechanisms of action in both in vitro and in vivo systems to develop new drugs with anticancer properties.

When discovering drugs based on plant products, attention should be paid to many important factors, including the availability and effectiveness of the plant material or the compound being tested, the ability to modify the structure, the molecule size, the stability of the compounds, and their toxicity [35]. Hence, molecular-level studies are important to determining the chemical components of plants, their chemical configuration, the process of biosynthesis and degradation, natural distribution, or bioactivity [36]. However, the main problem in the research on phytochemicals at the molecular level is the lack of a complete understanding of their interactions with various signaling molecules, which can be overcome by using techniques such as molecular docking, QSAR modeling (Quantitative structure–activity relationship model), or cross-linked pharmacology. Additionally, the use of LC-MS and LC-NMR techniques can significantly contribute to accelerating the identification of compounds [11], and thus the possibility of using phytochemicals as new drugs.

3. Conclusions

In this Special Issue of the journal *Current Issues in Molecular Biology*, the latest research on various phytochemicals with potential anticancer properties is collected and their mechanism of action is presented both in vitro and in vivo. We hope that the presented results and data included in the review articles will make a significant contribution to the development of modern phytotherapy and will encourage further research on the presented phytochemicals for their future use in oncology.

Author Contributions: Conceptualization, W.T. and E.T.; writing—original draft preparation, W.T., E.T. and A.W.-C.; writing—review and editing, W.T., E.T. and A.W.-C. All authors have read and agreed to the published version of the manuscript.

Conflicts of Interest: The authors declare no conflicts of interest.

References

1. Bray, F.; Laversanne, M.; Sung, H.; Ferlay, J.; Siegel, R.L.; Soerjomataram, I.; Jemal, A. Global cancer statistics 2022: GLOBOCAN estimates of incidence and mortality worldwide for 36 cancers in 185 countries. *CA Cancer J. Clin.* **2024**, *74*, 229–263. [CrossRef] [PubMed]
2. Marino, P.; Mininni, M.; Deiana, G.; Marino, G.; Divella, R.; Bochicchio, I.; Giuliano, A.; Lapadula, S.; Lettini, A.R.; Sanseverino, F. Healthy Lifestyle and Cancer Risk: Modifiable Risk Factors to Prevent Cancer. *Nutrients* **2024**, *16*, 800. [CrossRef] [PubMed]
3. Mandal, M.K.; Mohammad, M.; Parvin, S.I.; Islam, M.M.; Gazi, H.A.R. A Short Review on Anticancer Phytochemicals. *Phcog. Rev.* **2023**, *17*, 11–23. [CrossRef]
4. Khan, S.U.; Fatima, K.; Aisha, S.; Malik, F. Unveiling the mechanisms and challenges of cancer drug resistance. *Cell Commun. Signal.* **2024**, *22*, 109. [CrossRef]
5. Neophytou, C.M.; Trougakos, I.P.; Erin, N.; Papageorgis, P. Apoptosis Deregulation and the Development of Cancer Multi-Drug Resistance. *Cancers* **2021**, *13*, 4363. [CrossRef]
6. Zimmermann-Klemd, A.M.; Reinhardt, J.K.; Winker, M.; Grundemann, C. Phytotherapy in Integrative Oncology-An Update of Promising Treatment Options. *Molecules* **2022**, *27*, 3209. [CrossRef]
7. Lemonnier, N.; Zhou, G.-B.; Prasher, B.; Mukerji, M.; Chen, Z.; Brahmachari, S.K.; Noble, D.; Auffray, C.; Sagner, M. Traditional Knowledge-based Medicine: A Review of History, Principles, and Relevance in the Present Context of P4 Systems Medicine. *Progrevmed* **2017**, *2*, e0011. [CrossRef]
8. Cech, N.B.; Oberlies, N.H. From plant to cancer drug: Lessons learned from the discovery of taxol. *Nat. Prod. Rep.* **2023**, *40*, 1153–1157. [CrossRef]
9. Khaiwa, N.; Maarouf, N.R.; Darwish, M.H.; Alhamad, D.W.M.; Sebastian, A.; Hamad, M.; Omar, H.A.; Orive, G.; Al-Tel, T.H. Camptothecin's journey from discovery to WHO Essential Medicine: Fifty years of promise. *Eur. J. Med. Chem.* **2021**, *223*, 113639. [CrossRef]
10. Taub, J.W.; Buck, S.A.; Xavier, A.C.; Edwards, H.; Matherly, L.H.; Ge, Y. The evolution and history of Vinca alkaloids: From the Big Bang to the treatment of pediatric acute leukemia. *Pediatr. Blood Cancer* **2024**, *71*, e31247. [CrossRef]
11. Choudhari, A.S.; Mandave, P.C.; Deshpande, M.; Ranjekar, P.; Prakash, O. Phytochemicals in Cancer Treatment: From Preclinical Studies to Clinical Practice. *Front. Pharmacol.* **2019**, *10*, 1614. [CrossRef]
12. Belwal, T.; Bisht, A.; Devkota, H.P.; Ullah, H.; Khan, H.; Pandey, A.; Bhatt, I.D.; Echeverria, J. Phytopharmacology and Clinical Updates of Berberis Species Against Diabetes and Other Metabolic Diseases. *Front. Pharmacol.* **2020**, *11*, 41. [CrossRef] [PubMed]
13. Almatroodi, S.A.; Alsahli, M.A.; Rahmani, A.H. Berberine: An Important Emphasis on Its Anticancer Effects through Modulation of Various Cell Signaling Pathways. *Molecules* **2022**, *27*, 5889. [CrossRef] [PubMed]
14. Milek, M.; Dzugan, M.; Pienkowska, N.; Galiniak, S.; Molon, M.; Litwinczuk, W. Ornamental Barberry Twigs as an Underexploited Source of Berberine-Rich Extracts-Preliminary Research. *Curr. Issues Mol. Biol.* **2024**, *46*, 13193–13208. [CrossRef]
15. Kleszcz, R.; Dorna, D.; Stawny, M.; Paluszczak, J. Honokiol Is More Potent than Magnolol in Reducing Head and Neck Cancer Cell Growth. *Curr. Issues Mol. Biol.* **2024**, *46*, 10731–10744. [CrossRef]
16. Hull, R.; Mbele, M.; Makhafola, T.; Hicks, C.; Wang, S.M.; Reis, R.M.; Mehrotra, R.; Mkhize-Kwitshana, Z.; Kibiki, G.; Bates, D.O.; et al. Cervical cancer in low and middle-income countries. *Oncol. Lett.* **2020**, *20*, 2058–2074. [CrossRef]
17. Rostro-Alonso, G.O.; Castillo-Montoya, A.I.; Garcia-Acosta, J.C.; Aguilar-Llanos, E.F.; Quintas-Granados, L.I.; Villegas-Vazquez, E.Y.; Garcia-Aguilar, R.; Porras-Vazquez, S.A.; Bustamante-Montes, L.P.; Alvarado-Sansininea, J.J.; et al. Cacalol Acetate as Anticancer Agent: Antiproliferative, Pro-Apoptotic, Cytostatic, and Anti-Migratory Effects. *Curr. Issues Mol. Biol.* **2024**, *46*, 9298–9311. [CrossRef]
18. Alaouna, M.; Hull, R.; Molefi, T.; Khanyile, R.; Mbodi, L.; Luvhengo, T.E.; Chauke-Malinga, N.; Phakathi, B.; Penny, C.; Dlamini, Z. Exploring Water-Soluble South African Tulbaghia violacea Harv Extract as a Therapeutic Approach for Triple-Negative Breast Cancer Metastasis. *Curr. Issues Mol. Biol.* **2024**, *46*, 10806–10828. [CrossRef]
19. O'Reilly, D.; Sendi, M.A.; Kelly, C.M. Overview of recent advances in metastatic triple negative breast cancer. *World J. Clin. Oncol.* **2021**, *12*, 164–182. [CrossRef]
20. Perou, C.M.; Sorlie, T.; Eisen, M.B.; van de Rijn, M.; Jeffrey, S.S.; Rees, C.A.; Pollack, J.R.; Ross, D.T.; Johnsen, H.; Akslen, L.A.; et al. Molecular portraits of human breast tumours. *Nature* **2000**, *406*, 747–752. [CrossRef]
21. Kolodziejska, R.; Tafelska-Kaczmarek, A.; Pawluk, M.; Sergot, K.; Pisarska, L.; Wozniak, A.; Pawluk, H. Ashwagandha-Induced Programmed Cell Death in the Treatment of Breast Cancer. *Curr. Issues Mol. Biol.* **2024**, *46*, 7668–7685. [CrossRef]

22. Mikulska, P.; Malinowska, M.; Ignacyk, M.; Szustowski, P.; Nowak, J.; Pesta, K.; Szelag, M.; Szklanny, D.; Judasz, E.; Kaczmarek, G.; et al. Ashwagandha (*Withania somnifera*)-Current Research on the Health-Promoting Activities: A Narrative Review. *Pharmaceutics* **2023**, *15*, 1057. [CrossRef] [PubMed]
23. Abd El-Hack, M.E.; Abdelnour, S.; Alagawany, M.; Abdo, M.; Sakr, M.A.; Khafaga, A.F.; Mahgoub, S.A.; Elnesr, S.S.; Gebriel, M.G. Microalgae in modern cancer therapy: Current knowledge. *Biomed. Pharmacother.* **2019**, *111*, 42–50. [CrossRef] [PubMed]
24. Hamouda, R.A.; Abd El Latif, A.; Elkaw, E.M.; Alotaibi, A.S.; Alenzi, A.M.; Hamza, H.A. Assessment of Antioxidant and Anticancer Activities of Microgreen Alga Chlorella vulgaris and Its Blend with Different Vitamins. *Molecules* **2022**, *27*, 1602. [CrossRef]
25. Munir, N.; Sharif, N.; Naz, S.; Manzoor, F. Algae: A potent antioxidant source. *SJMR* **2013**, *1*, 22–31.
26. Fedorov, S.N.; Ermakova, S.P.; Zvyagintseva, T.N.; Stonik, V.A. Anticancer and cancer preventive properties of marine polysaccharides: Some results and prospects. *Mar. Drugs* **2013**, *11*, 4876–4901. [CrossRef] [PubMed]
27. Toshkova-Yotova, T.; Sulikovska, I.; Djeliova, V.; Petrova, Z.; Ognyanov, M.; Denev, P.; Toshkova, R.; Georgieva, A. Exopolysaccharides from the Green Microalga Strain Coelastrella sp. BGV-Isolation, Characterization, and Assessment of Anticancer Potential. *Curr. Issues Mol. Biol.* **2024**, *46*, 10312–10334. [CrossRef]
28. Naeema, H.; Momala, U.; Imranb, M.; Shahbaza, M.; Hussain, M.; Alsagabyd, S.A.; Abdulmoneme, W.A.; Umarc, M.; Mujtabaf, A.; El-Ghorabg, A.H.; et al. Anticancer perspectives of genistein: A comprehensive review. *Int. J. Food Prop.* **2023**, *26*, 3305–3341. [CrossRef]
29. Sharifi-Rad, J.; Quispe, C.; Imran, M.; Rauf, A.; Nadeem, M.; Gondal, T.A.; Ahmad, B.; Atif, M.; Mubarak, M.S.; Sytar, O.; et al. Genistein: An Integrative Overview of Its Mode of Action, Pharmacological Properties, and Health Benefits. *Oxid. Med. Cell Longev.* **2021**, *2021*, 3268136. [CrossRef]
30. Banys, K.; Jelinska, M.; Wrzosek, M.; Skrajnowska, D.; Wrzesien, R.; Bielecki, W.; Bobrowska-Korczak, B. Inflammation Factors and Genistein Supplementation in Cancer-Preliminary Research. *Curr. Issues Mol. Biol.* **2024**, *46*, 2166–2180. [CrossRef]
31. Ju, Y.H.; Allred, K.F.; Allred, C.D.; Helferich, W.G. Genistein stimulates growth of human breast cancer cells in a novel, postmenopausal animal model, with low plasma estradiol concentrations. *Carcinogenesis* **2006**, *27*, 1292–1299. [CrossRef] [PubMed]
32. Brodzicka, A.; Galanty, A.; Pasko, P. Modulation of Multidrug Resistance Transporters by Food Components and Dietary Supplements: Implications for Cancer Therapy Efficacy and Safety. *Curr. Issues Mol. Biol.* **2024**, *46*, 9686–9706. [CrossRef] [PubMed]
33. Hwang, H.J.; Nam, Y.; Jang, C.; Kim, E.; Jang, E.S.; Lee, Y.J.; Lee, S.R. Anticancer Ribosomally Synthesized and Post-Translationally Modified Peptides from Plants: Structures, Therapeutic Potential, and Future Directions. *Curr. Issues Mol. Biol.* **2024**, *47*, 6. [CrossRef] [PubMed]
34. Abutayeh, R.F.; Altah, M.; Mehdawi, A.; Al-Ataby, I.; Ardakani, A. Chemopreventive Agents from Nature: A Review of Apigenin, Rosmarinic Acid, and Thymoquinone. *Curr. Issues Mol. Biol.* **2024**, *46*, 6600–6619. [CrossRef]
35. Anywar, G.; Namukobe, J. Chapter 2—Factors affecting the choice for plant-based products in drug discoveries. In *Phytochemicals as Lead Compounds for New Drug Discovery*; Egbuna, C., Shashank Kumar, S.K., Eds.; Elsevier: Amsterdam, The Netherlands, 2020; pp. 15–24.
36. Sinha, D.; Odoh, U.E.; Ganguly, S.; Muhammad, M.; Chatterjee, M.; Chikeokwu, I.; Egbuna, C. Chapter 1—Phytochemistry, history, and progress in drug discovery. In *Phytochemistry, Computational Tools and Databases in Drug Discovery*; Elsevier: Amsterdam, The Netherlands, 2023; pp. 1–26.

current issues in
molecular biology

MDPI

Article

Ornamental Barberry Twigs as an Underexploited Source of Berberine-Rich Extracts—Preliminary Research

Michał Miłek [1], Małgorzata Dżugan [1,*], Natalia Pieńkowska [2], Sabina Galiniak [2], Mateusz Mołoń [3] and Wojciech Litwińczuk [4]

1 Department of Chemistry and Food Toxicology, Institute of Food Technology and Nutrition, University of Rzeszow, Ćwiklińskiej 1a, 35-601 Rzeszow, Poland; mmilek@ur.edu.pl
2 Institute of Medical Sciences, University of Rzeszow, Warzywna 1a, 35-310 Rzeszow, Poland; npienkowska@ur.edu.pl (N.P.); sgaliniak@ur.edu.pl (S.G.)
3 Institute of Biology, University of Rzeszow, Zelwerowicza 4, 35-601 Rzeszow, Poland; mmolon@ur.edu.pl
4 Department of Physiology and Plant Biotechnology, Institute of Agricultural Sciences, Environment Management and Protection, University of Rzeszow, Ćwiklińskiej 2, 35-601 Rzeszow, Poland; wlitwinczuk@ur.edu.pl
* Correspondence: mdzugan@ur.edu.pl; Tel.: +48-178721619

Abstract: Berberine is a natural substance obtained from the roots of common barberry which, due to its strong pharmacological activity, is a commonly tested ingredient of dietary supplements. However, ornamental barberries, which are widely available, have not been considered as a source of berberine so far. The research aimed to check whether the ornamental barberry leaves and twigs could be used as an easily accessible raw material for obtaining natural berberine-rich extract with biological activity. Twigs and leaves of seven cultivars of ornamental barberry extracts were assessed for their polyphenol content, antioxidant potential (FRAP and DPPH), and berberine content using high-performance thin layer chromatography (HPTLC). As a reference, commercially available roots of *Berberis vulgaris* were used. For the next step, selected extracts (two with high and two with low berberine content) were tested on three cell lines (HaCaT, A375, Caco-2) using neutral red assay, and pure berberine sulfate (1–100 μg mL^{-1}) was used as a control. Although the antioxidant potential of aqueous–methanol extracts of tested barberry was higher for the leaves than for the twigs, the berberine content was determined only in the twig extracts (from 42 to 676 mg 100 g^{-1}). Studies on cell lines have shown the general toxicity of barberry extracts, but the observed effect was not directly correlated with the content of the alkaloid. However, the extract showed greater activity compared to an analogous dose of pure berberine, suggesting a significant effect of the matrix composition. For the first time, it was shown that the twigs of selected cultivars of ornamental barberry can be considered as a promising berberine source for the pharmaceutical industry to develop new effective formulations. However, these findings require further studies.

Keywords: berberine; ornamental barberry; twigs; polyphenols; HPTLC; anticancer

1. Introduction

A large genus of barberry (*Berberis* sp.) includes approximately 400–450 species of deciduous and evergreen shrubs found in Europe, America, and Africa [1,2]. Only one species—European (common) barberry (*B. vulgaris* L.) grows wild in Poland. It is also common in Europe, North Africa, the Middle East, and Central Asia [2]. However, it is of no great importance in horticulture (and as an alternative crop) as it is susceptible to fungal diseases, including rust and powdery mildew. What is worse, it is the primary host of *Puccinia graminis* Pers. which causes a cereal disease called stalk rust of cereals and grasses [3,4]. Other species, among others Thunberg's barberry (*B. thunbergii* DC.), are not as susceptible to diseases and offered as ornamental plants in hundreds of cultivars with varied shapes, growth strength, and colorful leaves (different shades and combinations of yellow, green, and red). It is well known that the color of leaves is related to the presence of various polyphenols and carotenoids. Flavonoids and phenolic acids are present in leaves and flowers, while fruits are abundant in anthocyanins [5]. More than 20 alkaloids (including berberine, palmatine, oxyberberine, isocoridine, lambertine, berbamine, jatrrorhizine) were found in the barberry plant [2,5]. Chemically, they belong to the groups of protoberberine, isoquinoline, and bisbenzylisoquinoline alkaloids [5]. Both groups of secondary metabolites have various properties beneficial for medicinal uses. The main areas of ethnomedical applications were the territories of present-day China, India, Turkey, and Iran [6]. The traditionally used effects of barberry preparations include cholagogue, stomachic, laxative, diaphoretic, antipyretic, and antiseptic. They were also used for skin problems, hemorrhoids, and varicose veins [1,5]. Modern pharmacological studies confirm the antidiabetic, anti-inflammatory, wound-healing, anti-allergic, immunomodulatory, hepatoprotective, and anticancer effects of barberry. It also has strong antioxidant and antimicrobial effects [5,7]. Barberry also plays a role in the food industry as a source of fruit used to produce drinks, liqueurs, sauces, desserts, and jellies [6].

The main bioactive substance of barberry, named after this plant, is berberine (Figure 1). It is classified as an isoquinoline alkaloid. In addition to the *Berberis* genus, it is also present in other plants from the Annonaceae, Papaveraceae, Menispermaceae, Ranunculaceae, and Rutaceae families [8]. The other genera and species of plants containing this alkaloid include, among others, *Annickia* sp., *Jeffersonia diphylla*, *Mahonia* sp., *Tinospora sinensis*, *Agremone* sp., *Chelidonium majus*, *Corydalis* sp., *Papaver* sp., *Coptis* sp., *Hydrastis canadensis*, and *Phyllodendron* sp. [8]. Berberine can be extracted from plant material using various techniques, most commonly using methanol, ethanol, chloroform, and other solvent mixtures [8]. Pure berberine can be obtained from extracts by lowering the pH through the addition of concentrated acid (hydrochloric or sulfuric) and cooling to cause crystallization [9]. In dietary supplements, it is most often used in the salt form as chloride or sulfate, with better solubility in water [10]. Moreover, due to extremely low berberine bioavailability, various nano-carriers and enhancers are applied [10,11]. Various analytical techniques have been used to determine berberine in plant material or drug preparation (HPLC, TLC, Capillary electrophoresis, GC-MS, colorimetry), among them TLC is distinguished by low cost, ease of implementation, good accuracy and stability [10].

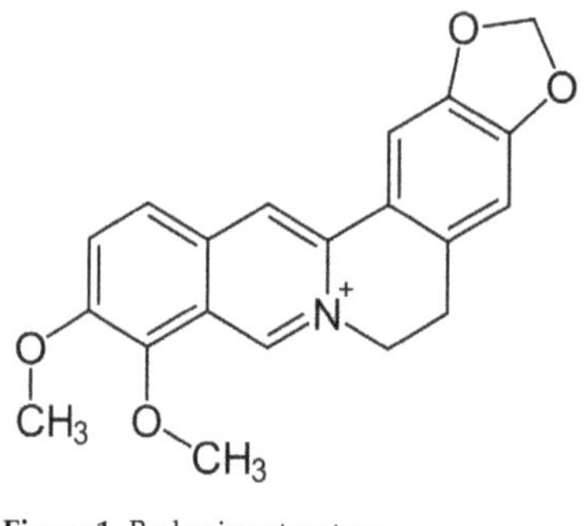

Figure 1. Berberine structure.

In addition to berberine and other alkaloids, polyphenols constitute an important group of barberry phytochemical components: flavonoids (luteolin, isorhamnetin and quercetin derivatives) as well as anthocyanins (peonidin, cyanidin, petunidin, malvidin, leonidin and their derivatives) [1]. Barberry fruits also contain carotenoids [1]. The HPTLC technique, a more advanced version of thin layer chromatography, is increasingly used to analyze phytochemical profiles of plant extracts, as it allows for direct comparison of up to 20 samples on one chromatographic plate [10,12,13].

Berberine, in addition to its antioxidant and antimicrobial effects, also exhibits immunomodulatory, cardioprotective, hepatoprotective, and renoprotective effects [8,14,15].

It is used in cardiovascular and digestive diseases, diabetes, and skin problems. Several possible mechanisms for lowering blood glucose levels have been identified [8]. Also, several mechanisms of the anticancer action of this alkaloid have been identified, including inducing cell cycle arrest, inhibition of telomerase, induction of apoptosis, induction of anti-inflammatory cytokines, inhibition of angiogenesis, and ROS-mediated mechanisms [8,16]. Great hopes are attached to its use in the treatment of neurodegenerative diseases [17,18]. Due to this, new sources of berberine are being sought, and attempts are being made to synthesize it and its analogs with potential pharmacological activity [19–23]. The bioactivity of berberine is assessed primarily in vitro on cell lines, but many clinical trials have already been conducted [24]. According to market reports, the global berberine market, mainly for dietary supplements, pharmaceutical and cosmetic industry, was estimated at USD 852.3 million in 2023 and is expected to grow to USD 1845.4 million in 2033, with a CAGR of 8.9% during the forecast period from 2024 to 2033 [25]. Taking into account such data, the search for new sources of this bioactive substance is economically justified.

The wealth of bioactive compounds is contained not only in easily accessible fruits but also in the leaves, twigs, and roots of barberries. More and more often, the acquisition of these raw materials is abandoned due to the significant reduction in the population of wild barberry [26]. The question arises whether the leafy twigs of ornamental barberry can be considered as good source of berberine as the roots of *B. vulgaris*. Thus, the work aimed to select ornamental cultivars of barberry that would be a more efficient and cheaper source of berberine, and at the same time, its cultivation would be safer for crops than common barberry. To our knowledge, this is the first time that twigs and leaves of selected ornamental barberry varieties have been studied. Initial studies have focused on assessing the bioactivity of full extracts from the tested plant materials.

2. Materials and Methods

2.1. Plant Material

The plant samples (several-month-old twigs, of 10–50 cm length and max 8 mm diameter) were manually collected from the central part of three healthy shrubs of each clone at the end of September (before mass fruit ripening). The 7-year barberry (*Berberis* sp.) shrubs were growing in the light shade in the private collection of Wiesław Więcek Nursery of Ornamental Trees and Shrubs (Stobierna 38, 36-002 Jasionka, Poland; 50.143, 22.072). Most of the clones belonged to the *Berberis thunbergii*, two to the *Berberis koreana*, and one was an interspecific (*B. thunbergii* × *B. vulgaris*) hybrid (Table 1). They differed in shrub growth intensity and shape, and mainly in the color of the leaves, from yellow through green, red to purple. The color of the leaves may have changed during the growing season.

Table 1. Characterization of used *Berberis* spp. plants.

No.	Cultivar	Species	Leaf Color
1	'Red Tears'	*Berberis koreana*	Green leaves, turning red in autumn
2	'NN'	*Berberis koreana*	Green leaves, turn purple in autumn. Seedlings of unknown origin selected and cloned in 'Więcek' nursery
3	'Superba'	*Berberis* × *ottawensis* (*B. thunbergii* × *B. vulgaris*)	Dark red leaves with a bluish tint
4	'Powwow'	*Berberis thunbergii*	The leaves are yellowish at the beginning of the vegetation period, later becoming green, some with lighter spots. in autumn they turn orange-red
5	'Golden Carpet'	*Berberis thunbergii*	Intense yellow leaves; in full sun the leaves may burn
6	'Red Pillar'	*Berberis thunbergii*	Greenish-red leaves
7	'Golden Ring'	*Berberis thunbergii*	Dark purple-red leaves with a greenish-yellow border

The collected leafy twigs were dried for 10 days in the open air at room temperature. Then, twigs and leaves were separated. The dry plant materials were stored in a dry place closed in paper bags protected from light until the analyzes (up to six months) in a controlled humidity (25–30%) and temperature (20–22 °C) chamber. Two samples of *Berberis vulgaris* root bark (conventional and organic) were purchased from Nat Vita (Długołęka, Poland) company as a control sample of a herbal source of berberine. Berberine sulfate (99% purity) was purchased from Aliness (Ostrówiec, Poland).

2.2. Extracts Preparation

Extracts were prepared according to a modified procedure of Alam et al. [27]. Briefly, 5 g of ground, dried plant material was flooded with 25 mL of 70% ethanol. Extraction was carried out in an ultrasonic bath (700 W; Sonic-10, Polsonic, Warsaw, Poland) twice for 20 min at a temperature of about 50 °C. Then, the extracts were filtered through paper and subjected to chemical analyses. For biological studies, they were concentrated to about 1/3 volume, removing ethanol in a vacuum rotary evaporator (RVC 2–18 CDPlus, Martin Christ, Osterode am Harz, Germany) and lyophilized (Alpha 1–2 LD plus, Martin Christ, Osterode am Harz, Germany) for 48 h to obtain a dry extract.

2.3. Total Phenolic Content

Total phenolic content in crude extracts was measured according to Dżugan et al. [27] using the Folin–Ciocalteu method. The results were expressed in mg of gallic acid equivalents per g of dry weight of raw material.

2.4. Antioxidant Potential

The antioxidant potential of crude extracts was assessed using FRAP and DPPH methods according to Dżugan et al. [28]. The results were expressed in μmol of Trolox equivalents per g of dry weight of raw material.

2.5. HPTLC Determination of Berberine

The berberine content in the extracts was assessed by HPTLC according to the modified procedure of Alam et al. [26]. Extracts in a volume of 2 μL were applied to HPTLC Silica Gel 60 F254 plates (20 cm × 10 cm) (Merck, Darmstadt, Germany) using a Linomat 5 automatic applicator (Camag, Muttenz, Switzerland). The chromatogram was developed using a mobile phase composed of n-propanol, formic acid, and water (90:1:9, *v*/*v*/*v*) in the automatic developing chamber (ADC2, Camag). After development, the plate was visualized under 366 nm UV light using a TLC Visualizer (Camag). Quantitative analysis was performed based on the standard curve for berberine sulfate (250 μg mL^{-1} in methanol) applied in a volume of 2 to 8 μL (0.5 to 2 μg of standard). A standard curve ($y = \frac{2.812\times10^{-2}x}{5.958\ 10^{-7}+x}$, $R^2 = 0.9906$) was constructed based on the peak area of the chromatograms generated by the software (Vision CATS, Camag). The analyses were conducted under constant conditions of temperature (22 °C) and relative humidity (33%). For the method, repeatability and accuracy were established by applying three selected standard concentrations on the same day (3 repetitions) and on 3 different days; both parameters did not exceed 0.3% RSD. Based on the signal-to-noise ratio (S/N), the limit of detection (LOD, S/N = 3) was established as 2.5 μg mL^{-1} and the limit of quantitation (LOQ, S/N = 10) as 12.5 μg mL^{-1}.

2.6. Cell Culture

Cytotoxicity was studied in three human cell lines—immortalized keratinocytes HaCaT, human malignant melanoma A375, and human colorectal adenocarcinoma cells Caco-2. All used cell lines were obtained from ATCC (American Type Culture Collection, Manassas, VA, USA). Cells were cultured in DMEM/F-12 with 10% heat-inactivated FBS (HaCaT and A-375) or 20% heat-inactivated FBS (Caco-2), 1% *v*/*v* penicillin-streptomycin and incubated at 37 °C under conditions of 5% CO_2, 95% humidity (Binder, Germany). The growth medium was changed twice a week, cells were passed at 80–90% confluence using 0.25% trypsin 0.03% EDTA in calcium and magnesium-free PBS.

2.7. Cytotoxicity Assay

Cells were seeded in a 96-well clear plate at a density of 7.5×10^3 cells/well (HaCaT) and 1×10^4 (A-375 and Caco-2) in 100 μL culture medium and allowed to attach for 24 h at 37 °C. The cells were treated with tested sterile extracts or berberine for 24 h. Non-treated cells were used as a control. After exposure, the cytotoxicity test—neutral red assay (NR)—was performed according to Repetto et al. [29]. Briefly, the medium with the compound tested was removed and replaced with a 2% neutral red solution in cell culture medium (100 μL/well), the plate was incubated at 37 °C for 1 h. The cells were then rinsed with warm PBS and a permeabilized solution (50% distilled water, 49% ethanol 96%, and 1% glacial acetic acid) (100 μL/well).

The plate was shaken (800 rpm) at room temperature for 25 min (Heidolph Inkubator 1000, Germany). Absorbance was measured at 540 nm against 620 nm using the TECAN Infinite 200 microplate reader (Tecan, Grödig, Austria). The results were presented as a percentage of control counted from 9 replicates.

2.8. Statistical Analysis

The results were presented as mean values ± SD (total phenolic content, antioxidant potential and berberine content) or interquartile range (IQR; 25%–75%) (cytotxicity assay). To evaluate the significance of differences between compared samples, one-way ANOVA and Tukey's test were performed after prior confirmation of the normality of the data distribution. To evaluate the differences between the control and the treated cells, one-way ANOVA and Dunnett's post hoc tests were utilized. A *p*-value of less than 0.05 was deemed to indicate statistical significance (for the confidence interval level of 95%). The statistical evaluations were performed using the Statistica 13.3 (Statsoft, Tulsa, OK, USA) software.

3. Results and Discussion

3.1. Total Phenolic Content and Antioxidant Potential of Extracts

The total phenolic content and antioxidant potential of the tested barberry twigs are summarized in Table 2.

Table 2. Total phenolic content and antioxidant potential of analyzed plant material.

Cultivar	TPC [mg GAE g^{-1} d.m]		FRAP [μmol TE g^{-1} d.m.]		DPPH [μmol TE g^{-1} d.m.]	
	Leaves	Twigs	Leaves	Twigs	Leaves	Twigs
'Red Tears'	63.91 ± 0.79 ^{b}	19.19 ± 0.30 ^{a}	293.47 ± 12.30 ^{a}	83.69 ± 13.20 ^{ab}	77.15 ± 11.88 ^{a}	39.38 ± 0.46 ^{a}
'NN'	107.61 ± 1.30 ^{c}	32.17 ± 2.33 ^{c}	494.52 ± 13.05 ^{bc}	152.87 ± 18.74 ^{d}	328.00 ± 42.14 ^{c}	98.02 ± 7.28 ^{c}
'Superba'	96.12 ± 5.87 ^{c}	25.63 ± 1.24 ^{b}	434.08 ± 9.97 ^{b}	112.93 ± 12.20 ^{c}	216.36 ± 44.63 ^{b}	66.44 ± 6.48 ^{b}
'Powwow'	49.25 ± 2.70 ^{a}	15.16 ± 1.09 ^{a}	223.83 ± 12.85 ^{a}	71.86 ± 1.90 ^{a}	50.96 ± 4.88 ^{a}	34.50 ± 0.38 ^{a}
'Golden Carpet'	104.24 ± 5.84 ^{c}	24.25 ± 0.67 ^{b}	500.22 ± 18.69 ^{c}	116.35 ± 6.35 ^{c}	314.58 ± 22.22 ^{c}	56.77 ± 4.34 ^{b}
'Red Pillar'	103.35 ± 3.29 ^{c}	19.76 ± 1.21 ^{ab}	528.91 ± 5.38 ^{c}	95.73 ± 6.35 ^{bc}	216.11 ± 5.42 ^{b}	43.76 ± 4.29 ^{ab}
'Golden Ring'	136.64 ± 6.12 ^{d}	25.82 ± 1.49	686.82 ± 30.57 ^{d}	113.09 ± 6.39 ^{c}	301.17 ± 17.27 ^{c}	67.87 ± 7.75 ^{b}
Berberis vulgaris root bark	8.21 ± 0.23		35.62 ± 1.82		14.11 ± 0.17	
Berberis vulgaris (organic) root bark	5.81 ± 0.65		25.84 ± 0.77		9.50 ± 0.29	

a,b,c,d—means marked with different letters are significantly different ($p < 0.05$).

Higher values of polyphenol content and correlated (Pearson's coefficients above 0.9) antioxidant capacity were found for barberry leaves (Table 3). The polyphenol content ranged from 49.25 mg GAE g^{-1} dry weight for *B. thunbergii* 'Powwow' to 136.64 for the 'Golden Ring' cultivars. This may be related to the leaf color; the 'Golden Ring' cultivar is characterized by dark red leaves, so the TPC index may also include anthocyanins present in them. In the case of twigs, the polyphenol content was lower but more even, between 15 and 32 mg GAE g^{-1} of raw material. Since barberry leaves and twigs, especially ornamental varieties, are not typical herbal raw materials, it is difficult to find data on the content of phenolic compounds and antioxidant potential. For *B. vulgaris*, the polyphenol content in leaves was reported at 58.5 mg GAE g^{-1}, similar to the stems—57.7 mg g^{-1} [14]. The bark of barberry roots examined for comparative purposes was characterized by a much lower content of phenolic compounds and antioxidant potential that was several times lower than that of other plant raw materials. This suggests that above-ground parts of these plants may be valuable sources of antioxidants. Previously, the roots, twigs, and leaves of two species of barberry growing in different locations in Croatia were compared. The content of phenolic compounds was of a similar order of magnitude as in our case; furthermore, the IC50 value for the DPPH method increased in the order: of root, twigs, leaves, which means that leaves have the highest antiradical potential [30]. This trend was observed for both *B. vulgaris* and *B. croatica*. This confirms the observations described above, regardless of the species and cultivar of the plant. Another study, for *B. vulgaris*, however, indicated that the root extract was a more potent free radical scavenger (44.3% inhibition) than the leaf extract (21.4%) [31]. A similar trend was described for other methods: ABTS scavenging and β-carotene bleaching. Some studies also indicate the antioxidant potential of berberine in vitro [9,32], although our studies did not confirm this.

Table 3. Correlation matrix for the studied parameters of antioxidant activity, polyphenols, and berberine content.

	TPC	FRAP	DPPH	Berberine Content
TPC	1.000	0.982 *	0.978 *	−0.430
FRAP	0.982 *	1.000	0.970 *	−0.321
DPPH	0.978 *	0.970 *	1.000	−0.446
Berberine content	−0.430	−0.321	−0.446	1.000

*—marked correlation coefficients are significant ($p < 0.05$).

3.2. Berberine Content

Berberine is usually determined by HPLC or UHPLC, but an attempt is being made to simplify the analysis by introducing the HPTLC method [13,33–35]. Figure 2 shows the results of the separation of ornamental barberry twig extracts and *B. vulgaris* root bark extract by the HPTLC method. The yellow band at Rf = 0.20 in UV 366 nm corresponds to berberine. This alkaloid was not detected in leaf extracts. For all extracts, an additional band at Rf = 0.12 was visible, which may be attributed to palmatine [35]. It is the second most abundant alkaloid determined in barberry [36]. In the case of samples of 'Powwow', 'Golden Carpet', 'Red Pilar', 'Golden Ring', and common barberry roots, bands from another alkaloid (Rf = 0.22) were visible above the berberine band.

Based on the fluorescence intensity of berberine bands in UV 366 nm, a standard curve was constructed and the alkaloid content in the extracts tested was calculated. The results for twigs of tested ornamental cultivars and *B. vulgaris* root bark are presented in Figure 3.

The lowest values for *B. koreana species* (0.042–0.067%) compared to *B. thunbergii* varieties (0.364–0.676%) were obtained. The intermediate value for the 'Superba' hybrid (0.103%) was also found. Compared to tested *B. vulgaris* root bark, the content found in all *B. thunbergii* cultivars was on average 66% higher. Berberine content has previously been studied mainly in the root bark, less frequently in the stem bark of various barberry species. A similar value, determined using HPLC-DAD-MS, for the roots of *B. vulgaris* was given by Vilinsky et al. [37] (0.426%); for *B. thunbergii* of an unspecified cultivar, these authors offered an even higher value (1.377%). For *B. lycium* roots, values in a similar range (0.203–1.134%) were reported by Chaudhary et al. [35] and even higher for *B. lycium* and *B. aristata* (2.6–3%) by Andola et al. [13]. For *B. aristata* stem bark, depending on the geographical origin of the plant, Ahamad et al. [34] reported a berberine content of as much as 6.14–9.44%. In turn, the berberine content (LC-MS/MS quantitation) in cortex from 0.058 mg g^{-1} (*B. gagnepainii*) to 1.15 mg g^{-1} (*B. pruinosa*) was reported by Tuzimski et al. [36]. In some cases, quantification of berberine in extracts was also carried out by the HPTLC technique [13,34,35]. The reported higher berberine contents in the roots and bark of barberry species other than *B. vulgaris* may suggest their potential use as a source of berberine, as well as the use of other parts of the plant.

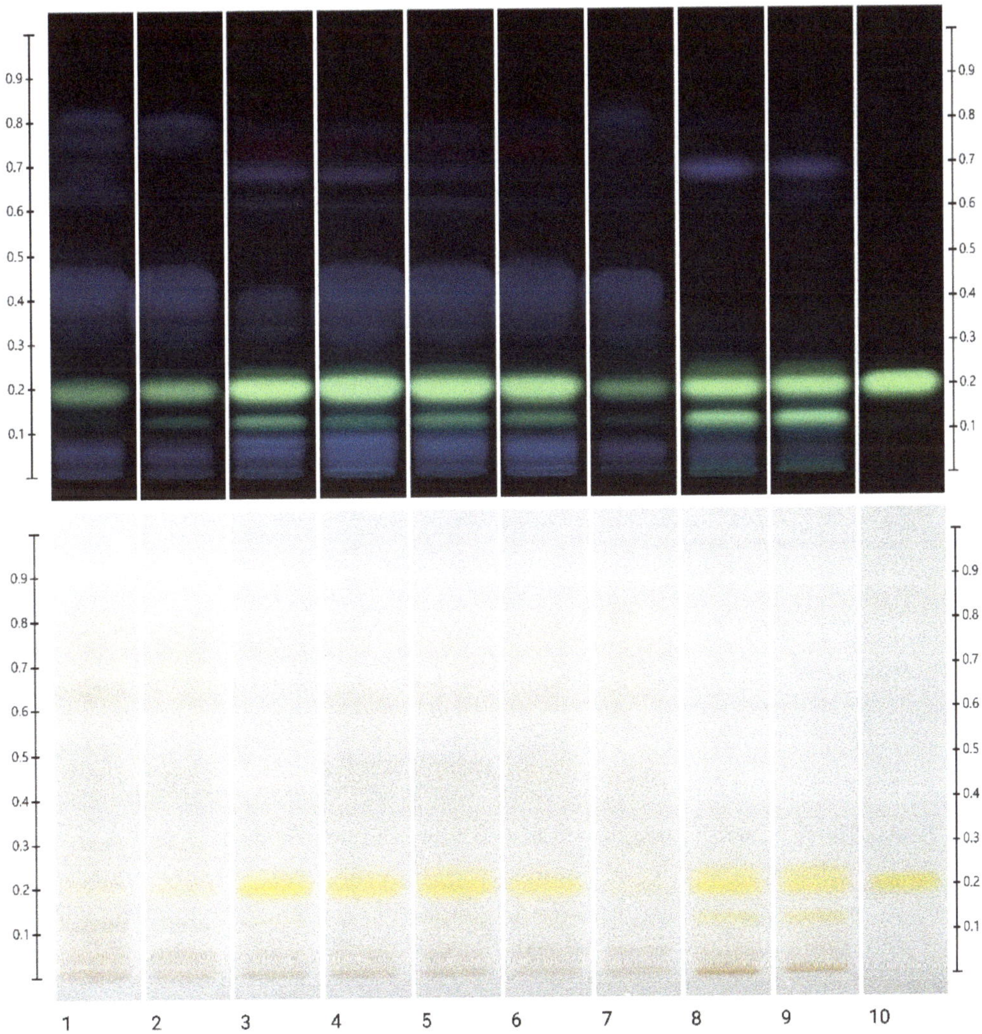

Figure 2. HPTLC analysis of berberine content in twig extracts. Top visible in 366 nm UV light, bottom in visible light. Tracks: 1—'NN', 2—'Superba', 3—'Powwow', 4—'Golden Carpet', 5—'Red Pillar', 6—'Golden Ring', 7—'Red Tears', 8—root bark, 9—*Berberis vulgaris* (organic) root bark, 10—berberine standard.

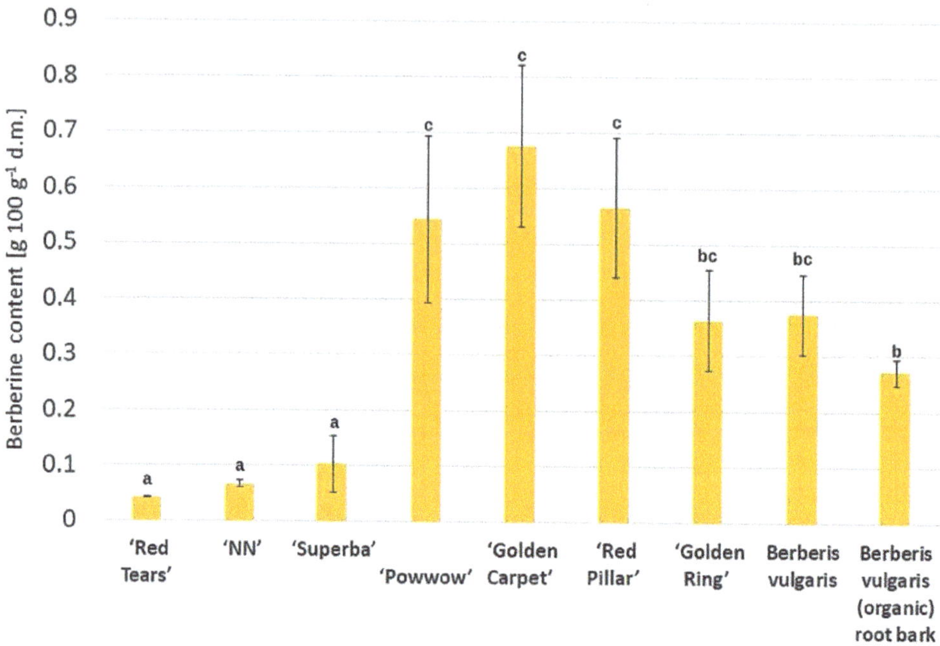

Figure 3. Berberine content in twigs of tested barberry cultivars compared to reference material (*B. vulgaris* root bark). The bars represent standard deviation; a,b,c—means marked with different letters are significantly different ($p < 0.05$).

3.3. Cytotoxic Effect of Ornamental Barberry Extracts

Discovering effective natural compounds with potent anticancer activity is a crucial area of research. Natural products have long been a rich source of novel chemotherapeutic agents, with many approved drugs and drug candidates originating from plant, marine, or microbial sources [38,39]. Cytotoxicity assays are a fundamental tool in this process, allowing researchers to assess the ability of natural extracts or purified compounds to selectively kill cancer cells [40,41]. One of the key advantages of natural products as a source of anticancer drugs is their diverse chemical structures and modes of action [42]. Many natural compounds exhibit cytotoxicity through different mechanisms, inducing oxidative stress, or modulating key signaling pathways in cancer cells [39]. Carefully designed cytotoxicity assays can help elucidate these mechanisms and guide the development of natural product-derived therapeutics.

Taking the above into account, selected extracts from ornamental barberry twigs were subjected to cytotoxicity studies using three cell lines. Two extracts with high ('Golden Carpet' and 'Golden Ring') and two with low ('Superba' and 'Red Tears') berberine content were tested with the use of three human cell lines—immortalized keratinocytes HaCaT, human malignant melanoma A375 and human colorectal adenocarcinoma cells Caco-2. In addition, based on cultivar differences an attempt was made to determine the mechanism of the observed effect and to identify key components of extracts.

As shown in Figure 4, only the 'Red Tears' extract did not have a statistically significant effect on HaCaT keratinocytes at concentrations up to 500 μg mL^{-1}. In contrast, the other three extracts analyzed, namely 'Superba', 'Golden Carpet', and 'Golden Ring', exhibited dose-dependent toxicity towards the treated keratinocyte cells. Interestingly, the absence of berberine in 'Red Tears' correlates with its ineffectiveness, suggesting that berberine is a key factor significantly limiting the viability of keratinocyte cells. Conversely, the high berberine content in 'Golden Carpet' and 'Golden Ring' and the associated negative effects at higher doses ($p < 0.001$) indicate the potential cytotoxic properties of this alkaloid at elevated concentrations. In addition to berberine, the extracts also contain numerous polyphenolic compounds, which can also affect the bioactivity of the extracts in vitro. The 'Red Tears' cultivar was characterized by a significantly lower TPC value than the others tested on the HaCaT line. The weaker effect of the extract of this variety, even at a high concentration of the extract, may result from a lower content of polyphenols or matrix effects, weaker synergy of this class of metabolites with berberine.

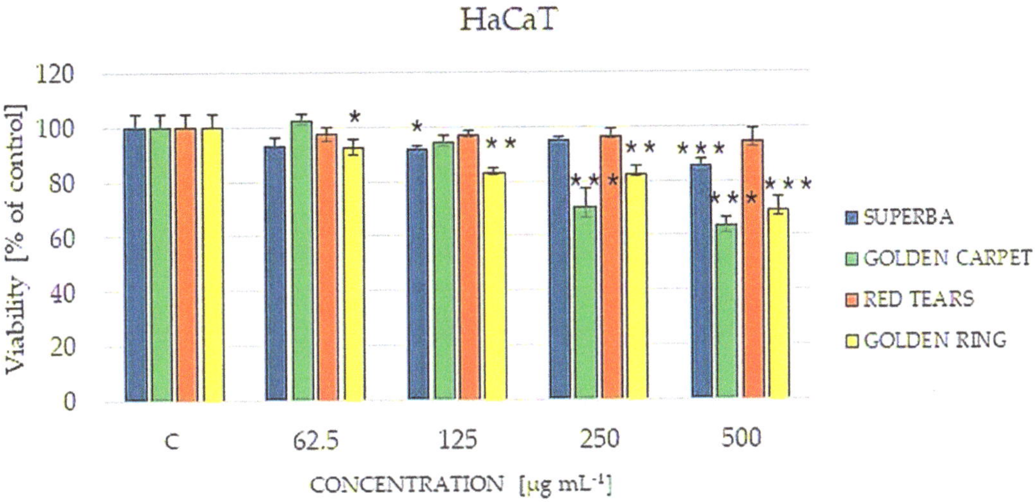

Figure 4. Cultivar-dependent effect of selected barberry extracts ('Superba', 'Golden carpet', 'Red Tears', 'Golden ring') on the viability of human keratinocytes HaCaT cells estimated by the Neutral Red assay. The cells were treated with extracts in concentrations of 62.5, 125, 250 and 500 μg mL^{-1}. Non-treated cells were used as a control (C). Data are expressed as median from at least three independent experiments. Error bars represent 25% and 75% percentiles. Statistical significance was assessed using one-way ANOVA and Dunnett's post hoc test (* $p < 0.05$, ** $p < 0.01$, *** $p < 0.001$).

Subsequently, the impact of the analyzed extracts on the viability of A375 melanoma cancer cells was investigated. As shown in Figure 5, the 'Superba' extract exhibited the strongest cytotoxic effect among the analyzed extracts. Even the lowest concentration of the 'Superba' extract had a statistically significant impact on the cytotoxicity of A375 cells ($p < 0.001$). At a concentration of 500 μg mL^{-1}, cell viability decreased to 44%. Interestingly, compared to HaCaT cells, A375 cells were sensitive to the 'Red Tears' extract, with viability dropping to 80% at concentrations of 250 and 500 μg mL^{-1} ($p < 0.001$). The extracts of 'Golden Carpet' and 'Golden Ring' abundant in berberine had the least impact on A375 cells, showing dose-dependent effects; at the highest concentrations analyzed, the cytotoxic impact on viability was statistically significant. Therefore, our preliminary research suggests that the use of barberry extracts in the treatment of melanoma may be reasonable, however, the observed cytotoxic effect does not seem to be directly related to the berberine content. However, a previous study reported the inhibitory effect of pure berberine on the migration of melanoma cancer cells [43].

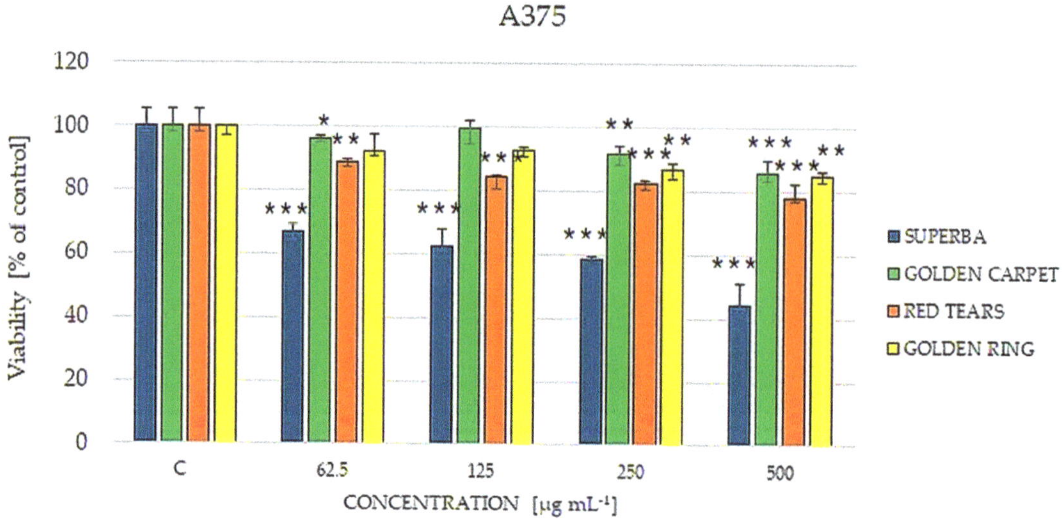

Figure 5. Cultivar-dependent effect of selected barberry extracts ('Superba', 'Golden carpet', 'Red Tears', 'Golden ring') on the viability of human malignant melanoma A375 cells estimated by the Neutral Red assay. The cells were treated with extracts in concentrations of 62.5, 125, 250, and 500 μg mL^{-1}. Non-treated cells were used as a control (C). Data are expressed as median from at least three independent experiments. Error bars represent 25% and 75% percentiles. Statistical significance was assessed using one-way ANOVA and Dunnett's post hoc test (* $p < 0.05$, ** $p < 0.01$, *** $p < 0.001$).

As Caco-2 colorectal cancer cells have been more frequently used in the examination of the mechanism of berberine activity, we also investigated the impact of the analyzed extracts on Caco-2 cells. As shown in Figure 6, the utilized concentration of 500 μg mL^{-1} had a toxic effect on these cells in the case of all analyzed extracts. A particularly significant impact was noted for berberine-rich 'Golden Carpet' and 'Golden Ring' extracts but also for 'Red Tears' extract. In conclusion, Caco-2 cells were sensitive to barberry twig extracts, but it has not been confirmed that it is dependent on the berberine content.

To confirm the tendency observed for barberry extracts cytotoxicity we have undertaken similar studies for pure berberine in the concentration range 0.001–0.25 mg mL^{-1} with the use of previously analyzed human cells. Taking into account the concentration of berberine in the extracts used (from 1 to 16 μg mL^{-1}) Table 3 shows the effect for comparable doses of pure berberine sulfate. The dose of 100 μg mL^{-1} unequivocally exhibited cytotoxic activity against keratinocytes and both cancer cells used in the study. Interestingly, this cytotoxic effect was significant in the case of the HaCaT and A375 cell lines for 10-fold lower dose.

No direct dependence of the polyphenols content in the extracts on the in vitro effects has been observed, but they are important components of the extract matrix and may shape the bioactivity of the entire extract through synergistic or antagonistic interactions.

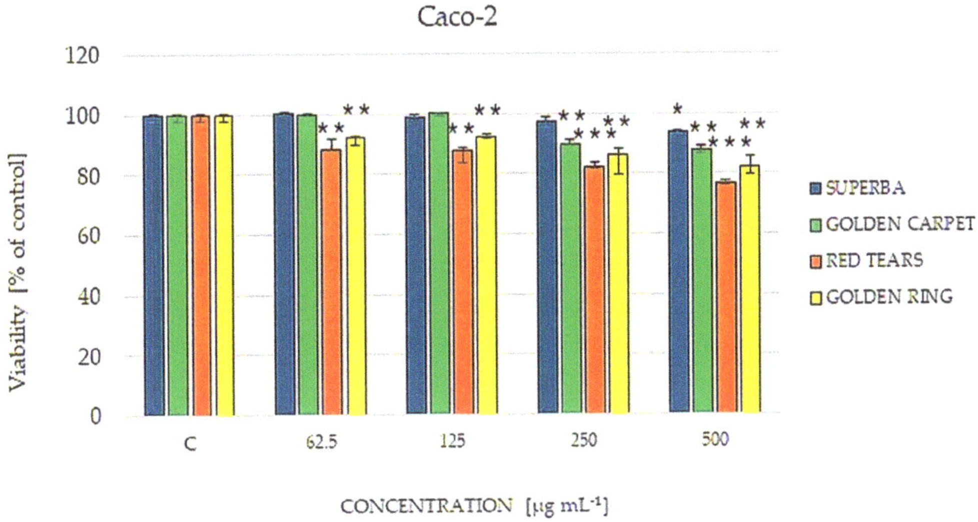

Figure 6. Cultivar-dependent effect of selected barberry extracts ('Superba', 'Golden carpet', 'Red Tears', 'Golden ring') on the viability of human colorectal adenocarcinoma cells Caco-2 estimated by the Neutral Red assay. The cells were treated with extracts in concentrations of 62.5, 125, 250 and 500 μg mL^{-1} Non-treated cells were used as a control (C). Data are expressed as median from at least three independent experiments. Error bars represent 25% and 75% percentiles. Statistical significance was assessed using one-way ANOVA and Dunnett's post hoc test (* $p < 0.05$, ** $p < 0.01$, *** $p < 0.001$).

Subsequently, calculations were performed to compare cytotoxicity effects taking into account the berberine content in the highest dose of extracts (500 mg mL^{-1}) (Table 4). The comparison carried out showed that tested extracts in general exhibited stronger cytotoxicity than comparable doses of pure berberine. Thus, it could be concluded that berberine in the composition of other phytochemicals that occurred in barberry extracts has a different cytotoxic effect compared to pure berberine. In this respect, the results obtained are promising and require continuation with higher doses of the extract in cytotoxicity assays on cell lines. It should be mentioned, however, that berberine and its derivatives can activate or enhance lysosomal activity in cells [44], hence the applied Neutral Red test may have certain limitations and the results should be confirmed using other procedures.

Table 4. The comparison of the cytotoxic effect of pure berberine and ornamental barberry twig extracts.

Tested Sample	Berberine Content [μg mL^{-1}]	Viability [%]		
		HaCat	A375	Caco-2
Ornamental barberry extracts (500 μg mL^{-1} dose)				
'Golden carpet'	16.3	63.59 ***	85.87 ***	87.55 **
'Golden Ring'	11.83	72.89 ***	84.79 **	82.20 **
'Superba'	3.9	85.24 ***	44.21 ***	93.66 *
'Red Tears'	1.06	94.10	77.93***	76.42 ***
Pure berberine	1	96.80 ***	95.89 **	96.88
	10	82.80 ***	79.70 ***	95.89
	100	58.64 ***	40.32 ***	74.68 ***

Statistical significance according to control cells was assessed using one-way ANOVA and Dunnett's post hoc test (* $p < 0.05$, ** $p < 0.01$, *** $p < 0.001$).

Recent studies have highlighted the potential of berberine as a promising anticancer agent, with the ability to inhibit the proliferation and induce the death of cancer cells [45]. Berberine has been shown to exert antiproliferative effects on a variety of cancer cell types, including hepatoma, colon, epithelial ovarian, and breast cancer cells [46,47]. In addition to its antiproliferative effects, berberine has also demonstrated proapoptotic properties [48–50]. Moreover, it has been reported to modulate the production of inflammatory mediators, such as tumor necrosis factor-α, in cancer cells [50]. In addition to its direct antiproliferative effects, berberine has also been reported to exhibit other beneficial properties that may contribute to its anticancer potential, like modulating epigenetic mechanisms [45].

However, many studies on the pharmacological potential of berberine have been performed for pure compound and do not take into account the influence of additional components contained in the barberry extract. Meanwhile, the positive matrix effect on phytochemical bioaccessibility can be considered as was shown in the case of organosulfur components of garlic [51]. This is especially important due to the low solubility and the low absorption of berberine itself which represent a limiting factor to its activity. The majority of efforts were addressed to improve those liabilities to reduce the high dosages that result in gastrointestinal adverse events [52,53]. The absorption of berberine from extracts of ornamental barberry twigs may be better due to enhancing the impact of the matrix, but this requires further research using in vitro digestion, analogously to the study of Petrangolini et al. [54].

There are known examples of extracts having a stronger effect than individual metabolites. In terms of antimicrobial properties, it has been previously found that the full plant extract containing berberine was more active than the isolated alkaloid [55]. Similarly, a stronger effect of crude barberry extract than berberine chloride was demonstrated in the α-glucosidase inhibition test, whereas the effect on acetylcholinesterase was the same [56]. Some research suggests that barberry extracts can have beneficial effects on the cardiovascular system. They may help in lowering blood pressure, reducing cholesterol levels, and improving overall heart health [57]. One of the most frequently studied biological effects, including clinical studies, is the antidiabetic effect of barberry extracts and berberine itself. Promising results have been obtained for berberine as an active substance, and the proposed mechanisms of action include increasing insulin sensitivity, modulating gut microbiota, activating the adenosine AMPK pathway, promoting intestinal glucagon-like protein-1 secretion, stimulating glycolysis, inhibiting gluconeogenesis in liver, and upregulating hepatic low-density lipoprotein receptor mRNA expression [58]. Moreover, extracts of *Berberis* sp. and other plants containing these alkaloids have also been studied in this field. However, the effects of the studies were not as directly promising as for pure berberine [58]. Numerous reports confirm the usefulness of both berberine and plant extracts rich in it in the treatment of the metabolic syndrome [58]. As confirmation of the positive effect of barberry extracts in the treatment of cancer in the studies by Rigillo et al., it was demonstrated that *B. aristata* extracts containing berberine and other protoberberine-type alkaloids inhibited the migration of cancer cells without any effect on healthy cells [59].

Overall, the available evidence suggests that ornamental barberry twig extract is a promising natural source of active berberine. Moreover, the full extract of twigs of selected ornamental barberry varieties seems to have greater activity compared to the analogous dose of the reference berberine sulfate. This may indicate the occurrence of a beneficial effect of the components of the complex matrix of the extract. The next step should be the confirmation of the bioactivity of pure berberine isolated from the tested raw materials. Well-evidenced ability of berberine to inhibit the proliferation of various cancer cell types, as well as its potential to modulate key signaling pathways and epigenetic mechanisms, make the studied raw material an intriguing target for further investigation and potential clinical trial. Moreover, due to the widespread and greater safety of ornamental barberry cultivation compared to *B. vulgaris*, the obtained results are promising and can be implemented.

4. Conclusions

Using quantitative thin-layer chromatography, it was shown for the first time that ornamental barberry twigs collected before fruit ripening contain berberine (from 0.042 to 0.676 g 100 g^{-1}), but its content differed between species and cultivars. Meanwhile, this alkaloid was not found in leaf extracts, despite the fact that they exhibited higher antioxidant potential compared to twig extracts. Particularly high berberine content was found for two golden-leafed cultivars: 'Golden carpet' and 'Golden Ring' of the *B. thunbergii* species.

Preliminary in vitro studies showed that ornamental barberry twig extracts, compared to pure berberine sulfate administered in an analogous dose, show greater cytotoxicity towards studied HaCaT, A375, and Caco-2 cells. It was suggested that matrix effects related to the presence of other phytochemical components may be responsible for the observed greater bioactivity of berberine-rich extracts. These findings seem to be innovative due to the health effects of berberine being well documented, whereas the effects of ornamental barberry extracts with a more complex composition are less understood and pose a research challenge. However, due to the fact that the composition of the extract complex mixture is not fully established, conclusions about the bioactivity of the berberine-containing extract should be treated with caution. They need confirmation in the future planned comparative research of the cytotoxic effect against used cell lines between selected twig barberry extracts and pure berberine isolated from them. Valuable clarifications could also be obtained from future studies of the bioavailability of berberine from the barberry twig extract using in vitro digestion.

Due to the fact that the use of the full barberry extract without the need for berberine purification seems to be more economically advantageous, the next step of research will be the scaling up of the extraction technology for industrial applications. However, since ornamental barberry twigs are easier to obtain in controlled cultivation of this plant than common barberry roots, promising results of preliminary studies may lead to the offer of a new raw material for the isolation of berberine for the pharmaceutical industry as well as the use of the full extract of ornamental barberry twigs as a new form of dietary supplement. However, this requires deeper research on the mechanisms of berberine and berberine-containing extract action using various biological models.

Author Contributions: Conceptualization, M.D. and W.L.; methodology, M.M. (Michał Miłek), N.P., S.G. and M.M. (Mateusz Mołoń); software, M.M. (Michał Miłek); validation, M.M. (Michał Miłek) and M.M. (Mateusz Mołoń); formal analysis, M.M. (Michał Miłek) and M.D.; investigation, M.M. (Michał Miłek), N.P. and S.G.; resources, W.L.; data curation, M.M. (Michał Miłek), M.D. and M.M. (Mateusz Mołoń); writing—original draft preparation, M.M. (Michał Miłek) and M.M. (Mateusz Mołoń); writing—review and editing, M.D.; visualization, M.M. (Michał Miłek) and M.M. (Mateusz Mołoń); supervision, M.D. and W.L.; project administration, M.D.; funding acquisition, M.D. All authors have read and agreed to the published version of the manuscript.

Funding: This work was supported by the Polish Ministry of Science and Higher Education research project within the University of Rzeszów PB/ZCHTZ/2024.

Institutional Review Board Statement: Not applicable.

Informed Consent Statement: Not applicable.

Data Availability Statement: Data are contained within the article.

Acknowledgments: We are grateful to Wiesław Więcek, the owner of Nursery of Ornamental Trees and Shrubs in Stobierna, Poland for providing plant samples for research.

Conflicts of Interest: The authors declare no conflicts of interest.

References

1. Rashmi, A.; Rajasekaran, A.; Pant, J. The genus Berberis Linn.: A review. *Pharmacogn. Rev.* **2008**, *2*, 369–385.
2. Salehi, B.; Selamoglu, Z.; Sener, B.; Kilic, M.; Kumar Jugran, A.; de Tommasi, N.; Sinisgalli, C.; Milella, L.; Rajkovic, J.; Flaviana, B.; et al. Berberis Plants—Drifting from Farm to Food Applications, Phytotherapy, and Phytopharmacology. *Foods* **2019**, *8*, 522. [CrossRef] [PubMed]

3. Wang, M.N.; Wan, A.M.; Chen, X.M. Barberry as alternate host is important for *Puccinia graminis* f. sp. tritici but not for *Puccinia striiformis* f. sp. tritici in the U.S. Pacific Northwest. *Plant Dis.* **2015**, *99*, 1507–1516. [CrossRef] [PubMed]
4. Villegas, D.; Bartaula, R.; Cantero-Martínez, C.; Luster, D.; Szabo, L.; Olivera, P.; Berlin, A.; Rodriguez-Algaba, J.; Hovmøller, M.S.; McIntosh, R.; et al. Barberry plays an active role as an alternate host of *Puccinia graminis* in Spain. *Plant Pathol.* **2022**, *71*, 1174–1184. [CrossRef] [PubMed]
5. Khan, I.; Najeebullah, S.; Ali, M.; Shinwari, Z. Phytopharmacological and ethnomedicinal uses of the Genus Berberis (Berberidaceae): A review. *Trop. J. Pharm. Res.* **2016**, *15*, 2047–2057. [CrossRef]
6. Sarraf, M.; Beig Babaei, A.; Naji-Tabasi, S. Investigating functional properties of barberry species: An overview. *J. Sci. Food Agric.* **2019**, *99*, 5255–5269. [CrossRef]
7. Srivastava, S.; Srivastava, M.; Misra, A.; Pandey, G.; Rawat, A.K.S. A review on biological and chemical diversity in Berberis (Berberidaceae). *EXCLI J.* **2015**, *14*, 247–267. [CrossRef]
8. Neag, M.A.; Mocan, A.; Echeverría, J.; Pop, R.M.; Bocsan, C.I.; Crisan, G.; Buzoianu, A.D. Berberine: Botanical Occurrence, traditional uses, extraction methods, and relevance in cardiovascular, metabolic, hepatic, and renal disorders. *Front. Pharmacol.* **2018**, *9*, 557. [CrossRef]
9. Jain, S.; Tripathi, S.; Tripathi, P.K. Antioxidant and antiarthritic potential of berberine: In vitro and in vivo studies. *Chin. Herb. Med.* **2023**, *15*, 549–555. [CrossRef]
10. Patel, P. A bird's eye view on a therapeutically 'wonder molecule': Berberine. *Phytomed. Plus* **2021**, *1*, 100070. [CrossRef]
11. Preeti, S.; Prabhat, U.; Shardendu, M.; Ananya, S.; Suresh, P. Berberine a Potent Substance for Researcher: A Review. *World J. Pharm. Pharm. Sci.* **2015**, *4*, 547–573.
12. Mazhar, M.; Agrawal, S.S. Standardization of *Berberis aristata* DC and *Nigella sativa* L. Using HPTLC and GCMS and Their Antineoplasia Activity in 7,12-Dimethylbenz[a]anthracene-Induced Mouse Models. *Front. Pharmacol.* **2021**, *12*, 642067. [CrossRef] [PubMed]
13. Andola, H.C.; Rawal, R.S.; Rawat, M.S.M.; Bhatt, I.D.; Purohit, V.K. Analysis of Berberine Content using HPTLC Fingerprinting of Root and Bark of Three Himalayan Berberis Species. *Asian J. Biotechnol.* **2010**, *2*, 239–245. [CrossRef]
14. Och, A.; Olech, M.; Bąk, K.; Kanak, S.; Cwener, A.; Cieśla, M.; Nowak, R. Evaluation of the Antioxidant and Anti-Lipoxygenase Activity of *Berberis vulgaris* L. Leaves, Fruits, and Stem and Their LC MS/MS Polyphenolic Profile. *Antioxidants* **2023**, *12*, 1467. [CrossRef] [PubMed]
15. Ai, X.; Yu, P.; Peng, L.; Luo, L.; Liu, J.; Li, S.; Lai, X.; Luan, F.; Meng, X. Berberine: A Review of its Pharmacokinetics Properties and Therapeutic Potentials in Diverse Vascular Diseases. *Front. Pharmacol.* **2021**, *12*, 762654. [CrossRef]
16. Song, D.; Hao, J.; Fan, D. Biological properties and clinical applications of berberine. *Front. Med.* **2020**, *14*, 564–582. [CrossRef] [PubMed]
17. Cheng, Z.; Kang, C.; Che, S.; Su, J.; Sun, Q.; Ge, T.; Guo, Y.; Lv, J.; Sun, Z.; Yang, W.; et al. Berberine: A Promising Treatment for Neurodegenerative Diseases. *Front. Pharmacol.* **2022**, *13*, 845591. [CrossRef]
18. Tian, E.; Sharma, G.; Dai, C. Neuroprotective Properties of Berberine: Molecular Mechanisms and Clinical Implications. *Antioxidants* **2023**, *12*, 1883. [CrossRef]
19. Gatland, A.E.; Pilgrim, B.S.; Procopiou, P.A.; Donohoe, T.J. Short and efficient syntheses of protoberberine alkaloids using palladium-catalyzed enolate arylation. *Angew. Chem.-Int. Ed.* **2014**, *53*, 14555–14558. [CrossRef]
20. Yang, Z.; Zhang, Y.; Chen, X.; Li, W.; Li, G.B.; Wu, Y. Total Synthesis and Evaluation of B-Homo Palmatine and Berberine Derivatives as p300 Histone Acetyltransferase Inhibitors. *Eur. J. Org. Chem.* **2018**, *2018*, 1041–1052. [CrossRef]
21. Filli, M.S.; Ibrahim, A.A.; Kesse, S.; Aquib, M.; Boakye-Yiadom, K.O.; Farooq, M.A.; Raza, F.; Zhang, Y.; Wang, B. Synthetic berberine derivatives as potential new drugs. *Braz. J. Pharm. Sci.* **2022**, *58*, e18835. [CrossRef]
22. Tajiri, M.; Yamada, R.; Hotsumi, M.; Makabe, K.; Konno, H. The total synthesis of berberine and selected analogues, and their evaluation as amyloid beta aggregation inhibitors. *Eur. J. Med. Chem.* **2021**, *215*, 113289. [CrossRef] [PubMed]
23. Han, J.; Li, S. De novo biosynthesis of berberine and halogenated benzylisoquinoline alkaloids in Saccharomyces cerevisiae. *Commun. Chem.* **2023**, *6*, 27. [CrossRef]
24. Och, A.; Och, M.; Nowak, R.; Podgórska, D.; Podgórski, R. Berberine, a Herbal Metabolite in the Metabolic Syndrome: The Risk Factors, Course, and Consequences of the Disease. *Molecules* **2022**, *27*, 1351. [CrossRef] [PubMed]
25. Berberine Supplement Market (by Product Type: Capsules, Tablets, Liquid and Powder; by Application: Dietary Supplements, Pharmaceuticals, Cosmetics, Others; by Distribution Channel)—Global Market Size, Share, Growth, Trends, Statistics Analysis Report, by Region, and Segment Forecasts 2024–2032. Available online: https://datahorizzonresearch.com/berberine-supplement-market-2960 (accessed on 12 November 2024).
26. Wojciechowska, I. European barberry—Ornamental nad medicinal plant. *Kosmos* **2017**, *66*, 487–490. (In Polish)
27. Alam, S.D.; Beg, M.A.; Bagadi, M.; Locatelli, M.; ALOthman, Z.A.; Mustaqeem, M.; Ali, I. Facile extraction of berberine from different plants, separation, and identification by thin-layer chromatography, high-performance liquid chromatography, and biological evaluation against Leishmaniosis. *J. Sep. Sci.* **2023**, *46*, 2300582. [CrossRef]
28. Dżugan, M.; Miłek, M.; Grabek-Lejko, D.; Hęclik, J.; Jacek, B.; Litwińczuk, W. Antioxidant activity, polyphenolic profiles and antibacterial properties of leaf extract of various paulownia spp. clones. *Agronomy* **2021**, *11*, 2001. [CrossRef]
29. Repetto, G.; del Peso, A.; Zurita, J.L. Neutral red uptake assay for the estimation of cell viability/cytotoxicity. *Nat. Protoc.* **2008**, *3*, 1125–1131. [CrossRef] [PubMed]

30. Zovko Končić, M.; Kremer, D.; Karlović, K.; Kosalec, I. Evaluation of antioxidant activities and phenolic content of *Berberis vulgaris* L. and *Berberis croatica* Horvat. *Food Chem. Toxicol.* **2010**, *48*, 2176–2180. [CrossRef]
31. El-Zahar, K.M.; Al-Jamaan, M.E.; Al-Mutairi, F.R.; Al-Hudiab, A.M.; Al-Einzi, M.S.; Mohamed, A.A.Z. Antioxidant, Antibacterial, and Antifungal Activities of the Ethanolic Extract Obtained from *Berberis vulgaris* Roots and Leaves. *Molecules* **2022**, *27*, 6114. [CrossRef]
32. Luo, A.; Fan, Y. Antioxidant activities of berberine hydrochloride. *J. Med. Plants Res.* **2011**, *5*, 3702–3707.
33. Satija, S.; Malik, S.; Garg, M. Development of a new, rapid, and sensitive validated high-performance thin-layer chromatographic method for the estimation of berberine in Tinospora cordifolia. *J. Planar Chromatogr.-Mod. TLC* **2016**, *29*, 209–215. [CrossRef]
34. Ahamad, J.; Kaskoos, R.A.; Amin, S.; Mir, S.R. Development and Validation of an HPTLC Method for Estimation of Berberine in *Berberis aristata*. *Res. J. Phytochem.* **2021**, *15*, 58–65. [CrossRef]
35. Chaudhary, M.K.; Misra, A.; Shankar, U.; Agnihotri, P.; Srivastava, S. Intra-specific Variation of Alkaloid Content in *Berberis lycium* from the Western Himalaya. *J. Herbs Spices Med. Plants* **2021**, *27*, 386–395. [CrossRef]
36. Tuzimski, T.; Petruczynik, A.; Kaproń, B.; Plech, T.; Makuch-Kocka, A.; Janiszewska, D.; Sugajski, M.; Buszewski, B.; Szultka-Młyńska, M. In Vitro and In Silico of Cholinesterases Inhibition and In Vitro and In Vivo Anti-Melanoma Activity Investigations of Extracts Obtained from Selected Berberis Species. *Molecules* **2024**, *29*, 2048. [CrossRef]
37. Villinski, J.R.; Dumas, E.R.; Chai, H.B.; Pezzuto, J.M.; Angerhofer, C.K.; Gafner, S. Antibacterial activity and alkaloid content of *Berberis thunbergii, Berberis vulgaris* and *Hydrastis canadensis*. *Pharm. Biol.* **2003**, *41*, 551–557. [CrossRef]
38. Bedi, A.; Adholeya, A.; Deshmukh, S.K. Novel Anticancer compounds from Endophytic fungi. *Curr. Biotechnol.* **2018**, *7*, 168–184. [CrossRef]
39. Prabhu, K.S.; Siveen, K.S.; Kuttikrishnan, S.; Jochebeth, A.; Ali, T.A.; Elareer, N.R.; Iskandarani, A.; Khan, A.Q.; Merhi, M.; Dermime, S.; et al. Greensporone A, a fungal secondary metabolite suppressed constitutively activated AKT via ROS generation and induced apoptosis in leukemic cell lines. *Biomolecules* **2019**, *9*, 126. [CrossRef] [PubMed]
40. John, J.E. Cytotoxic Natural Products and their Pharmacological Mode of Action: A Hypothesis on their Complexity and Spectrum of Activity. *Curr. Enzym. Inhib.* **2012**, *8*, 100–103. [CrossRef]
41. Asma, S.T.; Acaroz, U.; Imre, K.; Morar, A.; Shah, S.R.A.; Hussain, S.Z.; Arslan-Acaroz, D.; Demirbas, H.; Hajrulai-Musliu, Z.; Istanbullugil, F.R.; et al. Natural Products/Bioactive Compounds as a Source of Anticancer Drugs. *Cancers* **2022**, *14*, 6203. [CrossRef]
42. Dey, P.; Kundu, A.; Chakraborty, H.J.; Kar, B.; Choi, W.S.; Lee, B.M.; Bhakta, T.; Atanasov, A.G.; Kim, H.S. Therapeutic value of steroidal alkaloids in cancer: Current trends and future perspectives. *Int. J. Cancer* **2019**, *145*, 1731–1744. [CrossRef] [PubMed]
43. Liu, J.F.; Lai, K.C.; Peng, S.F.; Maraming, P.; Huang, Y.P.; Huang, A.C.; Chueh, F.S.; Huang, W.W.; Chung, J.G. Berberine inhibits human melanoma A375.S2 cell migration and invasion via affecting the FAK, uPA, and NF-κB signaling pathways and inhibits PLX4032 resistant A375.S2 cell migration in vitro. *Molecules* **2018**, *23*, 2019. [CrossRef]
44. Liu, X.; Zhang, N.; Liu, Y.; Liu, L.; Zeng, Q.; Yin, M.; Wang, Y.; Song, D.; Deng, H. MPB, a novel berberine derivative, enhances lysosomal and bactericidal properties via TGF-b-activated kinase 1-dependent activation of the transcription factor EB. *FASEB J.* **2019**, *33*, 1468–1481. [CrossRef]
45. Tillhon, M.; Guamán Ortiz, L.M.; Lombardi, P.; Scovassi, A.I. Berberine: New perspectives for old remedies. *Biochem. Pharmacol.* **2012**, *84*, 1260–1267. [CrossRef] [PubMed]
46. Eo, S.H.; Kim, J.H.; Kim, S.J. Induction of G2/M arrest by berberine via activation of PI3K/Akt and p38 in human chondrosarcoma cell line. *Oncol. Res.* **2014**, *22*, 147–157. [CrossRef]
47. Liu, D.; Meng, X.; Wu, D.; Qiu, Z.; Luo, H. A natural isoquinoline alkaloid with antitumor activity: Studies of the biological activities of berberine. *Front. Pharmacol.* **2019**, *10*, 9. [CrossRef]
48. Ortiz, L.M.G.; Lombardi, P.; Tillhon, M.; Scovassi, A.I. Berberine, an epiphany against cancer. *Molecules* **2014**, *19*, 12349–12367. [CrossRef]
49. Xie, W.; Zhang, Z.; Song, L.; Huang, C.; Guo, Z.; Hu, X.; Bi, S.; Yu, R. Cordyceps militaris Fraction induces apoptosis and G2/M Arrest via c-Jun N-Terminal kinase signaling pathway in oral squamous carcinoma KB Cells. *Pharmacogn. Mag.* **2018**, *14*, 116–123.
50. Parant, M. Effects of TNF in bacterial infections. *Ann. Inst. Pasteur Imm.* **1988**, *139*, 301–304. [CrossRef]
51. Torres-Palazzolo, C.A.; Ramírez, D.A.; Beretta, V.H.; Camargo, A.B. Matrix effect on phytochemical bioaccessibility. The case of organosulfur compounds in garlic preparations. *LWT* **2021**, *136*, 110301. [CrossRef]
52. Battu, S.K.; Repka, M.A.; Maddineni, S.; Chittiboyina, A.G.; Avery, M.A.; Majumdar, S. Physicochemical characterization of berberine chloride: A perspective in the development of a solution dosage form for oral delivery. *AAPS PharmSciTech* **2010**, *11*, 1466–1475. [CrossRef] [PubMed]
53. Sut, S.; Faggian, M.; Baldan, V.; Poloniato, G.; Castagliuolo, I.; Grabnar, I.; Perissutti, B.; Brun, P.; Maggi, F.; Voinovich, D.; et al. Natural Deep Eutectic Solvents (NADES) to enhance berberine absorption: An in vivo pharmacokinetic study. *Molecules* **2017**, *22*, 1921. [CrossRef] [PubMed]
54. Petrangolini, G.; Corti, F.; Ronchi, M.; Arnoldi, L.; Allegrini, P.; Riva, A. Development of an Innovative Berberine Food-Grade Formulation with an Ameliorated Absorption: In Vitro Evidence Confirmed by Healthy Human Volunteers Pharmacokinetic Study. *Evid.-Based Complement. Altern. Med.* **2021**, *2021*, 563889. [CrossRef] [PubMed]
55. Sami, F.J.; Nur, S. Cytotoxic Effect, Antibacterial Activity, and in Silico Evaluation of Berberine Compound from Methanolic Extract of Arcangelisia flava Merr Stems. *J. Kefarmasian Indones.* **2024**, *14*, 39–50.

56. Abd El-Wahab, A.E.; Ghareeb, D.A.; Sarhan, E.E.M.; Abu-Serie, M.M.; El Demellawy, M.A. In vitro biological assessment of berberis vulgaris and its active constituent, berberine: Antioxidants, anti-acetylcholinesterase, anti-diabetic and anticancer effects. *BMC Complement. Altern. Med.* **2013**, *13*, 218. [CrossRef]
57. Özgen, M.; Saraçoğlu, O.; Geçer, E.N. Antioxidant capacity and chemical properties of selected barberry (*Berberis vulgaris* L.) fruits. *Hortic. Environ. Biotechnol.* **2012**, *53*, 447–451. [CrossRef]
58. Imenshahidi, M.; Hosseinzadeh, H. *Berberis Vulgaris* and Berberine: An Update Review. *Phythoter. Res.* **2016**, *30*, 1745–1764. [CrossRef]
59. Rigillo, G.; Cappellucci, G.; Baini, G.; Vaccaro, F.; Miraldi, E.; Pani, L.; Tascedda, F.; Bruni, R.; Biagi, M. Comprehensive Analysis of *Berberis aristata* DC. Bark Extracts: In Vitro and In Silico Evaluation of Bioaccessibility and Safety. *Nutrients* **2024**, *16*, 2953. [CrossRef]

current issues in molecular biology

MDPI

Article

Exploring Water-Soluble South African *Tulbaghia violacea* Harv Extract as a Therapeutic Approach for Triple-Negative Breast Cancer Metastasis

Mohammed Alaouna [1,2], Rodney Hull [2], Thulo Molefi [2,3], Richard Khanyile [2,3], Langanani Mbodi [4], Thifhelimbilu Emmanuel Luvhengo [5], Nkhensani Chauke-Malinga [2,6], Boitumelo Phakathi [7], Clement Penny [1] and Zodwa Dlamini [2,*]

1 Department of Internal Medicine, Faculty of Health Sciences, University of the Witwatersrand, Johannesburg 2193, South Africa; ala3570@gmail.com (M.A.); clement.penny@wits.ac.za (C.P.)
2 SAMRC Precision Oncology Research Unit (PORU), DSI/NRF SARChI Chair in Precision Oncology and Cancer Prevention (POCP), Pan African Cancer Research Institute (PACRI), University of Pretoria, Pretoria 0084, South Africa; rodney.hull@up.ac.za (R.H.); thulo.molefi@up.ac.za (T.M.); richard.khanyile@up.ac.za (R.K.); nkhens@icloud.com (N.C.-M.)
3 Department of Medical Oncology, Steve Biko Academic Hospital, University of Pretoria, Pretoria 0084, South Africa
4 Gynaecologic Oncology Unit, Department of Obstetrics and Gynaecology, Charlotte Maxeke Johannesburg Academic Hospital, University of the Witwatersrand, Johannesburg 2193, South Africa; langanani.mbodi@wits.ac.za
5 Department of Surgery, Charlotte Maxeke Johannesburg Academic Hospital, University of the Witwatersrand, Parktown, Johannesburg 2193, South Africa; thifhelimbilu.luvhengo@wits.ac.za
6 Papillon Plastic Surgery, Suite 203B, 24 12th Avenue, Linksfield West, Johannesburg 2192, South Africa
7 Department of Surgery, Faculty of Health Sciences, University of Kwa-Zulu Natal, Durban 4041, South Africa; phakathib@ukzn.ac.za
* Correspondence: zodwa.dlamini@up.ac.za

Abstract: Triple-negative breast cancer (TNBC) accounts for approximately 20% of all breast cancer cases and is characterized by a lack of estrogen, progesterone, and human epidermal growth factor 2 receptors. Current targeted medicines have been unsuccessful due to this absence of hormone receptors. This study explored the efficacy of *Tulbaghia violacea*, a South African medicinal plant, for the treatment of TNBC metastasis. Extracts from *T. violacea* leaves were prepared using water and methanol. However, only the water-soluble extract showed anti-cancer activity and the effects of this water-soluble extract on cell adhesion, invasion, and migration, and its antioxidant activity were assessed using MCF-10A and MDA-MB-231 cells. The *T. violacea* extract that was soluble in water effectively decreased the movement and penetration of MDA-MB-231 cells through the basement membrane in scratch and invasion tests, while enhancing their attachment to a substance resembling an extracellular matrix. The sample showed mild-to-low antioxidant activity in the antioxidant assy. Nuclear magnetic resonance spectroscopy revealed 61 chemical components in the water-soluble extract, including DDMP, 1,2,4-triazine-3,5(2H,4H)-dione, vanillin, schisandrin, taurolidine, and α-pinene, which are known to have anti-cancer properties. An in-depth examination of the transcriptome showed alterations in genes linked to angiogenesis, metastasis, and proliferation post-treatment, with reduced activity in growth receptor signaling, angiogenesis, and cancer-related pathways, such as the Wnt, Notch, and PI3K pathways. These results indicate that *T. violacea* may be a beneficial source of lead chemicals for the development of potential therapeutic medicines that target TNBC metastasis. Additional studies are required to identify the precise bioactive chemical components responsible for the observed anti-cancer effects.

Keywords: migration; invasion; adhesion; oxidation; vanillin; schizandrin; taurolidine; alpha-pinene

1. Introduction

The subtype of breast cancer with the highest risk of spreading and the lowest survival rate is triple-negative breast cancer (TNBC) [1]. TNBC is the most aggressive form of breast cancer. In most countries and populations, ten to twenty percent of all breast cancers are TNBC cases [2] and as such, in the last 5 years, there has been an average of 170,000 TNBC cases per year worldwide [3]. TNBC is characterized by cellular mutations that lead to downregulated or absent expression of receptors for progesterone, estrogen, and human epidermal growth factor receptor 2 [4]. The absence of these receptors makes TNBC difficult to treat, since it is resistant to immune and hormone therapies [5]. Unlike other subtypes of breast cancer, the risk factors for TNBC include lifelong sensitivity to testosterone, shorter periods of breastfeeding, and giving birth to their first child at an older age [6]. TNBC is also found in younger patients diagnosed before the age of 39 [7]. Ethnicity is also an important risk factor for TNBC. People of African descent have a lower overall breast cancer risk than women of European descent, but they have higher mortality rates [8], with a higher incidence of TNBC. Additionally, black women tend to be diagnosed with TNBC at a younger age [9].

Genetic alterations commonly associated with TNBC include mutations in the *TP53* gene, which occurs in approximately 80–85% of patients [10]. *TP53* mutations are commonly associated with a lack of PR, ER, or HER2 expression [11]. Other genes that are commonly mutated in TNBC include RB1, BRCA1 and 2, PTEN, PIK3CA, USH2A, and MCL1; MYC expression is also increased in TNBC as is CCNE1 and FGFR2 expression [12].

Patients with TNBC are treated with non-specific cytotoxic multi-agent chemotherapy. The effectiveness of these treatments has been clinically demonstrated [13]. Despite their poor prognosis, TNBC tumors are particularly chemosensitive, albeit for a shorter duration than other breast cancers. Polychemotherapy has been shown to be effective in several trials; for example, taxane-containing regimens have demonstrated favorable effects on various disease-associated factors such as risk of recurrence, disease-free survival (DFS), and overall survival (OS) in TNBC [14].

Although antioxidant activity can prevent the development of cancer, antioxidants can promote tumorigenesis. One of the characteristics of cancer is an imbalance between ROS and antioxidants, which is normally defined as increased oxidative stress [15]. Cells that detach from the extracellular matrix (ECM) undergo apoptosis [16]. Apoptosis occurs through canonical apoptotic signaling and elevated ROS signaling pathways [17]. This means that any antioxidant process or compound that protects cells from ROS could also protect the cells from ROS-induced cell death. The survival of cells that detach from the ECM is promoted by antioxidant activity. This antioxidant activity can also promote cellular processes that promote tumor metastasis [18]. Small molecules that act as antioxidants, such as NAC (N-acetyl cysteine) and vitamin E, can reduce ROS levels and accelerate tumor metastasis [19].

Plants contain non-nutritive, bioactive, and diverse groups of organic chemicals known as phytochemicals [20]. Recently, phytochemicals isolated from green plants that have previously been used for medicinal purposes have become the focus of the search for new cancer-preventative and cancer therapeutic compounds [21]. Surprisingly, plants are the source of 47% of the FDA-approved drugs that can be used to treat cancer. Some of the recently synthesized anti-cancer compounds based on compounds isolated from plants include vinblastine and vincristine. These two anti-cancer drugs are derived from medicinal herbs such as comfrey [22]. Although several of these plant extracts have been explored as anti-cancer drugs in clinical trials, only a few affect the biochemical and molecular pathways that are actively involved in cancer/tumor formation and regulation, including cell cycle inhibitors, mitogenic signaling antagonists (to inhibit growth and proliferation), metastasis inhibitors, and immune system receptors [23]. One of the most common modes of action of phytochemicals in the treatment of cancer is the induction or modulation of autophagy and apoptosis [24]. In addition, phytochemicals may have antioxidant or pro-oxidant properties. Reactive oxygen species (ROS) are known to act as secondary messengers in a number of signaling cascades, including those directly related to cell proliferation. In this respect, ROS can be considered an important factor involved in the maintenance of cellular homeostasis. A mild increase in the generation of ROS, such as superoxide and hydrogen peroxide, has been shown to stimulate cell proliferation in several different cell types and may play a role in the carcinogenic process [25].

Tulbaghia violacea Harv. (Amaryllidaceae) is a small, bulbous plant native to South Africa. The plant is exclusively found in South Africa, namely, in the provinces of Natal, Gauteng, Northwest, Limpopo, Mpumalanga, and the Eastern Cape. The leaves are hairless and grow on slender, fleshy stems [26]. *T. violacea* (wild garlic) infusions in water have been used in traditional medicine in Southern Africa to cure a variety of ailments, including treating the symptoms associated with a variety of cancers. Many previous studies using this plant have indicated that it has verifiable effects on tumor cells.

Although *T. violacea* has been used in traditional medicine to treat various ailments, little scientific research has been conducted to validate its use. Previously *T. violacea* extracts using organic solvents have been shown to induce apoptosis in various cancer cell lines by inducing the overexpression of p53 [27–29]. It has also been shown that water-soluble extracts also induced apoptosis in cancer cells through increased expression of caspase 3 as well as through increased levels of ROS. The extracts were also shown to be selective for cancer cells, inducing cell death in these cells at a higher rate than in normal cells [30].

This study involved obtaining water- and methanol-soluble extracts from the leaves of *T. violacea* and testing their ability to inhibit the metastatic ability of triple-negative breast cancer cells by monitoring the effect of the extracts on cell adhesion, migration, and invasion. The antioxidant activity of the extracts was also measured using a DPPH antioxidant assay because of the link between antioxidant activity and the promotion of metastasis. Previously, IC_{50} values for these crude extracts were established using various cytotoxicity assays, which allowed us to test the effect of these extracts on the metastatic ability of a TNBC and normal breast cell lines at concentrations just below the IC_{50} as well at concentrations well below this value. In addition, the control breast cells were treated with the same concentration of the extract as the TNBC cells in further tests of the anti-cancer nature of these extracts.

2. Materials and Methods

2.1. Preparation of Plant Extracts

T. violacea plant extracts were prepared using aqueous extraction to obtain water-soluble extracts and methanol-based extraction to obtain non-water-soluble extracts. The species of the collected plants were confirmed by the staff at the C E Moss herbarium at the University of the Witwatersrand. The leaves of the plant were collected, rinsed with water, and cut into smaller pieces and dried for 120 h in a well-ventilated oven (Gallenkamp Genlab prime, Cambridges, UK) at 40 °C to ensure successful extraction. Once dried, the plant material was finely ground using an herb grinder (Fesh-Fesh) and passed through an 850-micron sieve. To extract water-soluble compounds, the dry powder was dissolved in 1 L of boiled water and allowed to cool for 24 h before filtering to obtain an aqueous extract. The filtrate was freeze-dried (Virtis Wizard 2.0, Warminster, PA, USA) to yield a dried aqueous plant extract, which was stored for 72 h.

In order to prepare a methanol extract containing compounds that are insoluble in water, the dried powder was dissolved in 250 mL of pure methanol. The filtrate was then placed in a Soxhlet extractor for 72 h. The crude methanol extract was then completely evaporated. The resulting powder was freeze-dried to form a dry powder.

Fresh solutions were prepared every day. For the aqueous extract, this involved taking 10 mg of powdered extract and dissolving it in either physiological saline, deionized water, or cell culture media, depending on the application. For the methanol extract, 10 mg of dried powdered extract was dissolved in a small amount of physiological saline, deionized water, or culture media; 25 µL of DMSO was added to all these solvents, giving a final concentration of 2.5% DMSO. Once the powder was dissolved, the volume was increased by adding 5 mL of physiological saline. This resulted in a final DMSO concentration of 0.5%. The diluted extract was applied to the cells for 24 h in fresh culture medium containing 10% FBS. Based on the high IC_{50} values for the methanol extract (820 μg/mL) and its inconsistent performance due to poor solubility, it was excluded from many metastasis assays and was only included in the antioxidant assay.

2.2. Cell Culture

MCF-10A (a non-tumorigenic breast epithelial cell line) and MDA-MB-231 (epithelial-like cells from a triple-negative breast cancer tumor) cell lines were used in this study. The cell lines were grown in culture flasks in DMEM media (Lonza, Basel, Switzerland, cat# BE15-604K) with penicillin/streptomycin (10,000 IU/mL) (Lonza, Basel, Switzerland, cat# 17-602E) and 10% FCS (Lonza, Basel, Switzerland cat#S711-001s), and incubated at 37 °C without CO_2.

2.3. Measuring the Effect of Active Plant Extract on Cell Adhesion

To determine the effect of the water-soluble extract on the ability of MDA-MB-231 and MCF-10A cells to adhere to the ECM, Geltrex™ (Thermo Fisher, Waltham, MA, USA, cat#A1413201, Invitrogen), an extracellular matrix (ECM) analog, was used to simulate the ECM in the assays. The surface of 12-well plates (Corning cat#3460, Corning, NY, USA) was coated with 250 μL of a neat Geltrex™ solution. The plate was incubated for 30 min at 37 °C. The wells were washed with blocking buffer (0.5% BSA in DMEM F12 (Lonza cat# 12719F)) for 30 min. The cells were treated with the water-soluble extract at a concentration of 300 μg/mL, as previously described. After 24 h, the cells were washed and suspended in serum-free medium, and were then added to the wells at a concentration of 1×10^5 cells/mL. The cells were incubated for 2 h, and the attached cells were washed and fixed for 10 min at room temperature. The cells were then washed and stained with crystal violet (Sigma-Aldrich, Burlington, MA, USA, cat# NC1635572) for 10 min. The dye was extracted from the stained cells using an SDS solution. Absorbance was measured at 550 nm (Spectramax multimodal plate reader). Control wells without cells were used as references. The absorbance was used as an indication of the number of cells that adhered to the ECM analogue.

2.4. Measuring the Effect the Active Plant Extract Had on Cell Invasion

A chemo-invasion assay was performed to determine the effect of the water-soluble extract on the ability of MDA-MB-231 and MCF-10A cells to invade other body tissues by penetrating an ECM analogue. Based on the original Boyden Assay [31], commercially available plastic inserts for multi-well plates, which possess a cell permeable membrane, as typified by Transwell® Permeable Supports (Corning cat#3460), were used to perform accurate repeatable invasion assays. When placed in the well of a multi-well tissue culture plate, these inserts create a two-chamber system separated by a cell-permeable membrane. The cells were serum-starved for 24 h and then transferred to pre-prepared plates containing transwell inserts. These plates contained media with FBS that served as a chemoattractant in the well. The transwell inserts were 6.5 mm thick with 8 μm pores (Sigma cat Cls3422). The inserts were coated with neat Geltrex and allowed to set at 37 °C for 30 min. Approximately 1×10^6 cells/mL were suspended in medium containing the *T. violacea* water-soluble extract at a concentration of 300 μg/mL, which was added to each insert. The cells were incubated at 37 °C for 24 h. The media was removed from the lower chamber, and the cells that had invaded into the lower chamber were fixed and stained with toluidine blue (Sigma cat#314) for 2 min. The dye was extracted from the cells using an SDS extraction solution for 1 h. The absorbance of the extracted dye at 620 nm was then measured using a SpectraMax M3 reader spectrophotometer (Molecular diagnostics, Sunnyvale, CA, USA).

2.5. Scratch Assay for Migration Analysis

A scratch/migration test was performed to investigate the effect of the plant extracts on the migration and proliferation rates of breast cancer and normal breast cells. The cells were grown in a cell culture plate until they formed a confluent cell monolayer. A cell-free zone was created by scoring the line through a confluent monolayer using a sterile pipette tip. The cells were then incubated with two concentrations of the *T. violacea* water-soluble plant extract, which were slightly lower than the IC_{50} (300 µg/mL) and half the IC_{50} (200 µg/mL). Cells were treated with 5FU were used as a positive control, while the other cells were left untreated. Cell migration and proliferation were monitored microscopically over a 48 h period. Measurements were taken every 2 h for the first 6 h, and then at the 24 and 48 h marks. Changes in the width of the gap (which decreased as the cells proliferated and migrated) indicated cell migration. The width of the scratch was plotted against time to analyze the effect of the extracts on the cells.

2.6. Antioxidant Assay

To determine whether the plant extracts had antioxidant activity, the 2,2-diphenyl-1-picrylhydrazyl (DPPH) assay was performed. The assay was performed according to the method described by Blois [32]. A standard solution of DPPH was prepared by dissolving the DPPH powder (Sigma-Aldrich, Burlington, MA, USA, Cat# 044150.03) in methanol to obtain a final concentration of 50 µg/mL. Various concentrations of the extracts were prepared based on the IC_{50} values. A 96-well plate was prepared with a methanol-only blank, a reference sample of the DPPH solution only, and then various concentrations of the extracts in triplicate with the DPPH solution added. The plate was then incubated for 30 min in the dark. The absorbance of the wells was measured at 515 nm using a plate reader to determine the number of neutralized radicals. The percentage of DPPH used was calculated using the following formula:

$$\frac{\text{A515 of tested compound} - \text{blank}}{}$$

$$100\% - \text{A515 initial DPPH methanol solution} - \text{blank} \times 100$$

The concentration required to neutralize 50% of the DPPH (EC50) was determined by plotting the natural logarithm of the %DPPH remaining versus the concentration of the sample.

2.7. Determining the Molecular Composition of the Water-Soluble Extract

An NMR analysis was performed on the water-soluble extract of *T. violacea* to identify the chemical constituents of this crude extract. The NMR tube was cleaned, and approximately 10 mg of the starting material was added. All substances were dissolved before the samples were gently shaken. To ensure that all the samples were exposed to a uniform magnetic field, the spinner was turned after it was placed in the magnet. To eliminate fingerprints and grime, 2-propanol and laboratory tissues were used to wipe the exterior of the NMR tube. The rotor of an autosampler-equipped Varian 600 MHz spectrometer was employed. After the NMR test was completed, the spectra were analyzed, and peaks were assigned. The NMR spectrum was interpreted using an appropriate application to analyze the spectrum (MestReNova v14.3.3, from Mesytalab Research, Santiago de Compostela, Spain).

2.8. Next-Generation Sequencing to Measure the Transcript Levels of Genes Involved in Proliferation and Metastasis

Next-generation sequencing was performed by Inqaba Biotechnology Industries (Pretoria, South Africa). RNA fragments were analyzed using a bioanalyzer. A sequencing library was prepared using the MiSeq RNA-0 rRNA reduction library kit (Illumina, San Diego, CA, USA, cat# 20020492). Sequencing was performed using a NextSeq300 system (Illumina, San Diego, CA, USA. Paired-end sequencing was performed at a depth of 10 million bases over 300 cycles. Following sequencing, the raw sequencing data were analyzed using the Galaxy platform (Galaxy Europe ver 22.05 (galaxyproject.eu)) with a pipeline consisting of the following tools: Trimmomatic, which was used to trim the reads, and FastQC, which was used to generate the quality control reports. HiSAT2 was used to align the reads. Differential gene expression was analyzed using the Limma package ver 3.52.4 (limma-voom). The HG38 human genome was used as the reference genome, and reference mapping was performed using bowtie2. PANTHER was used to identify genes involved in invasion, metastasis, and adhesion. The feature counts for the transcript levels were compared between the treated and untreated cell extracts.

2.9. Statistical Analysis

When comparing the means for the data obtained from the adhesion, migration, and invasion assays, one-way ANOVA with the Bonferroni post hoc multiple comparisons test was performed. Tukey's test was then used for pairwise mean comparisons. For the migration assay, due to the inconsistent response of the normal cell line to the initial scratching of the monolayer, we performed Levene's test for homogeneity of variance. The significant differences between the treated and untreated samples were tested using one-way ANOVA with Bonferroni correction.

3. Results

3.1. Effect of the Extract on Cell Adhesion

To assess the effect of the *T. violacea* water-soluble leaf extract on cell adhesion in the triple-negative breast cancer cell line MDA-MB-231 and the normal breast cell line MCF-10, an adhesion assay was performed using Geltrex^{TM} as an ECM analog and the number of cells able to adhere to the surface before and after treatment was determined. The number of cells was determined using a dye-absorption assay. As shown in Figure 1, the extract increased the number of MDA-MB-231 cells that adhered to the ECM analog, with greater numbers of these cells being found on the matrix compared to the treated and untreated normal breast cells. At the same time, it was observed that the treatment had no effect on the number of normal cells that adhered to the ECM. As expected, the untreated MDA-MB-231 cells had fewer cells adhering to the synthetic ECM than the normal breast cells. This indicates that the *T. violacea* crude water-soluble extract was able to increase cell adhesion in a population of TNBC cells.

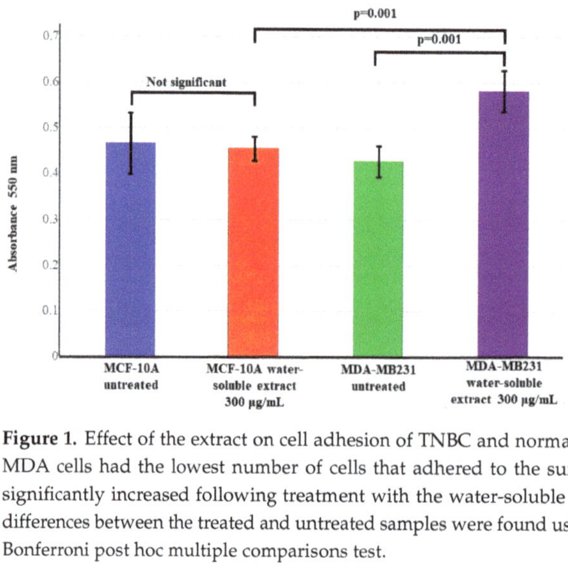

Figure 1. Effect of the extract on cell adhesion of TNBC and normal breast cell lines. The control MDA cells had the lowest number of cells that adhered to the surface of the matrix. This was significantly increased following treatment with the water-soluble *T. violacea* extract. Significant differences between the treated and untreated samples were found using one-way ANOVA with the Bonferroni post hoc multiple comparisons test.

3.2. Effect of the Extract on Cell Invasion

Since the ability of cells to penetrate and cross the ECM is vital for metastasis, an invasion assay was performed to test the effects of the water-soluble extract on the invasive properties of MDA-MB-231 and MCF-10A cells. Both cell lines were treated with concentrations of the extract just below the IC_{50}, which was determined in a previous study. The IC_{50} value determined for MDA-MB-231 cells was approximately 395 μg/mL after 72 h, while the IC_{50} value determined for MCF-10A cells was 537 μg/mL. The selected concentration of 300 μg/mL was predicted to kill approximately 40% of cells, and treatment of the TNBC cell line, MDA-MB-231, with the *T. violacea* water-soluble extract significantly decreased the ability of MDA-MB-231 cells to penetrate and cross the ECM analog ($p = 0.001$). This implies that it was able to decrease the ability of these cells to invade other tissues. It had no significant effect on the ability of MCF-10A cells to invade through an ECM analog, as the treated and untreated cells showed no significant difference in the number of cells that invaded through the ECM (Figure 2). The innate ability of MCF10A cells to invade the ECM was significantly less than that of untreated MDA-MB-231 cells ($p = 0.001$). The invasive ability of this TNBC cell line decreased below that of normal breast cells following treatment.

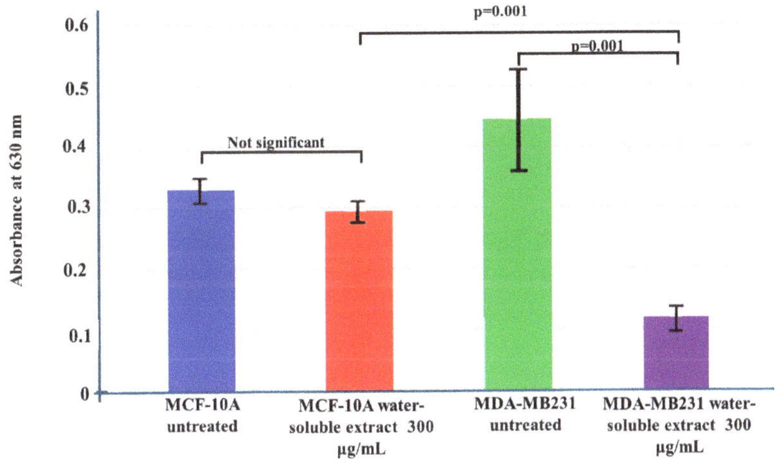

Figure 2. Effect of the extract on the invasive ability of TNBC and normal breast cell lines. The high absorbance for the untreated MDA-MB-231 samples indicates that many of these cells invaded through the ECM matrix, and so, the amount of dye absorbed was high. The treatment of these cells led to a large decrease in the number of invading cells. The extract had very little effect on the normal cells. The significant differences between the treated and untreated samples were tested using one-way ANOVA with the Bonferroni post hoc multiple comparisons test.

3.3. Measuring the Effect of the Active Plant Extract on Cell Migration

The wound-healing or scratch assay was one of the earliest methods developed to study cell migration in vitro [32]. This method is based on observations of cell migration into a "wound" that is created in a cell monolayer and to some extent mimics cell migration. This assay was performed to ascertain the potential effects of the crude extract on cell migration. Figure 3 displays the scratch area that was measured using Olympus EVOS M7000 imaging software version 1.0 and a light microscope (Olympus CKX41, Olympus, Hachioji, Tokyo, Japan) It can be seen from these plots that there was no significant difference in the area of the scratch between treated and untreated cells in either cell line ($p = 0.9969$ and $p = 0.9916$) at 0 h, indicating that the scratch size was the same between the treated and untreated cell lines. However, MCF10A cells showed large variances between replicates with large error bars for the standard error. Levene's test for variance of homogeneity showed that the MCF10A cells at 0 h did not meet the requirement for homogeneity (f-ratio = 16.07997, p-value = 0.002478). This indicated that the normal cell line reacted differently to the physical act of scratching the cell monolayer. Therefore, there does seem to be a significant difference between the treated and untreated MCF-10 cells at 0 h. As such, a logarithmic adjustment to the data was performed and the ANOVA was repeated

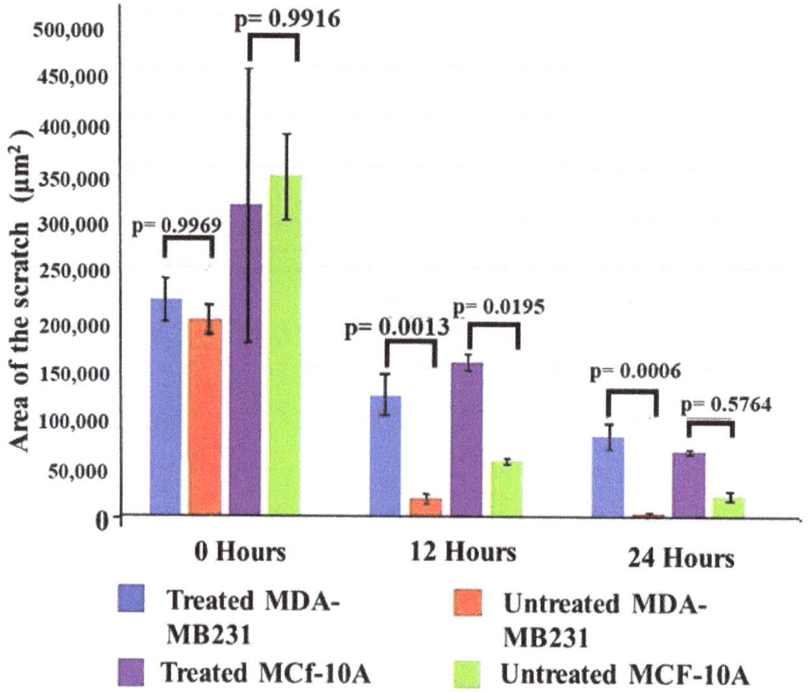

Figure 3. Effect of the extract on the migratory abilities of TNBC and normal breast cell lines. Changes in the scratch area following treatment with the extract were analyzed. Initially, there was no significant difference at 0 h, and no statistically significant difference was observed between the untreated and treated cells in either cell line. Treatment of either cell line with the extract for 12 h inhibited cell migration. This effect persisted in the MDA-MB-231 cells. However, the MCF-10A cells either recovered or were less affected by the extract. The significant differences between the treated and untreated samples were tested using one-way ANOVA with the Bonferroni post hoc multiple comparisons test. Due to the size of the error bars at 0 h, Levene's test for homogeneity of variance was performed. For the MCF-10A samples at 0 h, the homogeneity of variance assumption was not met (F-ratio = 16.07997, p-value = 0.002478).

After 12 h, there was nearly complete closure of the scratch in the untreated MDA-MB-231 cells, while the cells treated with *T. violacea* water-soluble extract showed a significantly larger cleared area where cell migration had not occurred (p = 0.0132). This lack of closure in the treated cells still persisted at the 24 h mark (p = 0.0006). A similar situation was observed in the normal MCF-10A breast cells, where there was a significant difference in the area of the scratch between treated and untreated cells at 12 h (p = 0.01953). However, after 24 h, there was no significant difference between treated and untreated MCF-10A cells (p = 0.5764). This indicates a weaker or shorter-lived effect of the extract on MCF-10A normal breast cells.

The effect of the various concentrations of the extract on the narrowing of the scratch in TNBC cell lines is shown in Figure 4. The untreated cells rapidly migrated to close the leading edges of the scratch after approximately 35 h. The highest concentration of the extract was as effective as 5FU at inhibiting cell migration. This concentration was previously established to kill 40% of MDA-MB-231 cells. A concentration of 200 µg/mL was previously shown to kill approximately 20% of cells. The lowest concentration of the extract (one-third of the IC_{50} value) was previously shown to kill less than 5% of MDA-MB-231 cells, and only delayed the closure of the scratch by approximately 25 h.

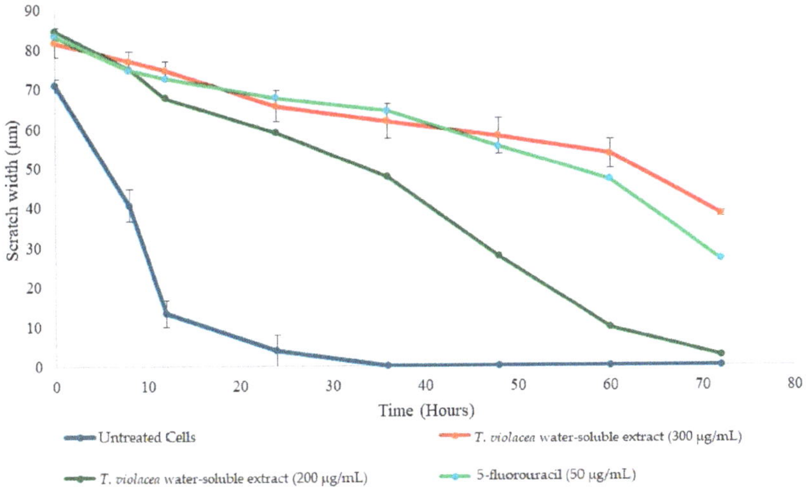

Figure 4. Effects of different concentrations of the water-soluble extract on the migratory abilities of TNBC cell lines. Changes in scratch width in μm^3 over time following treatment with the extract. The untreated cells migrated rapidly and by the 60th hour after treatment, the scratch was fully closed in the untreated cell line. The scratch in cells treated with lower concentrations of the water-soluble extract closed more rapidly and to a greater degree than the scratch in the positive control and cells treated with higher concentrations of water.

3.4. *Determination of Antioxidant Activity Using the 2,2-Diphenyl-1-picrylhydrazyl (DPPH) Radical-Scavenging Method*

Antioxidant activity was measured in terms of the hydrogen-donating ability or the radical-scavenging ability of the extracts using the stable radical DPPH. The experiments were performed according to the method described by Blois [33]. The amount of sample necessary to decrease the absorbance of DPPH by 50% (IC50) was calculated graphically for the water-soluble solutions of *T. violacea* at different concentrations. Figure 5 shows the results of this assay. The water-soluble extract showed antioxidant activity with a Y-intercept similar to that of the positive control, quercetin. However, as the concentration of quercetin increased, the antioxidant activity increased rapidly, whereas an increase in the concentration of the extract resulted in only a small increase in antioxidant activity. The IC_{50} value for the water-soluble extract was calculated to be 393 µg/mL. This value is much higher than that of classic antioxidants, as well as most of the many plant extracts, as presented in Table 1, implying that the antioxidant activity of the extract is very low and, as such, does not promote metastasis.

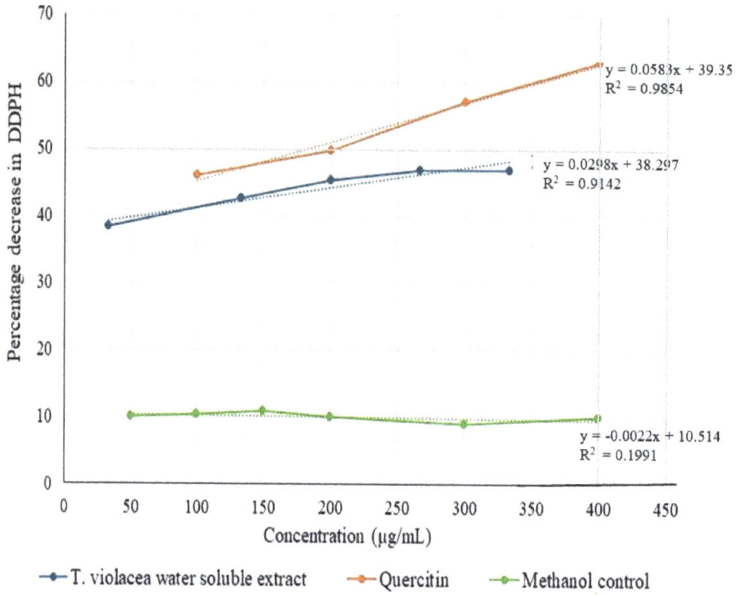

Figure 5. Antioxidant assay. The ability of the extract to scavenge DPPH free radicals is a reflection of its antioxidant activity. The activity of the water-soluble extract of *T. violacea* was similar to that of the positive control, quercetin. This implies that the water-soluble extract has antioxidant activity. The corresponding dotted trendlines give a clearer indication of the trend of antioxidant activity trend of each sample.

Table 1. Some IC50 values for well-known antioxidants.

Compound	IC_{50}	Ref(s).
Ascorbic acid	3.8 µg/mL	[34]
Astragalus Alopecurus var Maximus (Willd.)	115.5 µg/mL	[35]
Avocado (*Folium* perseae Mill.)	601 µg/mL	[36]
Caffeic acid	1.6 µg/mL	[37]
Cinnamon (*Cinnamomum verum* J. Presl)	21.3 µg/mL	[38]
Bindweed (*Convulvulus betonicifolia* Mill.)	346.5 µg/mL	[39]
Fennel (*Foeniculum vulgare* Mill.)	263.2 µg/mL	[40]
Tulbaghia violacea Harv.	393 µg/mL	This study
Verbascum speciousum Schrad.	173.3 µg/mL	[41]
Ginger (*Zingiber officinale* Roscoe)	16.2 µg/mL	[42]

3.5. Identification of Compounds Using NMR

An NMR analysis of the water-soluble extract indicated the presence of 61 compounds. A list of these compounds is provided in Table 2. The names of these compounds were used as queries to search PubChem in order to identify compounds with known anti-cancer activity. Eight compounds were identified that have known anti-cancer activity. These are 4H-pyran-4-one, 2,3-dihydro-3,5-dihydroxy-6-methyl-(DDMP), 1,2,4-triazine-3,5(2H,4H)-dione, benzaldehyde, 4-(1-methylethyl), vanillin, pyrrolidine, schizandrin, taurolidine, and alpha-pinene. Some of these compounds have known medical uses and applications, whereas others have known applications that are not related to medical applications. Finally, some of the identified compounds have no known uses. The structures of the eight compounds with known anti-cancer activity and their mass charge spectra are shown in Figure 6.

Table 2. Examples of compounds detected by NMR analysis of crude water-soluble *T. violacea* extracts.

Phytochemical Compound	Exact Mass	Formula	Ref.
4H-Pyran-4-one,2,3-dihydro-3,5-dihydroxy-6-methyl-(DDMP)	144.12	$C_6H_8O_4$	[43]
1,2,4-Triazine-3,5(2H,4H)-dione	113.08	$C_3H_3N_3O_2$	[44]
d-Glycero-d-galacto-heptose	210.18	$C_7H_{14}O_7$	[45]
Benzaldehyde, 4-(1-methylethyl)	148.20	$C_{10}H_{12}O$	[46]
Vanillin	152.15	$C_8H_8O_3$	[47]
Methoxy-phenyl oxime	151.16	$C_8H_9NO_2$	[48]
Pyrrolidine	71.12	C_4H_9N	[49]
Schizandrin	432.50	$C_{24}H_{32}O_7$	[50]
Taurolidine	284.40	$C_7H_{16}N_4O_4S_2$	[51]
Alpha-pinene	136.23	$C_{10}H_{16}$	[52]
Terbutaline,N-trifluoroacetyl-o,o,o-tris(trimethylsilyl)	537.80	$C_{23}H_{42}F_3NO_4Si_3$	[53]
Difenoxin	424.50	$C_{28}H_{28}N_2O_2$	[54]
Mephobarbital	246.26	$C_{13}H_{14}N_2O_3$	[55]
Benserazide	257.24	$C_{10}H_{15}N_3O_5$	[56]
Antipyrine	188.23	$C_{11}H_{12}N_2O$	[57]
Tricyclo [3.3.1.1(3,7)] decan-1-amine	151.25	$C_{10}H_{17}N$	[58]
Thymol	150.22	$C_{10}H_{14}O$	[59]
Cyclandelate	276.40	$C_{17}H_{24}O_3$	[60]
Benzene propanoic acid	150.17	$C_9H_{10}O_2$	[61]
Ethchlorvynol	144.60	C_7H_9ClO	[62]
Cycloserine	102.09	$C_3H_6N_2O_2$	[63]
Emylcamate	145.20	$C_7H_{15}NO_2$	[64]
2-Propen-1-amine	57.09	C_3H_7N	[65]
Methyl formate	60.05	$C_2H_4O_2$	[66]
Tetradecamethyl-cycloheptasiloxane	519.07	$C_{14}H_{42}O_7Si_7$	[67]
Cyanogen chloride	61.47	CNCl	[68]

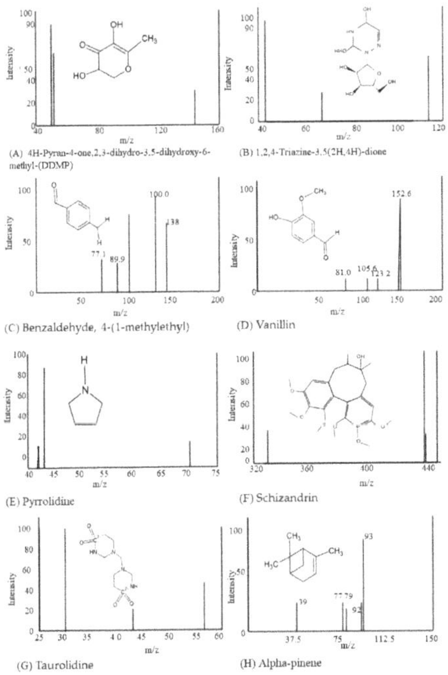

Figure 6. Compounds identified in the water-soluble extract with suspected antioxidant or anti-metastatic activity. Of the 61 compounds identified using NMR, these 8 compounds were identified as having either antioxidant activity or have published studies on their anti-metastatic activity.

3.6. Transcription Profiles of Genes Involved in Adhesion, Invasion, and Metastasis

Next-generation sequencing of RNA extracted from both MDA-MB231 and MCF-10A cells before and after treatment with the water-soluble *T. violacea* extract allowed us to establish the levels of transcripts (feature counts) in the transcriptomes of these cells. Using PANTHER to classify all the genes identified in this analysis based on their biological roles, all the genes that were involved in invasion, adhesion, and metastasis were identified and their levels of transcription before and after treatment were compared. Figure 7 shows the results of this analysis, with Figure 7A depicting the fold change in transcripts identified in the MDA-MB-231 TNBC cell line, while 7B depicts the fold change observed for these genes in MCF10A normal breast cells. Figure 7C shows the genes whose transcription was detected only after treatment in TNBC cells (red circle) or normal cells (blue circle). Additionally, the levels of the transcripts for some genes became undetectable in normal cells after treatment (green circle).

SNAI1 and 3 negatively regulate cell adhesion [69]. The transcription levels of both of these genes were increased in MDA-MB-231 cells following treatment. The same was true for Gli2. The inhibition of Gli2 has been associated with decreased migration and invasion [70]. DISP1, HHIPL1, SDCCAG8, and PTCH2 are components of the sonic hedgehog pathway that plays a role in stimulating invasion and metastasis [71]. The transcription of both of these genes increased following treatment with the water-soluble extract. CDON mediates cell adhesion, and its transcription increased following treatment with the extract [72]. LRP2BP is involved in cell migration and metastasis and was downregulated following treatment. The Ras signaling pathway is involved in cell migration and the transcription of components of this pathway (Grb2, Ras, and Sos [73]) remained largely unchanged. Several mitogen-activated protein kinase (MAPK) transcripts were detected. MAPKs are known to play a role in cell migration [74]. The transcript levels of most of these MAPKs remained unchanged following treatment, except for MAPK11, which increased following treatment. Components of the AKT pathway also play a role in cell migration and invasion [75]. The transcript levels of these genes remained largely unchanged. c-Fos knockdown results in decreased migration, invasion, and metastasis [76]. The only genes that showed major increases in transcription following treatment were c-fos, MAPK11, SNAIL1, CDON, and DISP1. In the MCF10A cell line, the treatment resulted in the absence of multiple transcripts, including those for multiple MAPKs, and AKT and Ras pathway components.

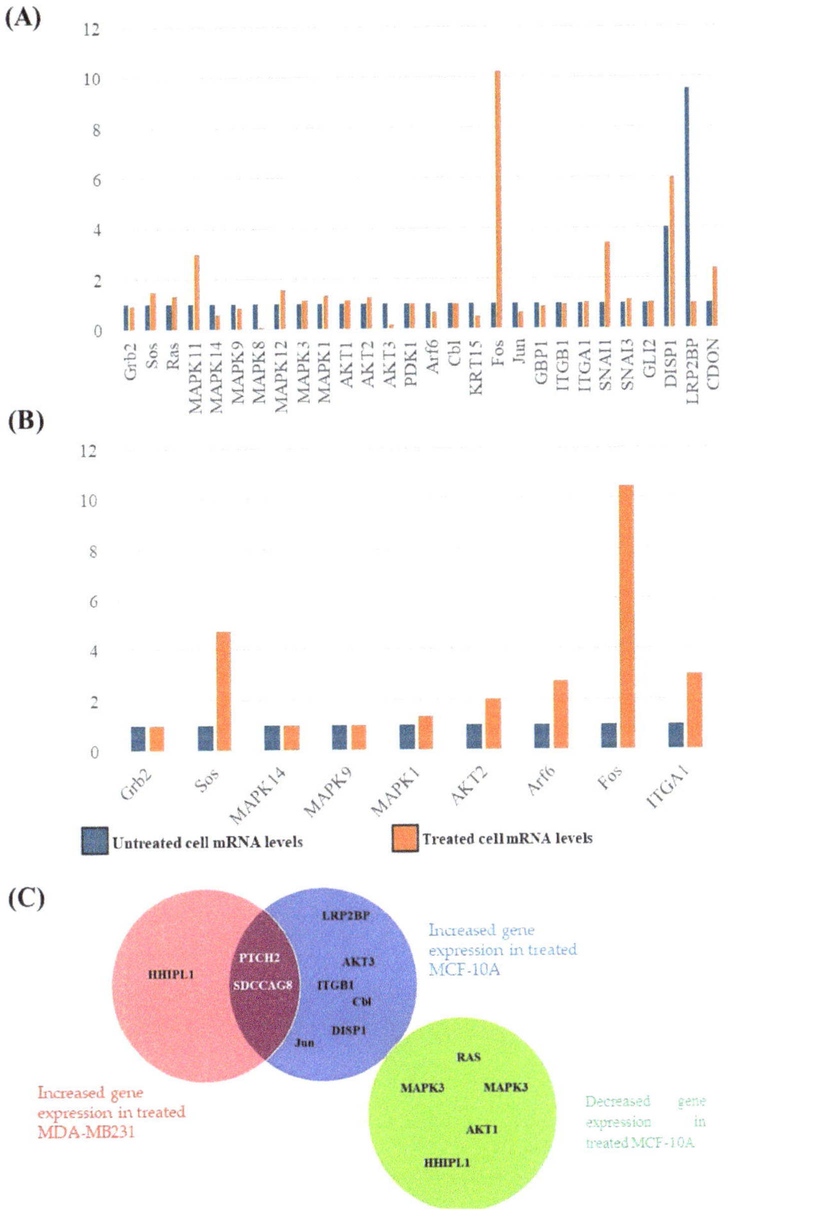

Figure 7. Levels of transcripts for genes involved in migration, invasion, and adhesion detected by NGS analysis of treated and untreated TNBC and normal breast cell lines. (**A**) Fold change in transcripts identified in MDA-MB-231 TNBC cells. The treatment resulted in an increase in the transcription of MAPK11, c-Fos, DISP1, and CDON. The levels of LRP2BP decreased following treatment. (**B**) The fold changes observed for these genes in MCF10A normal breast cells showed an increase in the transcription of Sos, AKT2, Arf6, c-Fos, and ITGA1. In both (**A**,**B**), red signifies the transcript level following treatment, while blue indicates the transcript level of untreated cells. (**C**) Genes whose transcription level was only detected after treatment in TNBC cells (red circle) or normal cells (blue circle). Additionally, the level of transcripts for some genes became undetectable in normal cells after treatment (green circle).

4. Discussion

The ability to invade tissues and penetrate the extracellular matrix of basement membranes and stromal compartments is a major reason why metastasis is the principal cause of cancer-related deaths [77,78]. Inhibition of cancer migration and invasion is an attractive target for the development of new therapies. The ability of cancer cells to metastasize depends on their adherence, ability to invade other tissues, and ability to move and migrate. The effect of the water-soluble extract on the ability of MDA-MB-231 cells to metastasize was assessed using various assays.

4.1. Cell Invasion, Migration, and Adhesion Assays

Cell differentiation, cell cycle, migration, and survival can all be stimulated by cell adhesion [79]. It also plays an essential role in cell communication, regulation, development, and the maintenance of tissues. Changes in cell adhesion can be a defining event in cancer [79,80]. In cancer cells, adhesiveness is generally reduced due to lower intercellular adhesion, allowing cancer cells to dissociate from other cells [80]. Tumor cells are characterized by changes in their adhesion to the ECM, which may be related to their invasive and metastatic potential. The ability of MDA-MB-231 cells to adhere to a synthetic analog of laminin ECM components was evaluated following treatment with the water-soluble extract and assessed using a toluene blue dye absorption assay. The water-soluble extract decreased the migration ability of these cells by increasing their adhesion to the ECM. At the same time, the extract had no effect on normal breast cell adherence to the ECM.

In vitro invasion assays were performed to better understand the effect of the *T. violacea* crude extract on the metastasis process. Neoplastic cells require the ability to invade the surrounding tissue or enter the blood or lymphatic system after adhering to cell membranes in vivo. Once attached to a target basement membrane, they are enzymatically digested by type IV collagenase, allowing for entry into the circulatory system, migration, and finally the establishment of a metastatic (secondary) tumor by re-attachment of the migrating cells to the blood vessel [81]. Invasion assays, which mimic this process, provide an indication of the ability of cells to pass through an ECM (laminin-1)-coated membrane similar to the basal lamina. Untreated MDA-MB-231 cells migrated through the matrix-coated membrane and attached to the underside. In contrast, the inclusion of the *T. violacea* crude water extracts in the assay significantly hampered cell invasion, resulting in far fewer cells traversing the membrane. These findings are consistent with those of the adhesion assays, as cell adhesion is required for invasion. Previous studies using breast, lung, cervical, prostate, and colon cancer cell lines found a positive correlation between adhesion and invasion [82].

The effect of the extracts on the migration ability of MDA-MB-231 cells was assessed using scratch or wound assays. The scratch assays showed that the scratch area decreased rapidly when the cells were left untreated, which was also observed when the distance between the two cell fronts was used as an indication of wound closure. The *T. violacea* water-soluble extract showed consistent effects on the migration of MDA-MB-231 cells at a concentration lower than the IC_{50} at 300 µg/mL, which was previously shown to kill less than 40% of cells. This effect occurred in the first 12 h following treatment and persisted for 24 h until approximately 35 h after treatment, when the effect began to decrease and cell migration increased. Since no further extract was added, this time indicates the active lifespan of the components within the extract or how long the cells take to recover. Using half of the IC_{50} concentration of the extract, it was observed that the inhibitory effect on cell migration ended after only 24 h. However, even at this lower concentration, the wound reached full closure after 72 h. This seems to indicate that the cells took time (approximately 24 h) to recover from the inhibitory effects of the extract on cell migration and it was not due to the continued activity of the extract. This effect of the *T. violacea* water-soluble extract was not exclusively due to increased cell death and seems to be due to the effect of the extract on the ability of cells to migrate by targeting the molecules or signaling pathways involved in migration. The migration of normal MCF-10A breast cells was negatively affected by the extract. However, the effect was not as strong or as long-lasting as that on TNBC cells. As expected, normal cells migrated at a slower rate than cancer cells.

4.2. Assay for Antioxidant Activity

Plants are rich in secondary metabolites that are natural antioxidants and their antioxidant activity is frequently linked to the presence of phenolic compounds. Polyphenolic compounds are the most potent natural antioxidants among the various plant secondary metabolites [83,84].

The water-soluble extract of *T. violacea* demonstrated weak-to-moderate antioxidant activity, particularly in reducing DPPH radicals [85]. However, the role of antioxidants in cancer progression and metastasis is intricate, as excessive antioxidant activity may potentially protect cancer cells from oxidative stress-induced cell death, thereby promoting tumor growth and metastasis [86]. Therefore, it is crucial to carefully evaluate the antioxidant properties of the *T. violacea* extract in the context of its potential anti-metastatic effects [27]. A balanced approach is necessary to understand the interplay between the extract's antioxidant and anti-cancer activities, as well as the underlying mechanisms involved [87]. Further research is warranted to elucidate the specific compounds responsible for these activities and their potential therapeutic applications [88] (Figure 5). The compounds that scavenge DPPH radicals are expected to be hydrophilic radical scavengers because of their presence in the water-soluble extract. One of the identified water-soluble radical scavengers was H-pyran-4-one, 2,3-dihydro-3,5-dihydroxy-6-methyl (DDMP). DDMP is a strong antioxidant [89] that can be formed non-enzymatically from hexose [90], and thermal degradation of D-glucose to form DDMP has been reported [91]. This study identified DDMP as a major water-soluble radical scavenger present in the *T. violacea* water-soluble extract. This may have contributed to the ability of the extract to act as a radical scavenger of DPPH radicals in the antioxidant assay. DDMP is known for its potent antioxidant properties [92]. The second relevant compound, pyrrolidine, is a nitroxide, a stable free radical with an unpaired electron in its nitroxyl group and therefore has antioxidant activity. Nitroxides can accept electrons from reactive oxygen species (ROS) and convert them into stable, non-radical forms. This process helps neutralize ROS and reduce oxidative stress, making nitroxides valuable as antioxidants and potentially useful in various medical and biological applications [48].

4.3. Effect of the Identified Compounds on Metastasis and Invasion

To achieve successful motility, cellular signaling networks are activated, which results in morphological changes [93]: cells lose their epithelial characteristics and adopt mesenchymal-like characteristics, such as E-cadherin expression. These signaling networks include the Wnt/β-catenin and Hh pathways [94]. Based on our findings, the *T. violacea* water crude extracts were able to disrupt the pathways involved in MDA-MB-231 migration and their ability to populate a cell-free zone. This implies that the crude *T. violacea* extracts are effective in promoting cell adhesion and impeding cell invasion and migration, thereby decreasing their metastatic ability.

Triazine-3,5(2H,4H)-dione (6-azauracil) is a pyrimidine analog that has demonstrated substantial antitumor effects against various transplantable mouse tumors [95]. The 1,2,4-triazine ring is a prominent structural motif in many naturally occurring and synthetically derived biologically active compounds. These include anti-cancer and anti-inflammatory agents [96]. Cytosine arabinoside is one of the three most important pyrimidine antimetabolites in cancer chemotherapy [97]. Well-established chemotherapeutic agents, such as 5-fluorouracil (5FU), 6-mercaptopurine (6MP), 6-thioguanine (6-TG), cytosine arabinoside (ARA-C), and methotrexate (MTX), inhibit cancer cell proliferation and survival by inhibiting DNA synthesis. These drugs target different aspects of cancer cell growth and replication, making them valuable tools for cancer chemotherapy [98]. Research performed on 6-azauridine (6AU) by the National Cancer Institute using animal models demonstrated that this compound led to hematological enhancements and could be used to treat newly diagnosed cancers [99]. The biological activities of azanucleosides, nucleoside analogs with a furanose ring replaced by a nitrogen-containing ring or chain, have been a subject of research interest [100]. 6AU is known to inhibit transcription by depleting the intracellular pool of guanosine monophosphate (GMP) and uridine monophosphate (UMP) [101].

Benzaldehyde, or 4-(1-methylethyl)-(cuminaldehyde), is known to cause lysosomal vacuolation, acidic compartment enlargement, cytotoxicity, and inhibition of topoisomerase I and II activities, thereby decreasing tumor size [102]. It is known as an agent capable of inhibiting cell growth [103].

Vanillin, chemically known as 4-hydroxy-3-methoxybenzaldehyde, has shown anti-cancer properties, mainly owing to its strong antimutagenic action [104]. The FDA considers vanillin safe for use in food and pharmaceutical products, due to its oral LD_{50} in rats ranging from 1.58 to 2.8 g/kg [105]. Vanillin has been demonstrated to decrease MMP-9, an enzyme responsible for extracellular matrix disintegration, which aids cancer cell invasion and metastasis. By inhibiting MMP-9, vanillin may further limit the invasive and metastatic potential of cancer cells via the downregulation of the nuclear factor-B (NF-κB) signaling pathway in human hepatocellular carcinoma cells [106]. The ability of vanillin to prevent cancer cell invasion and migration at non-lethal dosages may be due to its ability to inhibit DNA repair mechanisms. Vanillin also exhibits antioxidant activity. It inhibits DNA-dependent protein kinases, enhancing cancer cell sensitivity to cisplatin [107].

The structural similarities between vanillin and acetyl salicylic acid and their potential anti-invasive effects in different cancer cell lines call for further research into their therapeutic capabilities in impeding cancer cell invasiveness [107]. Previous studies have confirmed the anti-metastatic effectiveness of vanillin against breast cancer cells in laboratory and animal models [108]. Vanillin obstructs cell migration and the breakdown of the extracellular matrix (ECM), which is crucial for cancer invasion. This suggests that vanillin can effectively prevent cancer invasion in experimental models and may help reduce metastasis in living organisms. Furthermore, vanillin has been shown to decrease cell growth in vitro, indicating its potential as an improved anti-metastatic drug. Notably, the anti-metastatic effect of vanillin was evident in living organisms at a well-tolerated dosage in mice [104].

Another significant compound identified in the extract was schizandrin, which is known for its anti-cancer properties, including its ability to operate as a dual inhibitor of P-glycoprotein and multidrug resistance protein 1 (MRP1), contributing to its efficacy against cancer cells [109]. Schizandrin also inhibits ATR protein kinase, specifically its response to DNA damage [110]. Schizandrin has been shown to produce a remarkable reduction in 4T1 lung metastasis and prolonged survival in mice. It largely inhibits 4T1 cell metastasis at the local invasion stage and reduces epithelial–mesenchymal transition (EMT) in both 4T1 and primary human breast cancer cells, lowering their metastatic potential [111]. The involvement of schizandrin in suppressing cancer cell metastasis, as well as its advantages when combined with other anti-cancer medications, highlights its diverse pharmacological effects, including antioxidant, anti-asthmatic, anti-inflammatory, and anti-cancer properties [21].

Schisandrin inhibits glioma cell growth and invasion by modulating several signaling pathways [112] and inhibits TGF-1-induced epithelial–mesenchymal transition (EMT) in human A549 cells [113]. Cell migration, invasion, epithelial–mesenchymal transition (EMT), and cancer stem cell (CSC) properties are inhibited by schisandrin. Furthermore, it may regulate additional signaling pathways linked with EMT, including the SMAD, PI3K/AKT, Wnt, and Notch pathways, indicating that schisandrin has a larger regulatory impact on these cancer-related processes. Schisandrin causes cell cycle arrest in A549 cells by down-regulating cyclin D1, cyclin-dependent kinase (CDK) 4, and CDK6 while simultaneously upregulating p53 and p21 [114]. Schisandrin lowered SIRT1 protein expression, and there was a negative association between SIRT1 and the stimulation of SMURF2, which inhibits colon cancer cell proliferation and dissemination [115].

Taurolidine, another compound identified in the *T. violacea* extract, exhibits potent anti-neoplastic and cytotoxic activities, suggesting its potential as a chemotherapeutic agent [50].

Taurolidine exhibits anti-endotoxin, antimicrobial, anti-adhesive, and antifungal traits [116]. Taurolidine inhibited the growth of a rat metastatic colorectal tumor cell line in vitro and in vivo, indicating that it may be useful in preventing peritoneal metastases [117]. Taurolidine likely acts by directly diminishing IL-1 production in peritoneal macrophages, thereby obstructing the response of tumor cells to growth signals [118]. Consequently, taurolidine undergoes enzymatic hydrolysis and decomposes into methyloltaurultam and taurultam, which further breaks down into methyloltaurinamid, ultimately producing taurine and an active methylol group. However, the precise mechanism underlying the suppression of tumor growth by taurolidine in various cancers remains unclear [119]. In a Syrian hamster model of pancreatic adenocarcinoma, taurolidine effectively inhibited primary tumor growth and reduced metastases at both the chemotherapy port site and the liver [120]. The identification of a compound resembling the synthetic compound taurolidine implies that the *T. violacea* extract may contain one or more compounds that are natural product analogs with a similar anti-cancer activity. This possibility warrants further research in order to confirm the presence of these compounds and isolate them. Once isolated, their structural and functional similarity to taurolidine can be confirmed. These taurolidine-like compounds can then serve as lead compounds for the development of new therapeutic drugs to treat TNBC.

Alpha-pinene is a naturally occurring compound that exhibits anti-cancer characteristics [58]. Alpha-pinene was isolated from the water-soluble extract of *T. violacea*. Studies on human ovarian cancer cell lines and human hepatocellular liver carcinoma cell lines have shown that α-pinene has anti-cancer effects [52]. It has also been shown in tests on N2A neuroblastoma cells to have antioxidant, anti-cancer, and genotoxic effects [121]. The capacity of α-pinene to suppress tumor invasion was tested in a study employing highly metastatic MDA-MB-231 human breast cancer cells [122]. TNFα-induced matrix metalloproteinase-9 gene promoter activation and mRNA synthesis have been demonstrated to be inhibited by α-pinene in a dose-dependent manner [120]. NF-κB-dependent transcriptional activity was reduced by α-pinene treatment [123]. It can also suppress TNFα-induced MMP-9 gene expression and the invasive nature of MDA-MB-231 cells [124].

Finally, it is important to remember that when the extracts of *T. violacea* are used by traditional healers, they are using the entire extract and do not perform any purification methods that would isolate individual compounds. As such, the patient is treated with the entire mixture of compounds. We do not know what effect the compounds within the extract may have when working together as the complex mixture of compounds may result in certain compounds behaving very differently from how a pure version of that compound may behave. Perhaps it is the complex mixture of compounds which gives the extract its full ability and any attempt to make a treatment based on the extract should study the potential interactions between the compounds that make up the extract.

4.4. Transcript Analysis of Genes Involved in Migration, Invasion, and Adhesion

The analysis of the transcripts of genes involved in invasion, adhesion, and metastasis showed no clear pattern of changes in the pathways controlling these processes following treatment. Only a few genes in these pathways were altered after treatment with the water-soluble extract. Many genes showed insignificant changes in expression. The normal breast cell line had many genes whose transcripts were only detectable before or after treatment with the extract, which seemed to indicate that the extract induced greater changes in the normal cell line. The changes in the transcription levels of genes involved in migration, invasion, and adhesion did not reflect the changes in these processes that were observed following the treatment. Since the results of the assays seemed to indicate that the extract was able to inhibit migration and invasion while stimulating adhesion, we expected to observe a decrease in the level of transcription of genes involved in migration and invasion and an increase in the transcription of genes involved in adhesion.

The majority of previous studies on *T. violacea* extracts found anti-cancer activities in fractions obtained through the use of organic solvents. However, this study's results agree with those of the study carried out by Saibu et al. [29], which showed activity for the water-soluble extract. All the previous studies on *T. violacea* extracts focused on the cytotoxic nature of the extract and showed that the extract could increase the levels of apoptosis by increasing the expression of p53 and caspase 3 while increasing the levels of ROS. The transcriptome data in this study showed similar increases in the expression of pro-apoptotic genes; however, the focus of this study was on the ability of the extract to prevent the spread of cancer cells by inhibiting cancer cell metastasis and invasion, as well as increasing the cell adhesion to an ECM. The identification of different active compounds in the water and organic solvent fractions is likely due to differences in the extraction methods. This study could have been improved with the use of a "stronger" non-polar solvent than methanol, as there may be many compounds with activity which remained unextracted as they could not be dissolved in the methanol or water.

5. Conclusions

The ability of the water-soluble extract to inhibit cell invasion and metastasis and promote cell adhesion in a TNBC cell line implies that this extract can decrease the spread and progression of triple-negative breast cancer. The water-soluble extract also has moderate antioxidant activity and can prevent oxidative damage and protect tumor cells from death induced by ROS. However, this is an effect of the extract as a whole, and future work should involve activity studies to isolate individual compounds that give the extract its cytotoxic, anti-metastatic, and antioxidative properties. This would identify the compounds that give this extract its desirable cytotoxic and anti-metastatic activities that could be used for TNBC treatment. Therefore, the extract has potential as a basis for the development of new anti-cancer therapies for TNBC.

These results showed that in addition to the cytotoxic effects of the extract on cancer cells, the water-soluble extract was able to prevent metastasis and invasion as well as promote adhesion in a TNBC cell line.

Author Contributions: M.A.: investigation, formal analysis, and writing—original draft preparation. R.H.: investigation, supervision, and writing—review and editing. T.M.: writing—review and editing and validation. R.K.: writing—review and editing. L.M.: writing—review and editing. T.E.L.: writing—original draft preparation and writing—review and editing. N.C.-M.: writing—review and editing. B.P.: resources and writing—review and editing. C.P.: methodology, supervision, and writing—review and editing. Z.D.: conceptualization, writing—review and editing, supervision, and funding acquisition. All authors have read and agreed to the published version of the manuscript.

Funding: This research was funded by the South African Medical Research Council (SAMRC) (Grant Number 23108) and the National Research Foundation (NRF) (Grant Number 138139).

Institutional Review Board Statement: Not applicable.

Informed Consent Statement: Not applicable.

Data Availability Statement: The data presented in this study are available on request from the corresponding author.

Conflicts of Interest: The authors declare no conflicts of interest.

References

1. Shin, V.Y.; Siu, J.M.; Cheuk, I.; Ng, E.K.; Kwong, A. Circulating cell-free miRNAs as biomarker for triple-negative breast cancer. *Br. J. Cancer* **2015**, *112*, 1751–1759. [CrossRef] [PubMed]
2. Dent, R.; Hanna, W.M.; Trudeau, M.; Rawlinson, E.; Sun, P.; Narod, S.A. Pattern of metastatic spread in triple-negative breast cancer. *Breast Cancer Res. Treat.* **2009**, *115*, 423–428. [CrossRef] [PubMed]
3. Foulkes, W.D.; Smith, I.E.; Reis-Filho, J.S. Triple-negative breast cancer. *N. Engl. J. Med.* **2010**, *363*, 1938–1948. [CrossRef]
4. Carey, L.A.; Dees, E.C.; Sawyer, L.; Gatti, L.; Moore, D.T.; Collichio, F.; Ollila, D.W.; Sartor, C.I.; Graham, M.L.; Perou, C.M. The triple negative paradox: Primary tumor chemosensitivity of breast cancer subtypes. *Clin. Cancer Res. Off. J. Am. Assoc. Cancer Res.* **2007**, *13*, 2329–2334. [CrossRef] [PubMed]
5. Boyle, P. Triple-negative breast cancer: Epidemiological considerations and recommendations. *Ann. Oncol. Off. J. Eur. Soc. Med. Oncol.* **2012**, *23* (Suppl. S6), vi7–vi12. [CrossRef] [PubMed]

6. Lara-Medina, F.; Pérez-Sánchez, V.; Saavedra-Pérez, D.; Blake-Cerda, M.; Arce, C.; Motola-Kuba, D.; Villarreal-Garza, C.; González-Angulo, A.M.; Bargalló, E.; Aguilar, J.L.; et al. Triple-negative breast cancer in Hispanic patients: High prevalence, poor prognosis, and association with menopausal status, body mass index, and parity. *Cancer* **2011**, *117*, 3658–3669. [CrossRef]
7. Fostira, F.; Tsitlaidou, M.; Papadimitriou, C.; Pertesi, M.; Timotheadou, E.; Stavropoulou, A.V.; Glentis, S.; Bournakis, E.; Bobos, M.; Pectasides, D.; et al. Prevalence of BRCA1 mutations among 403 women with triple-negative breast cancer: Implications for genetic screening selection criteria: A Hellenic Cooperative Oncology Group Study. *Breast Cancer Res. Treat.* **2012**, *134*, 353–362. [CrossRef] [PubMed]
8. Bamidele, O.; Ali, N.; Papadopoulos, C.; Randhawa, G. Exploring factors contributing to low uptake of the NHS breast cancer screening programme among Black African women in the UK. *Divers. Equal. Health Care* **2017**, *14*, 212–219. [CrossRef]
9. Newman, L.A.; Stark, A.; Chitale, D.; Pepe, M.; Longton, G.; Worsham, M.J.; Nathanson, S.D.; Miller, P.; Bensenhaver, J.M.; Proctor, E.; et al. Association Between Benign Breast Disease in African American and White American Women and Subsequent Triple-Negative Breast Cancer. *JAMA Oncol.* **2017**, *3*, 1102–1106. [CrossRef]
10. Shah, S.P.; Roth, A.; Goya, R.; Oloumi, A.; Ha, G.; Zhao, Y.; Turashvili, G.; Ding, J.; Tse, K.; Haffari, G.; et al. The clonal and mutational evolution spectrum of primary triple-negative breast cancers. *Nature* **2012**, *486*, 395–399. [CrossRef]
11. Vagia, E.; Mahalingam, D.; Cristofanilli, M. The Landscape of Targeted Therapies in TNBC. *Cancers* **2020**, *12*, 916. [CrossRef] [PubMed]
12. Lee, K.M.; Giltnane, J.M.; Balko, J.M.; Schwarz, L.J.; Guerrero-Zotano, A.L.; Hutchinson, K.E.; Nixon, M.J.; Estrada, M.V.; Sánchez, V.; Sanders, M.E.; et al. MYC and MCL1 Cooperatively Promote Chemotherapy-Resistant Breast Cancer Stem Cells via Regulation of Mitochondrial Oxidative Phosphorylation. *Cell Metab.* **2017**, *26*, 633–647.e7. [CrossRef] [PubMed]
13. André, F.; Zielinski, C.C. Optimal strategies for the treatment of metastatic triple-negative breast cancer with currently approved agents. *Ann. Oncol. Off. J. Eur. Soc. Med. Oncol.* **2012**, *23* (Suppl. S6), vi46–vi51. [CrossRef] [PubMed]
14. Hayes, D.F.; Thor, A.D.; Dressler, L.G.; Weaver, D.; Edgerton, S.; Cowan, D.; Broadwater, G.; Goldstein, L.J.; Martino, S.; Ingle, J.N.; et al. HER2 and response to paclitaxel in node-positive breast cancer. *N. Engl. J. Med.* **2007**, *357*, 1496–1506. [CrossRef]
15. Luo, M.; Zhou, L.; Huang, Z.; Li, B.; Nice, E.C.; Xu, J.; Huang, C. Antioxidant Therapy in Cancer: Rationale and Progress. *Antioxidants* **2022**, *11*, 1128. [CrossRef] [PubMed]
16. Buchheit, C.L.; Weigel, K.J.; Schafer, Z.T. Cancer cell survival during detachment from the ECM: Multiple barriers to tumour progression. *Nat. Rev. Cancer* **2014**, *14*, 632–641. [CrossRef]
17. Schafer, Z.T.; Grassian, A.R.; Song, L.; Jiang, Z.; Gerhart-Hines, Z.; Irie, H.Y.; Gao, S.; Puigserver, P.; Brugge, J.S. Antioxidant and oncogene rescue of metabolic defects caused by loss of matrix attachment. *Nature* **2009**, *461*, 109–113. [CrossRef]
18. DeNicola, G.M.; Karreth, F.A.; Humpton, T.J.; Gopinathan, A.; Wei, C.; Frese, K.; Mangal, D.; Yu, K.H.; Yeo, C.J.; Calhoun, E.S.; et al. Oncogene-induced Nrf2 transcription promotes ROS detoxification and tumorigenesis. *Nature* **2011**, *475*, 106–109. [CrossRef]
19. Sayin, V.I.; Ibrahim, M.X.; Larsson, E.; Nilsson, J.A.; Lindahl, P.; Bergo, M.O. Antioxidants accelerate lung cancer progression in mice. *Sci. Transl. Med.* **2014**, *6*, 221ra215. [CrossRef]
20. Liu, M.M.; Huang, Y.; Wang, J. Developing phytoestrogens for breast cancer prevention. *Anti-Cancer Agents Med. Chem.* **2012**, *12*, 1306–1313. [CrossRef]
21. Zhang, Y.; Liu, X.; Ruan, J.; Zhuang, X.; Zhang, X.; Li, Z. Phytochemicals of garlic: Promising candidates for cancer therapy. *Biomed. Pharmacother. = Biomed. Pharmacother.* **2020**, *123*, 109730. [CrossRef] [PubMed]
22. Newman, D.J.; Cragg, G.M. Natural products as sources of new drugs over the 30 years from 1981 to 2010. *J. Nat. Prod.* **2012**, *75*, 311–335. [CrossRef] [PubMed]
23. Mans, D.R.; da Rocha, A.B.; Schwartsmann, G. Anti-cancer drug discovery and development in Brazil: Targeted plant collection as a rational strategy to acquire candidate anti-cancer compounds. *Oncologist* **2000**, *5*, 185–198. [CrossRef] [PubMed]
24. Yang, B.; Liu, Z.; Wang, Q.; Chai, Y.; Xia, P. Pharmacokinetic comparison of seven major bioactive components in normal and depression model rats after oral administration of Baihe Zhimu decoction by liquid chromatography-tandem mass spectrometry. *J. Pharm. Biomed. Anal.* **2018**, *148*, 119–127. [CrossRef]
25. Slika, H.; Mansour, H.; Wehbe, N.; Nasser, S.A.; Iratni, R.; Nasrallah, G.; Shaito, A.; Ghaddar, T.; Kobeissy, F.; Eid, A.H. Therapeutic potential of flavonoids in cancer: ROS-mediated mechanisms. *Biomed. Pharmacother. = Biomed. Pharmacother.* **2022**, *146*, 112442. [CrossRef]
26. Van Wyk, B.-E.; Oudtshoorn, B.v.; Gericke, N. *Medicinal Plants of South Africa*; Briza: Pretoria, South Africa, 1997.
27. Motadi, L.R.; Choene, M.S.; Mthembu, N.N. Anticancer properties of *Tulbaghia violacea* regulate the expression of p53-dependent mechanisms in cancer cell lines. *Sci. Rep.* **2020**, *10*, 12924. [CrossRef]
28. Takaidza, S.; Kumar, A.M.; Ssemakalu, C.C.; Natesh, N.S.; Karanam, G.; Pillay, M. Anticancer activity of crude acetone and water extracts of *Tulbaghia violacea* on human oral cancer cells. *Asian Pac. J. Trop. Biomed.* **2018**, *8*, 456–462.
29. Saibu, G.M.; Katerere, D.; Rees, J.; Meyer, M. Evaluation of the anti-cancer phytotherapeutic potential of *Tulbaghia violacea* plant. *FASEB J.* **2011**, *25*, 962.4. [CrossRef]
30. Saibu, G.M.; Katerere, D.R.; Rees, D.J.; Meyer, M. In vitro cytotoxic and pro-apoptotic effects of water extracts of *Tulbaghia violacea* leaves and bulbs. *J. Ethnopharmacol.* **2015**, *164*, 203–209. [CrossRef] [PubMed]
31. Boyden, S. The chemotactic effect of mixtures of antibody and antigen on polymorphonuclear leucocytes. *J. Exp. Med.* **1962**, *115*, 453–466. [CrossRef]

32. Todaro, G.J.; Lazar, G.K.; Green, H. The initiation of cell division in a contact-inhibited mammalian cell line. *J. Cell. Physiol.* **1965**, *66*, 325–333. [CrossRef] [PubMed]
33. Blois, M. Antioxidant determinations by the use of a stable free radical. *Nature* **1958**, *181*, 1199–1200. [CrossRef]
34. Sharma, G.; Sapkota, B.; Lamichhane, G.; Adhikari, M.; Kunwar, P. Antioxidant Activity of Selected Medicinal Plants of Nepal. *Int. J. Med. Biomed. Sci.* **2017**, *2*, 1–9. [CrossRef]
35. Güven, L.; Erturk, A.; Miloğlu, F.D.; Alwasel, S.; Gulcin, İ.J.P. Screening of antiglaucoma, antidiabetic, anti-alzheimer, and antioxidant activities of *Astragalus alopecurus* pall—Analysis of phenolics profiles by LC-MS/MS. *Pharmaceuticals* **2023**, *16*, 659. [CrossRef]
36. Polat Kose, L.; Bingol, Z.; Kaya, R.; Goren, A.C.; Akincioglu, H.; Durmaz, L.; Koksal, E.; Alwasel, S.H.; Gülçin, İ. Anticholinergic and antioxidant activities of avocado (*Folium perseae*) leaves–phytochemical content by LC-MS/MS analysis. *Int. J. Food Prop.* **2020**, *23*, 878–893. [CrossRef]
37. Cuvelier, M.-E.; Richard, H.; Berset, C. Comparison of the antioxidative activity of some acid-phenols: Structure-activity relationship. *Biosci. Biotechnol. Biochem.* **1992**, *56*, 324–325. [CrossRef]
38. Gulcin, I.; Kaya, R.; Goren, A.C.; Akincioglu, H.; Topal, M.; Bingol, Z.; Cetin Çakmak, K.; Ozturk Sarikaya, S.B.; Durmaz, L.; Alwasel, S. Anticholinergic, antidiabetic and antioxidant activities of cinnamon (*Cinnamomum verum*) bark extracts: Polyphenol contents analysis by LC-MS/MS. *Int. J. Food Prop.* **2019**, *22*, 1511–1526. [CrossRef]
39. Bingol, Z.; Kızıltaş, H.; Gören, A.C.; Kose, L.P.; Topal, M.; Durmaz, L.; Alwasel, S.H.; Gulcin, I.J.H. Antidiabetic, anticholinergic and antioxidant activities of aerial parts of shaggy bindweed (*Convulvulus betonicifolia* Miller subsp.)—Profiling of phenolic compounds by LC-HRMS. *Heliyon* **2021**, *7*, e06986. [CrossRef]
40. Oktay, M.; Gülçin, İ.; Küfrevioğlu, Ö.İ. Determination of in vitro antioxidant activity of fennel (*Foeniculum vulgare*) seed extracts. *LWT-Food Sci. Technol.* **2003**, *36*, 263–271. [CrossRef]
41. Kızıltas, H.; Bingol, Z.; Goren, A.; Alwasel, S.; Gulcin, I. Verbascum speciousum Schrad: Analysis of phenolic compounds by LC-HRMS and determination of antioxidant and enzyme inhibitory properties. *Rec. Nat. Prod* **2023**, *17*, 485–500.
42. Tohma, H.; Gülçin, İ.; Bursal, E.; Gören, A.C.; Alwasel, S.H.; Köksal, E. Antioxidant activity and phenolic compounds of ginger (*Zingiber officinale* Rosc.) determined by HPLC-MS/MS. *J. Food Meas. Charact.* **2017**, *11*, 556–566. [CrossRef]
43. Ban, J.O.; Hwang, I.G.; Kim, T.M.; Hwang, B.Y.; Lee, U.S.; Jeong, H.S.; Yoon, Y.W.; Kimz, D.J.; Hong, J.T. Anti-proliferate and pro-apoptotic effects of 2,3-dihydro-3,5-dihydroxy-6-methyl-4H-pyranone through inactivation of NF-kappaB in human colon cancer cells. *Arch. Pharmacal Res.* **2007**, *30*, 1455–1463. [CrossRef] [PubMed]
44. Sorm, F.; Jakubovic, A.; Slechta, L. The anticancerous action of 6-azauracil (3,5-dioxo-2,3,4,5-tetrahydro-1,2,4-triazine). *Experientia* **1956**, *12*, 271–272. [CrossRef] [PubMed]
45. Liang, L.; Wade Wei, T.Y.; Wu, P.Y.; Herrebout, W.; Tsai, M.D.; Vincent, S.P. Nonhydrolyzable Heptose Bis- and Monophosphate Analogues Modulate Pro-inflammatory TIFA-NF-κB Signaling. *Chembiochem. Eur. J. Chem. Biol.* **2020**, *21*, 2982–2990. [CrossRef]
46. Tsai, K.D.; Liu, Y.H.; Chen, T.W.; Yang, S.M.; Wong, H.Y.; Cherng, J.; Chou, K.S.; Cherng, J.M. Cuminaldehyde from Cinnamomum verum Induces Cell Death through Targeting Topoisomerase 1 and 2 in Human Colorectal Adenocarcinoma COLO 205 Cells. *Nutrients* **2016**, *8*, 318. [CrossRef]
47. Yan, Y.Q.; Xu, Q.Z.; Wang, L.; Sui, J.L.; Bai, B.; Zhou, P.K. Vanillin derivative 6-bromine-5-hydroxy-4-methoxybenzaldehyde-elicited apoptosis and G2/M arrest of Jurkat cells proceeds concurrently with DNA-PKcs cleavage and Akt inactivation. *Int. J. Oncol.* **2006**, *29*, 1167–1172. [CrossRef]
48. Ozma, M.A.; Ghotaslou, R.; Asgharzadeh, M.; Abbasi, A.; Rezaee, M.A.; Kafil, H.S. Cytotoxicity assessment and antimicrobial effects of cell-free supernatants from probiotic lactic acid bacteria and yeast against multi-drug resistant *Escherichia coli*. *Lett. Appl. Microbiol.* **2024**, *77*, ovae084. [CrossRef]
49. Sajjad, F.; You, Q.; Xing, D.; Fan, H.; Reddy, A.G.K.; Hu, W.; Dong, S. Synthesis and biological evaluation of substituted pyrrolidines and pyrroles as potential anticancer agents. *Arch. Pharm.* **2020**, *353*, e2000136. [CrossRef]
50. Lv, X.J.; Zhao, L.J.; Hao, Y.Q.; Su, Z.Z.; Li, J.Y.; Du, Y.W.; Zhang, J. Schisandrin B inhibits the proliferation of human lung adenocarcinoma A549 cells by inducing cycle arrest and apoptosis. *Int. J. Clin. Exp. Med.* **2015**, *8*, 6926–6936.
51. Baker, D.M.; Jones, J.A.; Nguyen-Van-Tam, J.S.; Lloyd, J.H.; Morris, D.L.; Bourke, J.B.; Steele, R.J.; Hardcastle, J.D. Taurolidine peritoneal lavage as prophylaxis against infection after elective colorectal surgery. *Br. J. Surg.* **1994**, *81*, 1054–1056. [CrossRef]
52. Aydin, E.; Türkez, H.; Geyikoğlu, F. Antioxidative, anticancer and genotoxic properties of α-pinene on N2a neuroblastoma cells. *Biologia* **2013**, *68*, 1004–1009. [CrossRef]
53. Duan, X.; Yang, Y.; Yang, A.; Zhao, Y.; Fan, F.; Niu, L.; Hao, N. Terbutaline attenuates LPS-induced injury of pulmonary microvascular endothelial cells by cAMP/Epac signaling. *Drug Dev. Res.* **2022**, *83*, 699–707. [CrossRef] [PubMed]
54. Paul, A. Antidiarrheal agents. In *Introduction to Basics of Pharmacology Toxicology: Volume 2: Essentials of Systemic Pharmacology: From Principles to Practice*; Springer: Singapore, 2021; pp. 605–611.
55. Matin, M.A.; Jaffery, F.N.; Kar, P.P. Role of striatal acetylcholine and free ammmonia in the central stimulatory effects of pp'DDT in rats. Protective effects of barbiturates. *Arch. Toxicol.* **1980**, *45*, 29–35. [CrossRef] [PubMed]
56. Ryan, M.; Slevin, J.T. Restless legs syndrome. *Am. J. Health-Syst. Pharm.* **2006**, *63*, 1599–1612. [CrossRef]

57. Refat, M.S.; Hamza, R.Z.; Adam, A.; Saad, H.A.; Gobouri, A.A.; Al-Salmi, F.A.; Altalhi, T.; El-Megharbel, S.M. Synthesis of N,N′-bis(1,5-dimethyl-2-phenyl-1,2-dihydro-3-oxopyrazol-4-yl) sebacamide that ameliorate osteoarthritis symptoms and improve bone marrow matrix structure and cartilage alterations induced by monoiodoacetate in the rat model: "Suggested potent anti-inflammatory agent against COVID-19". *Hum. Exp. Toxicol.* **2021**, *40*, 325–341. [CrossRef] [PubMed]
58. Parkes, J. Clinical pharmacology of amantadine and derivatives. In *Early Diagnosis and Preventive Therapy in Parkinson's Disease*; Springer: Vienna, Austria, 1989; pp. 335–341.
59. Hammoudi Halat, D.; Krayem, M.; Khaled, S.; Younes, S. A Focused Insight into Thyme: Biological, Chemical, and Therapeutic Properties of an Indigenous Mediterranean Herb. *Nutrients* **2022**, *14*, 2104. [CrossRef]
60. Ma, Y.-Z.; Qiang, G.-F.; Du, G.-H. Cyclandelate. In *Natural Small Molecule Drugs from Plants*; Du, G.-H., Ed.; Springer: Singapore, 2018; pp. 227–230.
61. Bu, R.; Xie, J.; Yu, J.; Liao, W.; Xiao, X.; Lv, J.; Wang, C.; Ye, J.; Calderón-Urrea, A. Autotoxicity in cucumber (*Cucumis sativus* L.) seedlings is alleviated by silicon through an increase in the activity of antioxidant enzymes and by mitigating lipid peroxidation. *J. Plant Biol.* **2016**, *59*, 247–259. [CrossRef]
62. Parker, F.S. Drugs, Pharmaceuticals, and Pharmacological Applications. In *Applications of Infrared Spectroscopy in Biochemistry, Biology, and Medicine*; Parker, F.S., Ed.; Springer: Boston, MA, USA, 1971; pp. 390–417.
63. van der Galiën, R.; Boveneind-Vrubleuskaya, N.V.; Peloquin, C.; Skrahina, A.; Touw, D.J.; Alffenaar, J.C. Pharmacokinetic Modeling, Simulation, and Development of a Limited Sampling Strategy of Cycloserine in Patients with Multidrug-/Extensively Drug-Resistant Tuberculosis. *Clin. Pharmacokinet.* **2020**, *59*, 899–910. [CrossRef]
64. Smith, J.M.; Misiak, H. Critical flicker frequency (CFF) and psychotropic drugs in normal human subjects-a review. *Psychopharmacologia* **1976**, *47*, 175–182. [CrossRef]
65. Arken, N. Schizandrol A reverses multidrug resistance in resistant chronic myeloid leukemia cells K562/A02. *Cell. Mol. Biol.* **2019**, *65*, 78–83. [CrossRef]
66. Stedjan, M.K.; Augspurger, J.D. Ring strain energy in ether-and lactone-containing spiro compounds. *J. Phys. Org. Chem.* **2015**, *28*, 298–303. [CrossRef]
67. Omoruyi, B.E.; Afolayan, A.J.; Bradley, G. The inhibitory effect of *Mesembryanthemum edule* (L.) bolus essential oil on some pathogenic fungal isolates. *BMC Complement. Altern. Med.* **2014**, *14*, 168. [CrossRef]
68. Zheng, A.; Dzombak, D.A.; Luthy, R.G. Formation of free cyanide and cyanogen chloride from chloramination of publicly owned treatment works secondary effluent: Laboratory study with model compounds. *Water Environ. Res. Res. Publ. Water Environ. Fed.* **2004**, *76*, 113–120. [CrossRef] [PubMed]
69. Neal, C.L.; McKeithen, D.; Odero-Marah, V.A. Snail negatively regulates cell adhesion to extracellular matrix and integrin expression via the MAPK pathway in prostate cancer cells. *Cell Adhes. Migr.* **2011**, *5*, 249–257. [CrossRef]
70. Chen, Q.; Xu, R.; Zeng, C.; Lu, Q.; Huang, D.; Shi, C.; Zhang, W.; Deng, L.; Yan, R.; Rao, H.; et al. Down-regulation of Gli transcription factor leads to the inhibition of migration and invasion of ovarian cancer cells via integrin β4-mediated FAK signaling. *PLoS ONE* **2014**, *9*, e88386. [CrossRef] [PubMed]
71. Chen, J.S.; Huang, X.H.; Wang, Q.; Huang, J.Q.; Zhang, L.J.; Chen, X.L.; Lei, J.; Cheng, Z.X. Sonic hedgehog signaling pathway induces cell migration and invasion through focal adhesion kinase/AKT signaling-mediated activation of matrix metalloproteinase (MMP)-2 and MMP-9 in liver cancer. *Carcinogenesis* **2013**, *34*, 10–19. [CrossRef]
72. Aravani, D.; Morris, G.E.; Jones, P.D.; Tattersall, H.K.; Karamanavi, E.; Kaiser, M.A.; Kostogrys, R.B.; Ghaderi Najafabadi, M.; Andrews, S.L.; Nath, M.; et al. HHIPL1, a Gene at the 14q32 Coronary Artery Disease Locus, Positively Regulates Hedgehog Signaling and Promotes Atherosclerosis. *Circulation* **2019**, *140*, 500–513. [CrossRef]
73. Drosten, M.; Dhawahir, A.; Sum, E.Y.; Urosevic, J.; Lechuga, C.G.; Esteban, L.M.; Castellano, E.; Guerra, C.; Santos, E.; Barbacid, M. Genetic analysis of Ras signalling pathways in cell proliferation, migration and survival. *EMBO J.* **2010**, *29*, 1091–1104. [CrossRef]
74. Huang, C.; Jacobson, K.; Schaller, M.D. MAP kinases and cell migration. *J. Cell Sci.* **2004**, *117*, 4619–4628. [CrossRef]
75. Singh, S.P.; Paschke, P.; Tweedy, L.; Insall, R.H. AKT and SGK kinases regulate cell migration by altering Scar/WAVE complex activation and Arp2/3 complex recruitment. *Front. Mol. Biosci.* **2022**, *9*, 965921. [CrossRef]
76. Wang, Q.; Liu, H.; Wang, Q.; Zhou, F.; Liu, Y.; Zhang, Y.; Ding, H.; Yuan, M.; Li, F.; Chen, Y. Involvement of c-Fos in cell proliferation, migration, and invasion in osteosarcoma cells accompanied by altered expression of Wnt2 and Fzd9. *PLoS ONE* **2017**, *12*, e0180558. [CrossRef] [PubMed]
77. Dorudi, S.; Hart, I.R. Mechanisms underlying invasion and metastasis. *Curr. Opin. Oncol.* **1993**, *5*, 130–135. [PubMed]
78. Gupta, G.P.; Massagué, J. Cancer metastasis: Building a framework. *Cell* **2006**, *127*, 679–695. [CrossRef] [PubMed]
79. Huang, S.; Ingber, D.E. The structural and mechanical complexity of cell-growth control. *Nat. Cell Biol.* **1999**, *1*, E131–E138. [CrossRef] [PubMed]
80. Okegawa, T.; Pong, R.C.; Li, Y.; Hsieh, J.T. The role of cell adhesion molecule in cancer progression and its application in cancer therapy. *Acta Biochim. Pol.* **2004**, *51*, 445–457. [CrossRef]
81. Hirohashi, S.; Kanai, Y. Cell adhesion system and human cancer morphogenesis. *Cancer Sci.* **2003**, *94*, 575–581. [CrossRef]
82. Omar, A.; Jovanovic, K.; Da Costa Dias, B.; Gonsalves, D.; Moodley, K.; Caveney, R.; Mbazima, V.; Weiss, S.F. Patented biological approaches for the therapeutic modulation of the 37 kDa/67 kDa laminin receptor. *Expert Opin. Ther. Pat.* **2011**, *21*, 35–53. [CrossRef]

83. Akula, U.S.; Odhav, B. In vitro 5-Lipoxygenase inhibition of polyphenolic antioxidants from undomesticated plants of South Africa. *J. Med. Plants Res.* **2008**, *2*, 207–212.
84. Hsu, C.Y.; Chan, Y.P.; Chang, J. Antioxidant activity of extract from Polygonum cuspidatum. *Biol. Res.* **2007**, *40*, 13–21. [CrossRef]
85. Olorunnisola, O.S.; Bradley, G.; Afolayan, A.J. Protective effect of *T. violacea* rhizome extract against hypercholesterolemia-induced oxidative stress in Wistar rats. *Molecules* **2012**, *17*, 6033–6045. [CrossRef]
86. Madike, L.N.; Takaidza, S.; Ssemakalu, C.; Pillay, M. Genotoxicity of aqueous extracts of *Tulbaghia violacea* as determined through an Allium cepa assay. *S. Afr. J. Sci.* **2019**, *115*, 1–6. [CrossRef] [PubMed]
87. Naidoo, V.; McGaw, L.J.; Bisschop, S.P.; Duncan, N.; Eloff, J.N. The value of plant extracts with antioxidant activity in attenuating coccidiosis in broiler chickens. *Vet. Parasitol.* **2008**, *153*, 214–219. [CrossRef] [PubMed]
88. Ncube, B.; Finnie, J.F.; Van Staden, J. In vitro antimicrobial synergism within plant extract combinations from three South African medicinal bulbs. *J. Ethnopharmacol.* **2012**, *139*, 81–89. [CrossRef] [PubMed]
89. Takara, K.; Otsuka, K.; Wada, K.; Iwasaki, H.; Yamashita, M. 1,1-Diphenyl-2-picrylhydrazyl radical scavenging activity and tyrosinase inhibitory effects of constituents of sugarcane molasses. *Biosci. Biotechnol. Biochem.* **2007**, *71*, 183–191. [CrossRef]
90. Yu, X.; Zhao, M.; Liu, F.; Zeng, S.; Hu, J. Identification of 2,3-dihydro-3, 5-dihydroxy-6-methyl-4H-pyran-4-one as a strong antioxidant in glucose–histidine Maillard reaction products. *Food Res. Int.* **2013**, *51*, 397–403. [CrossRef]
91. Mills, F.; Weisleder, D.; Hodge, J. 2,3-Dihydro-3,5-dihydroxy-6-methyl-4H-pyran-4-one, a novel nonenzymatic browning product. *Tetrahedron Lett.* **1970**, *11*, 1243–1246. [CrossRef]
92. Ibrahim, D.; Abdelfattah-Hassan, A.; Badawi, M.; Ismail, T.A.; Bendary, M.M.; Abdelaziz, A.M.; Mosbah, R.A.; Mohamed, D.I.; Arisha, A.H.; El-Hamid, M.I.A. Thymol nanoemulsion promoted broiler chicken's growth, gastrointestinal barrier and bacterial community and conferred protection against Salmonella Typhimurium. *Sci. Rep.* **2021**, *11*, 7742. [CrossRef]
93. Magi, S.; Tashiro, E.; Imoto, M. A chemical genomic study identifying diversity in cell migration signaling in cancer cells. *Sci. Rep.* **2012**, *2*, 823. [CrossRef]
94. Todaro, M.; Gaggianesi, M.; Catalano, V.; Benfante, A.; Iovino, F.; Biffoni, M.; Apuzzo, T.; Sperduti, I.; Volpe, S.; Cocorullo, G.; et al. CD44v6 is a marker of constitutive and reprogrammed cancer stem cells driving. *Cell Stem Cell* **2014**, *14*, 342–356. [CrossRef]
95. Hin, N.; Duvall, B.; Ferraris, D.; Alt, J.; Thomas, A.G.; Rais, R.; Rojas, C.; Wu, Y.; Wozniak, K.M.; Slusher, B.S.; et al. 6-Hydroxy-1,2,4-triazine-3,5(2H,4H)-dione Derivatives as Novel D-Amino Acid Oxidase Inhibitors. *J. Med. Chem.* **2015**, *58*, 7258–7272. [CrossRef]
96. John, V.; Raju, G.P.; Lakshmi, G.; Rani, B.L.; Bollikolla, H.B. Developments on 1,2,4-triazine scaffold substitutions for possible anticancer agents. *Caribb. J. Sci.* **2020**, *8*, 060–081. [CrossRef]
97. Harris, A.; Grahame-Smith, D.; Potter, C.; Bunch, C. Cytosine arabinoside deamination in human leukaemic myeloblasts and resistance to cytosine arabinoside therapy. *Clin. Sci.* **1981**, *60*, 191–198. [CrossRef] [PubMed]
98. Krynetski, E.Y.; Schuetz, J.D.; Galpin, A.J.; Pui, C.H.; Relling, M.V.; Evans, W.E. A single point mutation leading to loss of catalytic activity in human thiopurine S-methyltransferase. *Proc. Natl. Acad. Sci. USA* **1995**, *92*, 949–953. [CrossRef] [PubMed]
99. He, S.; Zhang, C.; Shafi, A.A.; Sequeira, M.; Acquaviva, J.; Friedland, J.C.; Sang, J.; Smith, D.L.; Weigel, N.L.; Wada, Y.; et al. Potent activity of the Hsp90 inhibitor ganetespib in prostate cancer cells irrespective of androgen receptor status or variant receptor expression. *Int. J. Oncol.* **2013**, *42*, 35–43. [CrossRef] [PubMed]
100. Hernández, D.; Boto, A. Nucleoside analogues: Synthesis and biological properties of azanucleoside derivatives. *Eur. J. Org. Chem.* **2014**, *2014*, 2201–2220. [CrossRef]
101. Abdelnabi, R.; Delang, L. Antiviral Strategies against Arthritogenic Alphaviruses. *Microorganisms* **2020**, *8*, 1365. [CrossRef]
102. Sankar, M.; Nowicka, E.; Carter, E.; Murphy, D.M.; Knight, D.W.; Bethell, D.; Hutchings, G.J. The benzaldehyde oxidation paradox explained by the interception of peroxy radical by benzyl alcohol. *Nat. Commun.* **2014**, *5*, 3332. [CrossRef]
103. Ahmed, W.; Sala, C.; Hegde, S.R.; Jha, R.K.; Cole, S.T.; Nagaraja, V. Transcription facilitated genome-wide recruitment of topoisomerase I and DNA gyrase. *PLoS Genet.* **2017**, *13*, e1006754. [CrossRef]
104. Bezerra, D.P.; Soares, A.K.; de Sousa, D.P. Overview of the Role of Vanillin on Redox Status and Cancer Development. *Oxidative Med. Cell. Longev.* **2016**, *2016*, 9734816. [CrossRef]
105. Ho, K.; Yazan, L.S.; Ismail, N.; Ismail, M. Toxicology study of vanillin on rats via oral and intra-peritoneal administration. *Food Chem. Toxicol. Int. J. Publ. Br. Ind. Biol. Res. Assoc.* **2011**, *49*, 25–30. [CrossRef]
106. Liang, J.A.; Wu, S.L.; Lo, H.Y.; Hsiang, C.Y.; Ho, T.Y. Vanillin inhibits matrix metalloproteinase-9 expression through down-regulation of nuclear factor-kappaB signaling pathway in human hepatocellular carcinoma cells. *Mol. Pharmacol.* **2009**, *75*, 151–157. [CrossRef]
107. Gallage, N.J.; Hansen, E.H.; Kannangara, R.; Olsen, C.E.; Motawia, M.S.; Jørgensen, K.; Holme, I.; Hebelstrup, K.; Grisoni, M.; Møller, B.L. Vanillin formation from ferulic acid in Vanilla planifolia is catalysed by a single enzyme. *Nat. Commun.* **2014**, *5*, 4037. [CrossRef] [PubMed]
108. Marton, A.; Kúsz, E.; Kolozsi, C.; Tubak, V.; Zagotto, G.; Buzás, K.; Quintieri, L.; Vizler, C. Vanillin Analogues o-Vanillin and 2,4,6-Trihydroxybenzaldehyde Inhibit NFκB Activation and Suppress Growth of A375 Human Melanoma. *Anticancer Res.* **2016**, *36*, 5743–5750. [CrossRef] [PubMed]
109. Panossian, A.; Wikman, G. Pharmacology of Schisandra chinensis Bail.: An overview of Russian research and uses in medicine. *J. Ethnopharmacol.* **2008**, *118*, 183–212. [CrossRef]

110. Hammond, E.M.; Denko, N.C.; Dorie, M.J.; Abraham, R.T.; Giaccia, A.J. Hypoxia links ATR and p53 through replication arrest. *Mol. Cell. Biol.* **2002**, *22*, 1834–1843. [CrossRef] [PubMed]
111. Zhang, Y.; Weinberg, R.A. Epithelial-to-mesenchymal transition in cancer: Complexity and opportunities. *Front. Med.* **2018**, *12*, 361–373. [CrossRef]
112. Lin, X.; Attar, R.; Mobeen, I.; Yulaevna, I.M.; Aras, A.; Butt, G.; Farooqi, A.A. Regulation of cell signaling pathways by Schisandrin in different cancers: Opting for "Swiss Army Knife" instead of "Blunderbuss". *Cell. Mol. Biol.* **2021**, *67*, 25–32. [CrossRef]
113. Zhuang, W.; Li, Z.; Dong, X.; Zhao, N.; Liu, Y.; Wang, C.; Chen, J. Schisandrin B inhibits TGF-β1-induced epithelial-mesenchymal transition in human A549 cells through epigenetic silencing of ZEB1. *Exp. Lung Res.* **2019**, *45*, 157–166. [CrossRef]
114. Zhang, Z.; Guo, S.; Liu, X.; Gao, X. Synergistic antitumor effect of α-pinene and β-pinene with paclitaxel against non-small-cell lung carcinoma (NSCLC). *Drug Res.* **2015**, *65*, 214–218. [CrossRef]
115. Pu, Z.; Zhang, W.; Wang, M.; Xu, M.; Xie, H.; Zhao, J. Schisandrin B Attenuates Colitis-Associated Colorectal Cancer through SIRT1 Linked SMURF2 Signaling. *Am. J. Chin. Med.* **2021**, *49*, 1773–1789. [CrossRef]
116. Vernon-Roberts, A.; Lopez, R.N.; Frampton, C.M.; Day, A.S. Meta-analysis of the efficacy of taurolidine in reducing catheter-related bloodstream infections for patients receiving parenteral nutrition. *JPEN J. Parenter. Enter. Nutr.* **2022**, *46*, 1535–1552. [CrossRef] [PubMed]
117. McCourt, M.; Wang, J.H.; Sookhai, S.; Redmond, H.P. Taurolidine inhibits tumor cell growth in vitro and in vivo. *Ann. Surg. Oncol.* **2000**, *7*, 685–691. [CrossRef] [PubMed]
118. Wouters, Y.; Mennen, G.R.H.; Te Morsche, R.H.M.; Roelofs, H.M.J.; Wanten, G.J.A. The Antiseptic and Antineoplastic Agent Taurolidine Modulates Key Leukocyte Functions. *In Vivo* **2022**, *36*, 2074–2082. [CrossRef] [PubMed]
119. Ogura, T.; Tanaka, Y.; Tamaki, H.; Harada, M. Docetaxel induces Bcl-2- and pro-apoptotic caspase-independent death of human prostate cancer DU145 cells. *Int. J. Oncol.* **2016**, *48*, 2330–2338. [CrossRef]
120. Wenger, F.A.; Kilian, M.; Braumann, C.; Neumann, A.; Ridders, J.; Peter, F.J.; Guski, H.; Jacobi, C.A. Effects of taurolidine and octreotide on port site and liver metastasis after laparoscopy in an animal model of pancreatic cancer. *Clin. Exp. Metastasis* **2002**, *19*, 169–173. [CrossRef]
121. Abe, M.; Asada, N.; Kimura, M.; Fukui, C.; Yamada, D.; Wang, Z.; Miyake, M.; Takarada, T.; Ono, M.; Aoe, M.; et al. Antitumor activity of α-pinene in T-cell tumors. *Cancer Sci.* **2024**, *115*, 1317–1332. [CrossRef] [PubMed]
122. Salehi, B.; Upadhyay, S.; Erdogan Orhan, I.; Kumar Jugran, A.; L.D. Jayaweera, S.; A. Dias, D.; Sharopov, F.; Taheri, Y.; Martins, N.; Baghalpour, N.; et al. Therapeutic Potential of α- and β-Pinene: A Miracle Gift of Nature. *Biomolecules* **2019**, *9*, 738. [CrossRef]
123. Matsuda, T.; Shimada, M.; Sato, A.; Akase, T.; Yoshinari, K.; Nagata, K.; Yamazoe, Y. Tumor necrosis factor-alpha-nuclear factor-kappa B-signaling enhances St2b2 expression during 12-O-tetradecanoylphorbol-13-acetate-induced epidermal hyperplasia. *Biol. Pharm. Bull.* **2011**, *34*, 183–190. [CrossRef]
124. Neves, A.; Rosa, S.; Gonçalves, J.; Rufino, A.; Judas, F.; Salgueiro, L.; Lopes, M.C.; Cavaleiro, C.; Mendes, A.F. Screening of five essential oils for identification of potential inhibitors of IL-1-induced Nf-kappaB activation and NO production in human chondrocytes: Characterization of the inhibitory activity of alpha-pinene. *Planta Medica* **2010**, *76*, 303–308. [CrossRef]

current issues in molecular biology

MDPI

Article

Honokiol Is More Potent than Magnolol in Reducing Head and Neck Cancer Cell Growth

Robert Kleszcz [1], Dawid Dorna [2], Maciej Stawny [3] and Jarosław Paluszczak [1,*]

1 Department of Pharmaceutical Biochemistry, Poznan University of Medical Sciences, 60-806 Poznań, Poland; kleszcz@ump.edu.pl

2 Department of Pharmaceutical Biochemistry, Doctoral School, Poznan University of Medical Sciences, 60-806 Poznań, Poland; dawid.dorna97@gmail.com

3 Department of Pharmaceutical Chemistry, Poznan University of Medical Sciences, 60-806 Poznań, Poland; mstawny@ump.edu.pl

* Correspondence: paluszcz@ump.edu.pl; Tel.: +48-61-641-8473

Abstract: The efficacy of treatment of head and neck squamous cell carcinoma (HNSCC) patients is still unsatisfactory, and there is an ongoing search for novel therapies. Locoregionally advanced HNSCC cases, which frequently require combined surgery and chemoradiotherapy, are especially difficult to treat. Natural compounds, like *Magnolia*-derived lignans—honokiol (HON) and magnolol (MAG)—can reduce cancer cell growth but retain a good safety profile and thus may show benefit as adjuvant therapeutics. The aim of this study was to evaluate the anti-cancer effects of HON and MAG in HNSCC cell lines and compare their effects between cisplatin-sensitive and cisplatin-tolerant cells. Cell viability was evaluated in FaDu and SCC-040 cells growing as monolayers and as spheroids. The effect of HON and MAG on the cell cycle, apoptosis, and gene expression was compared between wild-type FaDu cells and cisplatin persister FaDu cells. We observed that HON and MAG were more potent in reducing cell viability in cisplatin persister FaDu cells, although this effect was not directly followed by increased rates of apoptosis. Thus, HON's and MAG's capacity to affect cisplatin persister cells needs further studies. In general, we observed that HON exerted stronger cytotoxic effects than MAG in HNSCC cells, and the difference in their anti-cancer activity was especially pronounced in cells cultured in 3D.

Keywords: honokiol; magnolol; cisplatin; head and neck cancer; cisplatin persister cells; spheroids

1. Introduction

Cancer is the second leading cause of death worldwide, and head and neck squamous cell carcinoma (HNSCC) is fatal for more than 400,000 people per year [1]. Primary surgery treatment turns out to be insufficient or even impossible in a considerable number of patients; thus, it must be supported by chemo- and/or radiotherapy. Standard chemotherapeutics used to treat HNSCC are represented by cisplatin, 5-fluorouracil, and docetaxel, although currently targeted therapy regimens are also introduced, namely monoclonal antibodies against epithelial growth factor receptor (EGFR)—cetuximab, or programmed death receptor 1 (PD-1)—nivolumab and pembrolizumab [2]. For instance, to reach an overall survival rate above 50% for locally advanced HNSCC, concurrent chemoradiotherapy should be combined with targeted therapy or induction chemotherapy [3]. Approximately half of the patients recur and are single chemotherapy-resistant [4]. Thus, new concepts of adjuvant therapy for HNSCC are necessary to achieve progress in the overall survival time of HNSCC patients. Importantly, natural products are a rich source of biologically active compounds with anti-cancer activities [5], and their use provides possible benefits for patients, which requires further validation and confirmation.

Honokiol (HON), IUPAC Name 2-(4-hydroxy-3-prop-2-enylphenyl)-4-prop-2-enylphenol [6], is a lignan isolated from the bark, seed cones, and leaves of the *Mag-*

nolia officinalis tree, being a traditional Chinese bioactive compound [7,8]. HON presents pleiotropic pharmacological activities, including antioxidant, anti-inflammatory, neuro-, hepato-, and cardio-protective, or anti-microbial effects [7–13]. What is essential is that the anti-cancer properties of HON against breast, colon, liver, lung, and ovarian cancer or glioblastoma were also observed [7,8,13–15].

Magnolol (MAG), IUPAC Name 2-(2-hydroxy-5-prop-2-enylphenyl)-4-prop-2-enylphenol [16], is a structural isomer of HON (Figure 1), also isolated from *Magnolia officinalis*. Similarly to HON, MAG also exerts pleiotropic pharmacological effects, including anti-cancer effects [17–19]. However, some slight activity disparity can be observed, e.g., the difference in the position of one hydroxyl group is the cause of weaker antioxidant properties of MAG due to the formation of intramolecular hydrogen bonds between *ortho*-hydroxyl groups, which prevents the hydrogen atom from being abstracted by radicals [20,21]. This small structural difference between HON and MAG results in variation in their activities in various types of cancer cells [21].

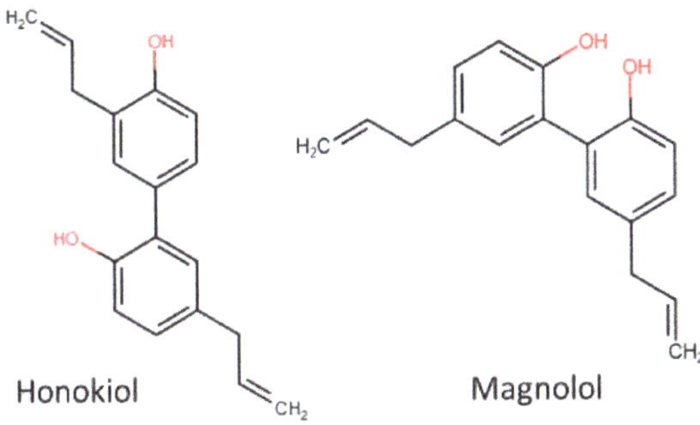

Figure 1. The chemical structure of honokiol and magnolol. Source: www.pol-aura.pl, accessed on 21 August 2024.

The induction of apoptosis is a frequent consequence of effective anti-cancer therapy. HON and MAG were reported to activate the extrinsic (death receptor-mediated) and intrinsic (mitochondria-mediated) pathways of apoptotic cell death via similar molecular mechanisms [22]. However, comparable concentrations of HON and MAG provoke unequal effects on cancer cell viability and apoptosis. For instance, HON is a much stronger viability reducer in glioblastoma [23] and bladder [24] cancer cells compared to MAG. In turn, the pro-apoptotic effect of HON was more potent than MAG in glioblastoma cancer cells, while both HON and MAG used alone were insufficient to induce apoptosis in the second case [23,24].

The data describing the effects of HON and MAG in head and neck carcinoma cells are limited. Most reports concern the anti-cancer properties of HON or the effect of *Magnolia* extracts containing HON and MAG [25–27]. A direct comparison of these properties between HON and MAG in HNSCC cells is lacking. In addition, resistance to standard therapy represents a significant problem of HNSCC therapy. HON combined with 5-fluorouracil (5-FU) synergistically improved the anti-cancer effect in HSC-3 and HSC-4 oral cancer cell lines [28]. Based on a model of acquired resistance to cetuximab, HON also improved the efficacy of this EGFR receptor-targeted treatment [29]. MAG increased chemosensitivity to cisplatin in oral cancer cells by affecting interleukin 6 (IL-6) and STAT3 [30]. Thus, it is also interesting to evaluate the effect of HON and MAG in cisplatin-resistant HNSCC cells.

To fill the information gap mentioned above, this study aimed to compare the effects of HON and MAG on the viability of HNSCC cells grown as monolayer or 3D spheroids. Moreover, in order to evaluate the possible effects of HON and MAG in resistant HNSCC cells, we compared their effects in wild-type (wt) and cisplatin persister FaDu cells.

2. Materials and Methods

2.1. Chemicals and Cell Culture Conditions

Honokiol and magnolol were purchased from Pol-Aura (Olsztyn, Poland), and stock solutions (20 mM) were prepared in DMSO and stored in aliquots at −20 °C. The experiments were performed using two commercially available HNSCC cell lines: FaDu hypopharyngeal cancer cells (American Type Culture Collection, ATCC, Manassas, VA, USA) and SCC-040 tongue cancer cells (German Collection of Microorganisms and Cell Cultures, DSMZ, Braunschweig, Germany). As previously described [31], the cells were grown using high-glucose Dulbecco's Modified Eagle's Medium (DMEM, Biowest, Nuaillé, France) supplemented with 5% Fetal Bovine Serum (FBS, EURx, Gdańsk, Poland), and 1% antibiotic solution (penicillin and streptomycin; Biowest, Nuaillé, France) under standard conditions (37 °C, 5% CO_2, 90% humidity) in a Memmert CO_2 incubator (Schwabach, Germany).

To generate cisplatin persister FaDu cells, a stepwise treatment regimen was applied. Initially, the wt FaDu cells were exposed to three doses of cisplatin at the IC25 concentration (1.12 μM, established during our previous study [31]), with each dose administered three days apart. Following this initial treatment phase, the cells underwent a one-week recovery period in a drug-free medium to mitigate acute cytotoxic effects and enable cellular recovery. After the recovery period, the cells were subjected to a second phase of treatment, consisting of three doses of cisplatin at the IC50 concentration (2.89 μM), again administered three days apart. Persister cells that survived the treatment were considered cisplatin-tolerant and were subsequently cultured with a constant presence of cisplatin at the IC25 concentration (IC25 of wt FaDu cells) for the entire experimental period to maintain the tolerant phenotype.

2.2. Cell Viability Assay

To assess the impact of HON and MAG on cell viability, the resazurin assay was performed. Cells (6×10^3/well) were seeded onto black 96-well plates. The following day, fresh medium containing HON or MAG (at the concentration range of 10–40 μM) was added. The control cells were treated with the vehicle (DMSO). After 48 h of incubation, cells were washed with pre-warmed PBS buffer. Subsequently, resazurin (Sigma-Aldrich, St. Louis, MO, USA) solution was added to wells, and cells were incubated for an additional 90 min. Fluorescence (excitation λ = 530 nm, emission λ = 590 nm) was measured using the Infinite M200 multiplate reader (Tecan, Grödig, Austria). Each experiment was conducted independently at least three times, with at least six replicates per variant each time.

2.3. The Analysis of Cell Viability in 3D Culture

The cells (6×10^3/well) were seeded into wells of ultra-low attachment 96-well plates (Corning, NY, USA). After the initial four days necessary for spheroid formation and growth, fresh medium containing the studied compounds was added into wells. Cell viability and cell death were measured after 72 h using the Cyto3D Live-Dead Assay kit (The Well Bioscience, North Brunswick, NJ, USA), according to the manufacturer's protocol. The assay was based on the use of two nucleus staining dyes—acridine orange (AO, leading to green fluorescence reflecting the presence of live cells) and propidium iodide (PI, leading to red fluorescence reflecting the presence of dead cells). Images of spheroids in the bright field and stained with AO were taken using the JuliFL microscope (NanoEntek, Seoul, Republic of Korea). The experiment was repeated twice, with five replicates each time.

2.4. The Analysis of the Cell Cycle

The analysis of the cell cycle was performed using Muse® Cell Cycle Kit (Luminex, Austin, TX, USA) according to the manufacturer's recommendations. Briefly, 1×10^5/well of cells were seeded in a 12-well plate and pre-incubated for 24 h in a complete culture medium. Afterward, fresh medium containing the tested compounds was added, and cells were incubated for an additional 48 h. Cells treated with topotecan were used as a positive control of cell cycle arrest. Then, cells were collected by trypsinization, washed with PBS buffer, fixed in 70% ethanol, and stored at −20 °C overnight. For analysis, cells were stained with propidium iodide solution in the presence of RNase A, and the fluorescence of cells was analyzed with Muse Cell Analyzer (Merck, Darmstadt, Germany) after 30 min incubation in the dark at room temperature. Data analysis was performed using Muse 1.5 Analysis software (Merck, Darmstadt, Germany). The experiment was repeated three times.

2.5. The Evaluation of Apoptosis

The induction of apoptosis was analyzed using Muse Annexin V & Dead Cell Kit (Luminex, Austin, TX, USA) according to the manufacturer's recommendations. Briefly, 1×10^5/well of cells were seeded in a 12-well plate and pre-incubated for 24 h in a complete culture medium. Afterward, fresh medium containing the tested compounds was added, and cells were incubated for an additional 48 h. Cells treated with topotecan were used as a positive control of apoptosis induction. Then, cells were collected by trypsinization, and after centrifugation, the cell pellet was re-suspended in complete culture medium containing Annexin V for phosphatidylserine staining and 7-amino actinomycin D (7-AAD) for the detection of dead cells, in order to discriminate early and late apoptotic cells. After 20 min incubation in the dark at room temperature, flow cytometric assessment was performed with the Muse Cell Analyzer (Merck, Darmstadt, Germany). Data analysis was conducted using Muse 1.5 Analysis software (Merck, Darmstadt, Germany). The experiment was repeated three times.

2.6. The Evaluation of Gene Expression

The effect of the compounds on the expression of genes associated with the regulation of the cell cycle and apoptosis (*BAX, BIRC5, CCND1, CDKN1A*) was performed as previously described [31]. Briefly, FaDu cells (wild-type and cisplatin persister cells) were exposed to the compounds for 48 h, and RNA was extracted from cells using RNA Extracol (EURx, Gdańsk, Poland). The experiment was repeated twice. Reverse transcription was performed using smART First Strand cDNA Synthesis Kit (EURx, Gdańsk, Poland), according to the manufacturer's protocol. Amplification was performed using SG qPCR Master Mix (EURx, Gdańsk, Poland) and the previously described gene-specific starters [31]. The mean expression of two reference genes (*PBGD, TBP*) was used to calculate the relative change in gene expression level (fold–change) in comparison to DMSO-treated cells.

2.7. Statistical Analysis

The statistically significant differences ($p \leq 0.05$) between experimental and control groups were detected using Student's *t*-test (GraphPad.com, accessed on 30 June 2024).

3. Results

3.1. FaDu Cisplatin Persister Cells Are More Sensitive to Viability Reduction by HON and MAG than FaDu wt Cells

Initially, we performed cell viability analyses to assess the anti-cancer properties of HON and MAG. In the 10–25 μM concentration range of HON, the SCC-040 cells were more affected than FaDu wt cells (Figure 2A). However, the activity of HON was similar at 30 μM and 40 μM concentrations, where both cell lines were almost totally affected. In turn, FaDu wt cells were more sensitive to MAG (Figure 2B). In this case, the viability curves showed weaker effects than for HON in both cell lines and reached approximately 73% and 62% reduction at 40 μM in FaDu wt and SCC-040 cells, respectively.

In addition, we established FaDu cisplatin persister cells to evaluate the potential activity of HON and MAG toward cisplatin-tolerant cells. HON and MAG reduced the viability of FaDu cisplatin persister cells more remarkably compared to FaDu wt cells. At the highest concentration used, the viability was close to 0%.

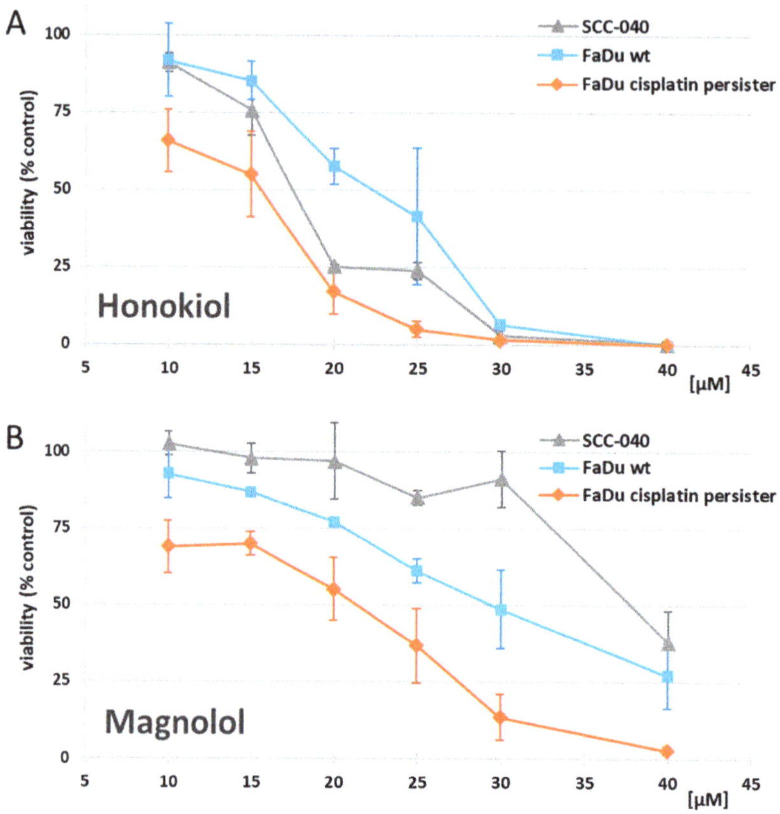

Figure 2. The effect of (**A**) honokiol and (**B**) magnolol on SCC-040, FaDu wt, and FaDu cisplatin persister cells viability based on the resazurin assay. Cells were treated with increasing concentrations of the compounds for 48 h. The results represent mean values ± SD from at least three independent experiments. Cells treated with the vehicle only were used as the control (100% viability).

3.2. HON Reduces the Viability of HNSCC Cells Growing in Spheroid Form

In the next step, we wanted to assess whether HON and MAG could induce anticancer effects in the spheroids of FaDu and SCC-040 cells, which constitute a better model for predicting in vivo activity. The results, which show the detection of both viable and dead cells, confirmed the potency of HON against FaDu cells (Figure 3A). As presented in the exemplary microscopic images, HON caused the collapse of the compact spheroid structure at the highest concentration. In turn, MAG had no significant impact on FaDu cell spheroids. In the 3D culture of SCC-040 cells, HON reduced the percentage of viable cells at higher concentrations, but the effects did not reach statistical significance (Figure 3B). Moreover, HON did not affect the proportion of dead cells. However, the destabilization of spheroids structure was observed at higher concentrations. SCC-040 cell spheroids were resistant to MAG, contrary to 2D results, where MAG at 40 μM reduced the viability below 50%.

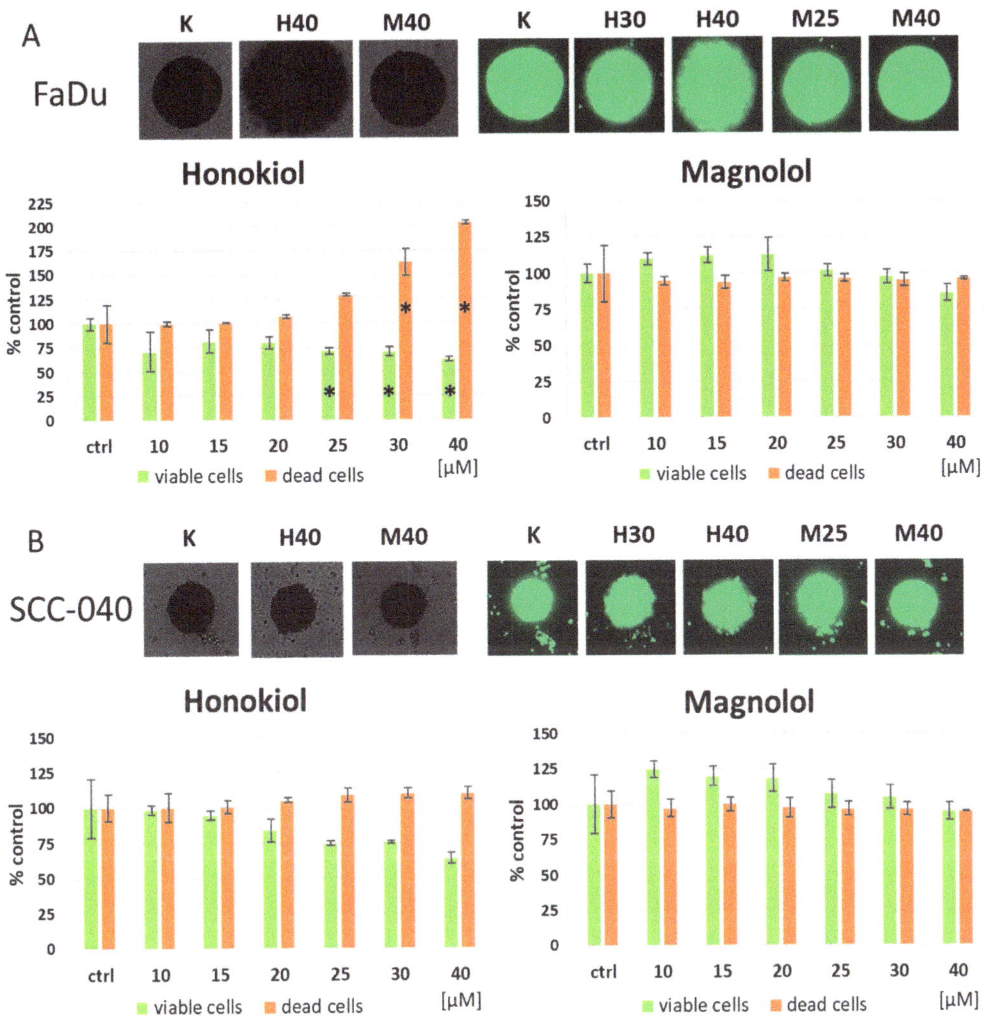

Figure 3. The effect of honokiol and magnolol on the viability of (**A**) FaDu and (**B**) SCC-040 cells grown in the form of spheroids. Cells were treated with increasing concentrations of the compounds for 72 h. Exemplary bright field images and images of stained cells (green fluorescence reflecting the presence of acridine orange in the nucleus of viable cells) are shown. The results in the graphs represent mean values ± SD from two experiments with five independent replicates each. The asterisk (*) denotes statistically significant differences in comparison to DMSO control (ctrl), $p \leq 0.05$.

Based on 2D and 3D viability analyses, it was shown that the activity of HON and MAG was more potent in FaDu cells. Moreover, FaDu cisplatin persister cells were more affected by these natural compounds. Thus, we performed additional functional and mechanistic analyses using wild-type and cisplatin persister FaDu cells to further characterize the action of HON and MAG.

3.3. HON and MAG Induce Cell Cycle Arrest in G1/G0 Phases in FaDu Cells

The cell cycle analysis was introduced to evaluate the possible differences in HON and MAG activity between FaDu wt and FaDu cisplatin persister cells (Figure 4). In

FaDu wt cells, the typical change observed was the cell cycle arrest in G1/G0 phases with a concomitant reduction in cell percentage in the S phase. Only with MAG at 15 μM concentration a slight enrichment of G2/M cell cycle phases was observed instead. In turn, cisplatin, along with the positive control, topotecan, presented a potent cell cycle arrest in the S and G2/M phases (Figure 4A).

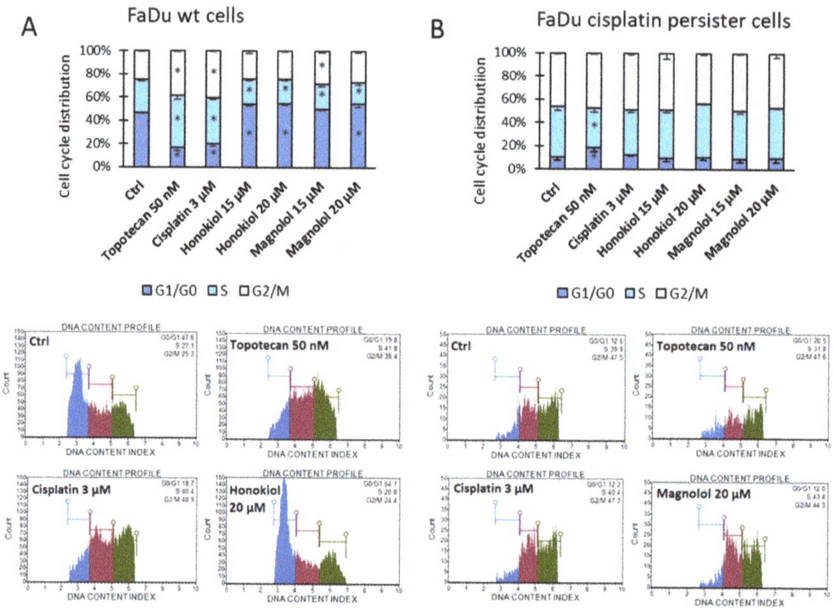

Figure 4. Cell cycle distribution analysis after propidium iodide (PI) staining in (**A**) FaDu wild-type (wt) cells and (**B**) FaDu cisplatin persister cells. The cells were incubated with cisplatin, honokiol, or magnolol for 48 h. Topotecan was used as the positive control of cell cycle arrest. Exemplary flow cytometry plots are shown. The blue area denotes the G1/G0 phases, the red area denotes the S phase, and the green area denotes the G2/M phases of the cell cycle. The results represent mean values ± SD from three independent experiments. The asterisk (*) denotes statistically significant differences in comparison to DMSO control (Ctrl) for each cell cycle phase, $p \leq 0.05$.

In FaDu cisplatin persister cells, due to the lengthy exposure of cells to cisplatin, the cell cycle distribution was similar to the effect of cisplatin in wt FaDu cells, with an even smaller percentage of cells in G1/G0 phases (Figure 4B). HON and MAG were unable to trigger additional effects. In these cells, only topotecan was able to change the proportion between the G1/G0 and S phases.

3.4. HON and MAG Are Weaker Apoptosis Inducers than Cisplatin in FaDu Cells

Annexin V-based flow cytometry analysis revealed a concentration-dependent increase in total apoptotic FaDu wt cells for topotecan (positive control) and cisplatin (Figure 5A). The results for HON and MAG were similar, and an approximately 50% increase in total apoptotic cell population was found for the chemicals at 20 μM concentration. In the case of MAG, an increase in the rate of late apoptotic cells was also present.

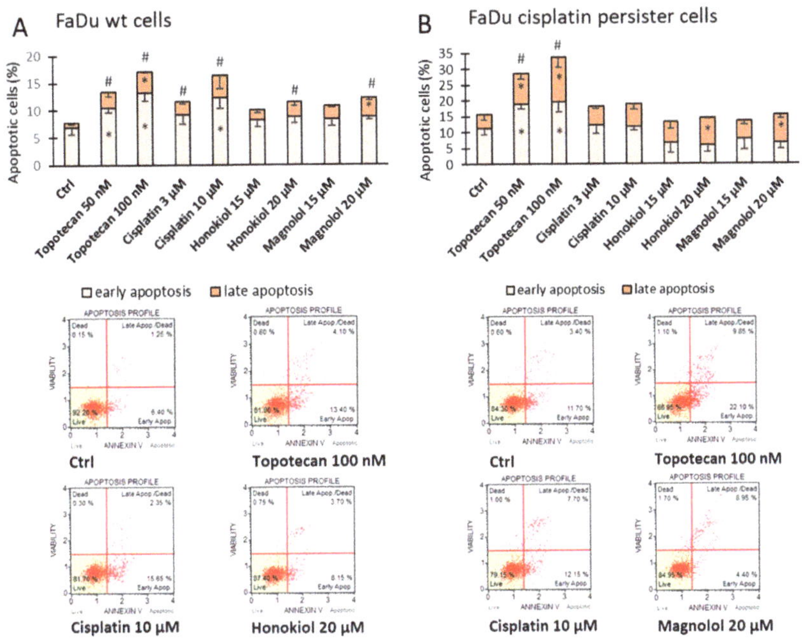

Figure 5. Apoptosis induction analysis after Annexin V and 7-amino actinomycin D staining in (**A**) FaDu wild-type (wt) cells and (**B**) FaDu cisplatin persister cells. The cells were incubated with cisplatin, honokiol, or magnolol for 48 h. Topotecan was used as the positive control. Exemplary flow cytometry plots are shown. The results represent mean values ± SD from three independent experiments. Statistically significant differences in comparison to DMSO control (Ctrl) for early and late apoptosis are represented by an asterisk (*), while for total apoptotic cells, the hash (#) was used, $p \leq 0.05$.

In FaDu cisplatin persister cells, an increase in total apoptotic cell population was shown only in topotecan-treated cells (Figure 5B). The lack of effects after treatment of cells with cisplatin confirmed their cisplatin persister status. Interestingly, although there was no enrichment in total apoptotic rate after incubation of cells with HON or MAG, the proportions between early and late apoptosis were modified with a doubled amount of late apoptotic cells for the chemicals at 20 µM concentration.

3.5. HON and MAG Act by Altering the Level of Expression of BIRC5 and CDKN1A Genes

In an attempt to explain the mechanism of action of HON and MAG in FaDu cells, we evaluated their effect on the level of expression of genes associated with the regulation of cell cycle and apoptosis, and we compared it to the effect exerted by cisplatin. In general, the effect of cisplatin was related to the tendency to decrease the level of expression of *CCND1* (which encodes the cell cycle stimulatory cyclin D1) and to increase the expression of *CDKN1A* (which encodes the cell cycle inhibitory p21 protein) in a dose-dependent manner in both cell populations, although the change reached statistical significance only in the case of *CCND1* reduction in FaDu wt cells at 10 µM concentration (Figure 6). On the other hand, HON and MAG acted by decreasing the level of expression of *BIRC5* (which encodes the pro-survival protein survivin) and by increasing the expression of *CDKN1A*, which was more pronounced in FaDu wt cells.

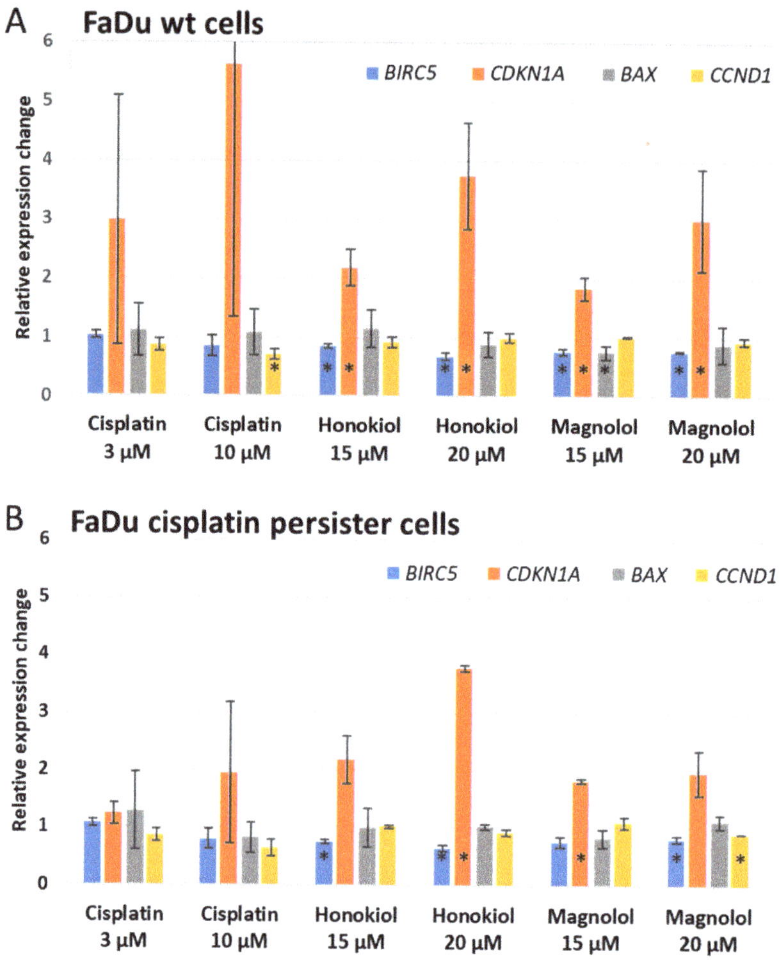

Figure 6. The results of the analysis of the changes in the level of expression of *BIRC5*, *CDKN1A*, *BAX*, and *CCND1* genes in (**A**) Fadu wt and (**B**) FaDu cisplatin persister cells. The cells were incubated with cisplatin, honokiol, or magnolol for 48 h. The results represent fold–change mean values ± SD from two independent experiments. The asterisk (*) inside bars denotes statistically significant differences in comparison to DMSO control, $p \leq 0.05$.

4. Discussion

Magnolia tree is a source of two compounds, honokiol, and magnolol, which have a pleiotropic activity that supports human health. In this study, we particularly focused on HON and MAG anti-cancer properties. Thus far, their potency against cancer cell growth has been evaluated in many tumor types, including colon, breast, liver, lung, and brain cancer, to name a few [21,32]. On the other hand, research on HNSCC has mainly concerned HON, and the influence of MAG has been poorly described so far.

Initially, we analyzed the influence of HON and MAG on the viability of HNSCC cells. It was shown that HON in concentrations reaching 40 µM demonstrated more substantial effects against SCC-040, FaDu wt, and FaDu cisplatin persister cells than its structural isomer MAG. A total of 30 µM HON reduced the viability below 10% of the control value, and 40 µM HON was entirely toxic. Based on other studies, the activity of HON in HNSCC is cell line-dependent. On the one hand, HON within the concentration range of 30–40 µM similarly affected OC2 and OCSL cell lines [25] or the HN-22 cell line at the concentration of 10 μg/mL (approximately 38 μM) [33]. On the other hand, the viability of several other HNSCC cells was significantly inhibited only at higher concentrations, e.g., HSC-3 and HSC-4 cell lines [28,34] or SCC-1 and SCC-5 cell lines [35]. Concerning MAG, our results confirmed its dose-dependent potential to diminish the viability of FaDu cells, with almost 75% reduction in the highest 40 μM concentration. In turn, SCC-040 cells were not meaningfully affected within the range of 10–30 μM MAG, but at 40 μM, the viability decreased below 50%. Other available data indicated even weaker activity of MAG in HSC-3 and SCC-9 cell lines, where at least 75 μM concentration was needed to achieve a decrease in cell viability below 50% [36].

In addition to 2D cell cultures, we also analyzed the influence of HON and MAG on the viability of FaDu and SCC-040 cells grown in 3D in the form of spheroids. Fluorescence analysis with concomitant microscopic observation of spheroids confirmed the anti-cancer activity of HON. However, the activity of MAG in HNSCC cells grown in 3D form was not potent enough. Therefore, based on viability analyses, HON presented more beneficial anti-cancer effects. The reason could be related to the mechanism of action of HON. For instance, Singh et al. (2015) [35] detected decreased EGFR, mTOR, and downstream targets expression after the exposure of HNSCC cells and their xenografts in athymic nude mice to HON. Moreover, molecular docking analysis proved the ability of HON to bind the EGFR active site with greater potency than the commonly used EGFR tyrosine-kinase (TK) domain inhibitor gefitinib. In our previous research, erlotinib, another EGFR TK domain inhibitor, reduced the viability of CAL 27 and FaDu cell spheroids even better than in 2D models or compounds with different mechanisms of action [37]. Therefore, HNSCC cell spheroids are possibly a good model for detecting sensitivity to anti-EGFR therapy, and from the two analyzed *Magnolia*-derived compounds, only HON affects EGFR signaling. In xenografts of HNSCC cells, a combination of HON with erlotinib [38] and HON with cetuximab (monoclonal antibody against the extracellular domain of EGFR) [29] caused a more significant reduction in tumor volume in comparison to those chemicals used individually. Thus, HON is promising as an adjuvant for treatments targeting EGFR in HNSCC cells, but other HON modes of action should be taken into account as well.

In this study, we also compared the sensitivity of FaDu wt and FaDu cisplatin persister cells to HON and MAG. Both compounds demonstrated a more pronounced decrease in viability in cisplatin persister cells, which may suggest the appearance of sensitization of FaDu cisplatin persister cells to HON and MAG. Therefore, in further experimental steps, we used these two populations of FaDu cells to assess the influence of HON and MAG on the cell cycle distribution and potential induction of apoptosis. We chose the same concentrations for HON and MAG (15 μM and 20 μM) to compare their activity and keep the concentration within values possible to reach in vivo [39]. In addition, cisplatin was tested in parallel as the reference of cellular response to standard chemotherapy.

Changes in the percentage of cells in each cell cycle phase were observed in FaDu wt cells. Cisplatin caused a typical increase in S and G2/M phases related to its mechanism of action [40]. In turn, HON and MAG provoked an increase in the G1 phase. This result is in line with the reports of other researchers and is related to decreased proliferation of cancer cells. Particularly, G1 cell cycle arrest was observed in OC2 and OCSL cell lines for HON [25] and HSC-3 and SCC-9 cell lines for MAG [36]. The flow cytometric analysis of apoptosis revealed an approximately 50% increase in apoptotic cell population as compared to control by HON and MAG in FaDu wt cells, while cisplatin doubled the apoptotic rate. The results of our study suggest that FaDu wt cells can be considered sensitive to the pro-apoptotic effect of HON and MAG applied at lower concentrations (≤20 μM). In contrast, the induction of apoptosis by HON was detected at significantly higher concentrations, 40 μM and 30 μM, in OC2 and OCSL cell lines, respectively [25]. For HSC-3 and HSC-4 cell lines, similar potency was shown for 10 μg/mL (ca. 38 μM) concentration of HON and extensive apoptosis for 15 μg/mL (ca. 56 μM) and 20 μg/mL (ca. 75 μM) [34]. Also, 75 μM MAG was needed to induce apoptosis in HSC-3 and SCC-9 cell lines [36].

FaDu cisplatin persister cells, due to lengthy exposure to cisplatin, were characterized by changes in the cell cycle distribution, similar to the effect of 48 h incubation of FaDu wt cells with cisplatin. Thus, the additional incubation of persister cells with cisplatin did not further change the distribution of cells across phases. HON and MAG did not exert any effects either. The basal apoptotic rate in FaDu cisplatin persister cells was higher than in FaDu wt cells. Nevertheless, topotecan (positive control) could still lead to a significant increase in the apoptotic cell population. Importantly, cisplatin had no significant impact on apoptosis, confirming the resistance of these persister cells to cisplatin. In parallel, HON and MAG lacked the potency to increase the rate of apoptotic cells. Nevertheless, HON and MAG doubled the percentage of late apoptotic cells, which may suggest a partly different mechanism of HON and MAG activity in FaDu cisplatin persister cells.

In order to assess the possible mechanisms responsible for the observed effects, we evaluated the level of expression of genes related to cell cycle and apoptosis control. The impact of HON and MAG on the expression of anti-apoptotic and pro-proliferative genes supports the observations from cytometric analyses. Survivin (encoded by the *BIRC5* gene) is a member of the inhibitor of apoptosis (IAP) family but can also promote cell cycle progression. Another protein, p21 (*CDKN1A*), is promoted by p53 to inhibit cell cycle progression. In HN-22 and HSC-4 cell lines, HON decreased the expression of survivin and increased the level of p21, which was related to the downregulation of the transcription factor specificity protein 1 (Sp1) [33]. Our results for FaDu wt and FaDu cisplatin persister cells confirm this observation. Another pro-apoptotic gene, *BAX*, was affected only by MAG 15 μM in FaDu wt cells, while the expression of cyclin D1 (*CCND1*), which promotes cell cycle progression, was slightly downregulated by MAG 20 μM in FaDu cisplatin persister cells. Survivin is known as an adverse prognostic factor for HNSCC patients and is involved in DNA damage repair induced by radiotherapy. HON improved the effects of radiotherapy by targeting survivin, as shown in the in vitro and xenograft models of HNSCC [41]. Therefore, the lowered expression of survivin upon treatment with HON and MAG highlights their usefulness as anti-cancer compounds.

Our study confirmed the anti-cancer activity of HON and MAG in HNSCC cells. The compounds reduced the viability of SCC-040, FaDu wt, and FaDu cisplatin persister cells. Moreover, FaDu cisplatin persister cells were the most susceptible to the influence of HON and MAG on viability. The potency of HON and MAG in assays evaluating their effect on cell cycle and apoptosis was similar; however, slight differences in the ability to modulate the expression of genes related to those processes were found. On the other hand, the anti-cancer effects against HNSCC cells observed in this study appeared at relatively high concentrations, which may limit the in vivo effectiveness of HON and MAG. Yet, while this study was limited to in vitro experiments, reports from other researchers, including in vivo xenograft studies [25,26,28,29,35,38], indirectly confirm the beneficial activity of HON and MAG in treating HNSCC. Moreover, these natural-derived compounds can also be valuable for the prevention of oral cancer development. In this regard, fibrotic buccal mucosal fibroblasts (fBMF) were much more affected by HON than normal BMF, and the progression of oral fibrogenesis into cancer was inhibited [42]. Interestingly, the safety profile of HON is also beneficial. HON can even prevent cisplatin ototoxicity without compromising its activity against tumor cells of different origins [43]. Yet, while showing a generally favorable safety profile, HON and MAG may still cause significant side effects, including hemorrhage due to the anti-thrombotic activity. In addition, they have been shown to affect the activity of enzymatic systems responsible for glucuronidation or sulfation reactions, which may lead to altered drug metabolism [44]. Thus, further research on the anti-cancer properties of HON and MAG is necessary.

5. Conclusions

This study confirmed that honokiol and magnolol can limit head and neck cancer cell viability. These effects are contributed to by the regulation of the cell cycle and apoptosis, which may be mechanistically related to alterations in the level of expression of *BIRC5* (encoding survivin) and *CDKN1A* (encoding p21) induced by HON and MAG. Although HON and MAG showed much higher potency against wild-type FaDu cells, the chemicals were able to reduce the viability and increase the late apoptosis rate in FaDu cisplatin-persister cells. This implies the potential applicability of HON and MAG in tackling chemoresistance, although this requires further, more detailed studies.

Author Contributions: Conceptualization, J.P. and M.S.; methodology, R.K. and J.P.; validation, R.K. and J.P.; formal analysis, R.K. and J.P.; investigation, D.D., R.K. and J.P.; resources, M.S. and J.P.; data curation, R.K. and J.P.; writing—original draft preparation, R.K. and J.P.; writing—review and editing, R.K., D.D., M.S. and J.P.; visualization, R.K. and J.P.; supervision, J.P.; project administration, J.P.; funding acquisition, M.S. and J.P. All authors have read and agreed to the published version of the manuscript.

Funding: This research received no external funding.

Institutional Review Board Statement: Not applicable.

Informed Consent Statement: Not applicable.

Data Availability Statement: The data generated in the present study are available from the corresponding author upon reasonable request.

Conflicts of Interest: The authors declare no conflicts of interest.

References

1. Sung, H.; Ferlay, J.; Siegel, R.L.; Laversanne, M.; Soerjomataram, I.; Jemal, A.; Bray, F. Global Cancer Statistics 2020: GLOBOCAN Estimates of Incidence and Mortality Worldwide for 36 Cancers in 185 Countries. *CA A Cancer J. Clin.* **2021**, *71*, 209–249. [CrossRef] [PubMed]
2. Sindhu, S.K.; Bauman, J.E. Current Concepts in Chemotherapy for Head and Neck Cancer. *Oral Maxillofac. Surg. Clin. N. Am.* **2019**, *31*, 145–154. [CrossRef] [PubMed]
3. Yuan, J.; Shi, K.; Chen, G.; Xu, W.; Qiu, L.; Fei, Y.; Zhu, Y.; Wu, M.; Li, Y.; Sun, X.; et al. A Network Meta-Analysis of the Systemic Therapies in Unresectable Head and Neck Squamous Cell Carcinoma. *Cancer Control* **2024**, *31*, 10732748241255535. [CrossRef] [PubMed]
4. Smussi, D.; Mattavelli, D.; Paderno, A.; Gurizzan, C.; Lorini, L.; Romani, C.; Bignotti, E.; Grammatica, A.; Ravanelli, M.; Bossi, P. Revisiting the Concept of Neoadjuvant and Induction Therapy in Head and Neck Cancer with the Advent of Immunotherapy. *Cancer Treat. Rev.* **2023**, *121*, 102644. [CrossRef]
5. Naeem, A.; Hu, P.; Yang, M.; Zhang, J.; Liu, Y.; Zhu, W.; Zheng, Q. Natural Products as Anticancer Agents: Current Status and Future Perspectives. *Molecules* **2022**, *27*, 8367. [CrossRef]
6. PubChem Honokiol. Available online: https://pubchem.ncbi.nlm.nih.gov/compound/72303 (accessed on 19 July 2024).
7. Pan, C.; Li, Q.; Xiong, S.; Yang, Y.; Yang, Y.; Huang, C.; Wang, Z.-P. Delivery Strategies, Structural Modification, and Pharmacological Mechanisms of Honokiol: A Comprehensive Review. *Chem. Biodivers.* **2024**, *21*, e202302032. [CrossRef]
8. Li, X.; Yuan, Z.; Wang, Y.; Wang, W.; Shi, J. Recent Advances of Honokiol: Pharmacological Activities, Manmade Derivatives and Structure-Activity Relationship. *Eur. J. Med. Chem.* **2024**, *272*, 116471. [CrossRef] [PubMed]
9. Faysal, M.; Khan, J.; Zehravi, M.; Nath, N.; Singh, L.P.; Kakkar, S.; Perusomula, R.; Khan, P.A.; Nainu, F.; Asiri, M.; et al. Neuropharmacological Potential of Honokiol and Its Derivatives from Chinese Herb Magnolia Species: Understandings from Therapeutic Viewpoint. *Chin. Med.* **2023**, *18*, 154. [CrossRef] [PubMed]
10. Huang, A.-L.; Yang, F.; Cheng, P.; Liao, D.; Zhou, L.; Ji, X.-L.; Peng, D.-D.; Zhang, L.; Cheng, T.-T.; Ma, L.; et al. Honokiol Attenuate the Arsenic Trioxide-Induced Cardiotoxicity by Reducing the Myocardial Apoptosis. *Pharmacol. Res. Perspect.* **2022**, *10*, e00914. [CrossRef]
11. Liao, K.-S.; Lee, Y.-R.; Chao, W.-Y.; Huang, Y.-J.; Chung, H.-C.; Chen, S.-H.; Li, Y.-Z.; Zhao, P.-W.; Chang, H.-Y. Honokiol Suppresses Cell Proliferation and Tumor Migration through ROS in Human Anaplastic Thyroid Cancer Cells. *Endocr. Metab. Immune Disord.-Drug Targets* **2024**, *24*, 1–9. [CrossRef]
12. Ochoa, C.; Roenfanz, H.F.; Kozlowski, M.C. Modification of Biphenolic Anti-Bacterial to Achieve Broad-Spectrum Activity. *ChemMedChem* **2022**, *17*, e202100783. [CrossRef] [PubMed]
13. Rauf, A.; Olatunde, A.; Imran, M.; Alhumaydhi, F.A.; Aljohani, A.S.M.; Khan, S.A.; Uddin, M.S.; Mitra, S.; Emran, T.B.; Khayrullin, M.; et al. Honokiol: A review of its pharmacological potential and therapeutic insights. *Phytomed. Int. J. Phytother. Phytopharm.* **2021**, *90*, 153647. [CrossRef]
14. Dominiak, K.; Gostyńska, A.; Szulc, M.; Stawny, M. The Anticancer Application of Delivery Systems for Honokiol and Magnolol. *Cancers* **2024**, *16*, 2257. [CrossRef]

15. Prasher, P.; Fatima, R.; Sharma, M.; Tynybekov, B.; Alshahrani, A.M.; Ateşşahin, D.A.; Sharifi-Rad, J.; Calina, D. Honokiol and its analogues as anticancer compounds: Current mechanistic insights and structure-activity relationship. *Chem.-Biol. Interact.* **2023**, *386*, 110747. [CrossRef]
16. PubChem Magnolol. Available online: https://pubchem.ncbi.nlm.nih.gov/compound/72300 (accessed on 19 July 2024).
17. Ranaware, A.M.; Banik, K.; Deshpande, V.; Padmavathi, G.; Roy, N.K.; Sethi, G.; Fan, L.; Kumar, A.P.; Kunnumakkara, A.B. Magnolol: A Neolignan from the Magnolia Family for the Prevention and Treatment of Cancer. *Int. J. Mol. Sci.* **2018**, *19*, 2362. [CrossRef] [PubMed]
18. Zhang, J.; Chen, Z.; Huang, X.; Shi, W.; Zhang, R.; Chen, M.; Huang, H.; Wu, L. Insights on the Multifunctional Activities of Magnolol. *Biomed. Res. Int.* **2019**, *2019*, 1847130. [CrossRef] [PubMed]
19. Lin, Y.; Li, Y.; Zeng, Y.; Tian, B.; Qu, X.; Yuan, Q.; Song, Y. Pharmacology, Toxicity, Bioavailability, and Formulation of Magnolol: An Update. *Front. Pharm.* **2021**, *12*, 632767. [CrossRef]
20. Zhao, C.; Liu, Z.-Q. Comparison of Antioxidant Abilities of Magnolol and Honokiol to Scavenge Radicals and to Protect DNA. *Biochimie* **2011**, *93*, 1755–1760. [CrossRef]
21. Wang, X.; Liu, Q.; Fu, Y.; Ding, R.-B.; Qi, X.; Zhou, X.; Sun, Z.; Bao, J. Magnolol as a Potential Anticancer Agent: A Proposed Mechanistic Insight. *Molecules* **2022**, *27*, 6441. [CrossRef]
22. Xu, H.L.; Tang, W.; Du, G.H.; Kokudo, N. Targeting Apoptosis Pathways in Cancer with Magnolol and Honokiol, Bioactive Constituents of the Bark of Magnolia Officinalis. *Drug Discov.* **2011**, *5*, 202–210. [CrossRef]
23. Cheng, Y.-C.; Hueng, D.-Y.; Huang, H.-Y.; Chen, J.-Y.; Chen, Y. Magnolol and Honokiol Exert a Synergistic Anti-Tumor Effect through Autophagy and Apoptosis in Human Glioblastomas. *Oncotarget* **2016**, *7*, 29116–29130. [CrossRef] [PubMed]
24. Wang, H.-H.; Chen, Y.; Changchien, C.-Y.; Chang, H.-H.; Lu, P.-J.; Mariadas, H.; Cheng, Y.-C.; Wu, S.-T. Pharmaceutical Evaluation of Honokiol and Magnolol on Apoptosis and Migration Inhibition in Human Bladder Cancer Cells. *Front. Pharm.* **2020**, *11*, 549338. [CrossRef] [PubMed]
25. Huang, K.-J.; Kuo, C.-H.; Chen, S.-H.; Lin, C.-Y.; Lee, Y.-R. Honokiol Inhibits in Vitro and in Vivo Growth of Oral Squamous Cell Carcinoma through Induction of Apoptosis, Cell Cycle Arrest and Autophagy. *J. Cell Mol. Med.* **2018**, *22*, 1894–1908. [CrossRef] [PubMed]
26. Huang, J.-S.; Yao, C.-J.; Chuang, S.-E.; Yeh, C.-T.; Lee, L.-M.; Chen, R.-M.; Chao, W.-J.; Whang-Peng, J.; Lai, G.-M. Honokiol Inhibits Sphere Formation and Xenograft Growth of Oral Cancer Side Population Cells Accompanied with JAK/STAT Signaling Pathway Suppression and Apoptosis Induction. *BMC Cancer* **2016**, *16*, 245. [CrossRef]
27. Zhang, Q.; Cheng, G.; Pan, J.; Zielonka, J.; Xiong, D.; Myers, C.R.; Feng, L.; Shin, S.S.; Kim, Y.H.; Bui, D.; et al. Magnolia Extract Is Effective for the Chemoprevention of Oral Cancer through Its Ability to Inhibit Mitochondrial Respiration at Complex I. *Cell Commun. Signal.* **2020**, *18*, 58. [CrossRef]
28. Ji, N.; Jiang, L.; Deng, P.; Xu, H.; Chen, F.; Liu, J.; Li, J.; Liao, G.; Zeng, X.; Lin, Y.; et al. Synergistic Effect of Honokiol and 5-Fluorouracil on Apoptosis of Oral Squamous Cell Carcinoma Cells. *J. Oral Pathol. Med.* **2017**, *46*, 201–207. [CrossRef]
29. Pearson, H.E.; Iida, M.; Orbuch, R.A.; McDaniel, N.K.; Nickel, K.P.; Kimple, R.J.; Arbiser, J.L.; Wheeler, D.L. Overcoming Resistance to Cetuximab with Honokiol, A Small-Molecule Polyphenol. *Mol. Cancer* **2018**, *17*, 204–214. [CrossRef]
30. Peng, C.-Y.; Yu, C.-C.; Huang, C.-C.; Liao, Y.-W.; Hsieh, P.-L.; Chu, P.-M.; Yu, C.-H.; Lin, S.-S. Magnolol Inhibits Cancer Stemness and IL-6/Stat3 Signaling in Oral Carcinomas. *J. Formos. Med. Assoc.* **2022**, *121*, 51–57. [CrossRef]
31. Dorna, D.; Kleszcz, R.; Paluszczak, J. Triple Combinations of Histone Lysine Demethylase Inhibitors with PARP1 Inhibitor–Olaparib and Cisplatin Lead to Enhanced Cytotoxic Effects in Head and Neck Cancer Cells. *Biomedicines* **2024**, *12*, 1359. [CrossRef]
32. Ong, C.P.; Lee, W.L.; Tang, Y.Q.; Yap, W.H. Honokiol: A Review of Its Anticancer Potential and Mechanisms. *Cancers* **2019**, *12*, 48. [CrossRef]
33. Kim, D.-W.; Ko, S.M.; Jeon, Y.-J.; Noh, Y.-W.; Choi, N.-J.; Cho, S.-D.; Moon, H.S.; Cho, Y.S.; Shin, J.-C.; Park, S.-M.; et al. Anti-Proliferative Effect of Honokiol in Oral Squamous Cancer through the Regulation of Specificity Protein 1. *Int. J. Oncol.* **2013**, *43*, 1103–1110. [CrossRef] [PubMed]
34. Chen, X.; Lu, R.; Dan, H.; Liao, G.; Zhou, M.; Li, X.; Ji, N. Honokiol: A Promising Small Molecular Weight Natural Agent for the Growth Inhibition of Oral Squamous Cell Carcinoma Cells. *Int. J. Oral Sci.* **2011**, *3*, 34–42. [CrossRef] [PubMed]
35. Singh, T.; Gupta, N.A.; Xu, S.; Prasad, R.; Velu, S.E.; Katiyar, S.K. Honokiol Inhibits the Growth of Head and Neck Squamous Cell Carcinoma by Targeting Epidermal Growth Factor Receptor. *Oncotarget* **2015**, *6*, 21268–21282. [CrossRef] [PubMed]
36. Chen, Y.-T.; Lin, C.-W.; Su, C.-W.; Yang, W.-E.; Chuang, C.-Y.; Su, S.-C.; Hsieh, M.-J.; Yang, S.-F. Magnolol Triggers Caspase-Mediated Apoptotic Cell Death in Human Oral Cancer Cells through JNK1/2 and P38 Pathways. *Biomedicines* **2021**, *9*, 1295. [CrossRef] [PubMed]
37. Kleszcz, R.; Skalski, M.; Krajka-Kuźniak, V.; Paluszczak, J. The Inhibitors of KDM4 and KDM6 Histone Lysine Demethylases Enhance the Anti-Growth Effects of Erlotinib and HS-173 in Head and Neck Cancer Cells. *Eur. J. Pharm. Sci.* **2021**, *166*, 105961. [CrossRef]
38. Leeman-Neill, R.J.; Cai, Q.; Joyce, S.C.; Thomas, S.M.; Bhola, N.E.; Neill, D.B.; Arbiser, J.L.; Grandis, J.R. Honokiol Inhibits Epidermal Growth Factor Receptor Signaling and Enhances the Antitumor Effects of Epidermal Growth Factor Receptor Inhibitors. *Clin. Cancer Res.* **2010**, *16*, 2571–2579. [CrossRef]
39. Arora, S.; Singh, S.; Piazza, G.A.; Contreras, C.M.; Panyam, J.; Singh, A.P. Honokiol: A Novel Natural Agent for Cancer Prevention and Therapy. *Curr. Mol. Med.* **2012**, *12*, 1244–1252. [CrossRef]

40. Velma, V.; Dasari, S.R.; Tchounwou, P.B. Low Doses of Cisplatin Induce Gene Alterations, Cell Cycle Arrest, and Apoptosis in Human Promyelocytic Leukemia Cells. *Biomark Insights* **2016**, *11*, 113–121. [CrossRef]
41. Wang, X.; Beitler, J.J.; Huang, W.; Chen, G.; Qian, G.; Magliocca, K.; Patel, M.R.; Chen, A.Y.; Zhang, J.; Nannapaneni, S.; et al. Honokiol Radiosensitizes Squamous Cell Carcinoma of the Head and Neck by Downregulation of Survivin. *Clin. Cancer Res.* **2018**, *24*, 858–869. [CrossRef]
42. Chen, P.-Y.; Ho, D.C.-Y.; Liao, Y.-W.; Hsieh, P.-L.; Lu, K.-H.; Tsai, L.-L.; Su, S.-H.; Yu, C.-C. Honokiol Inhibits Arecoline-Induced Oral Fibrogenesis through Transforming Growth Factor-β/Smad2/3 Signaling Inhibition. *J. Formos. Med. Assoc.* **2021**, *120*, 1988–1993. [CrossRef]
43. Tan, X.; Zhou, Y.; Agarwal, A.; Lim, M.; Xu, Y.; Zhu, Y.; O'Brien, J.; Tran, E.; Zheng, J.; Gius, D.; et al. Systemic Application of Honokiol Prevents Cisplatin Ototoxicity without Compromising Its Antitumor Effect. *Am. J. Cancer Res.* **2020**, *10*, 4416–4434. [PubMed]
44. Sarrica, A.; Kirika, N.; Romeo, M.; Salmona, M.; Diomede, L. Safety and Toxicology of Magnolol and Honokiol. *Planta Med.* **2018**, *84*, 1151–1164. [CrossRef] [PubMed]

current issues in molecular biology

MDPI

Article

Exopolysaccharides from the Green Microalga Strain *Coelastrella* sp. BGV—Isolation, Characterization, and Assessment of Anticancer Potential

Tanya Toshkova-Yotova [1], Inna Sulikovska [2], Vera Djeliova [3], Zdravka Petrova [2], Manol Ognyanov [4], Petko Denev [4], Reneta Toshkova [2] and Ani Georgieva [2,*]

[1] Department of Plant Ecophysiology, Institute of Plant Physiology and Genetics, Bulgarian Academy of Sciences, Acad. G. Bonchev Str., 21, 1113 Sofia, Bulgaria; t_toshkova_yotova@abv.bg
[2] Department of Pathology, Institute of Experimental Morphology, Pathology and Anthropology with Museum, Bulgarian Academy of Sciences, Acad. G. Bonchev Str., 25, 1113 Sofia, Bulgaria; inna_sulikovska@ukr.net (I.S.); zdr.z1971@abv.bg (Z.P.); reneta.toshkova@gmail.com (R.T.)
[3] Department of Molecular Biology of Cell Cycle, Institute of Molecular Biology "Acad. R. Tsanev", Bulgarian Academy of Sciences, Acad. G. Bonchev Str., 21, 1113 Sofia, Bulgaria; vera@bio21.bas.bg
[4] Laboratory of Biologically Active Substances, Institute of Organic Chemistry with Centre of Phytochemistry, Bulgarian Academy of Sciences, 139 Ruski Blvd., 4000 Plovdiv, Bulgaria; manol.ognyanov@orgchm.bas.bg (M.O.); petko.denev@orgchm.bas.bg (P.D.)
* Correspondence: georgieva_any@abv.bg

Abstract: Algal metabolites have been extensively studied as potential anticancer therapeutics. Among them, polysaccharides have attracted much attention because of their beneficial biological effects and safety. In the present research, the chemical characteristics, antitumor, and proapoptotic activities of extracellular polysaccharides (EPS) isolated from a new Bulgarian strain of the green microalga *Coelastrella* sp. BGV were investigated. A fast and convenient method of precipitation with cold ethanol was used to isolate EPS from the culture medium. The chemical characteristics of the isolated EPS were examined by colorimetric and spectrophotometric analyses, HPSEC-RID and HPLC-UV chromatography, and FT-IR spectroscopy. The results showed that the isolated EPS sample consists of three carbohydrate fractions with different molecular weights (11.5×10^4 Da, 30.7×10^4 Da, and 72.4×10^4 Da, respectively) and contains 7.14 ($w/w\%$) protein. HPLC-UV analysis revealed the presence of galactose and fucose. The total uronic acid content in the sample was 4.5 ($w/w\%$). The IR-FT spectrum of EPS revealed the presence of various functional groups typical of a polysaccharide (or proteoglycan) composed primarily of neutral sugars. The anticancer potential of the obtained EPS was assessed using cell lines with cancerous and non-cancerous origins as in vitro experimental models. The results of the performed MTT assay showed that EPS reduced the viability of the cervical and mammary carcinoma cell lines HeLa and MCF-7, while the control non-cancer cell lines BALB/3T3 and HaCaT were less affected. The HeLa cell line showed the highest sensitivity to the effects of EPS and was therefore used for further studies of its anticancer potential. The ability of EPS to inhibit cancer cell migration was demonstrated by wound-healing (scratch) assay. The cell cycle FACS analysis indicated that the EPS treatment induced significant increases in the sub G1 cell population and decreases of the percentages of cells in the G1, S, and G2-M phases, compared to the control. The fluorescent microscopy studies performed using three different staining methods in combination with Annexin V-FITC flow cytometric analysis clearly demonstrate the ability of EPS to induce cancer cell death via the apoptosis pathway. Moreover, an altered pattern and intensity of the immunocytochemical staining for the apoptosis- and proliferation-related proteins p53, bcl2, and Ki67 was detected in EPS-treated HeLa cancer cells as compared to the untreated controls. The obtained results characterize the new local strain of green microalgae *Coelastrella* sp. BGV as a producer of EPS with selective antitumor activity and provide an opportunity for further studies of its pharmacological and biotechnological potential.

Keywords: *Coelastrella* sp. BGV; antitumor activity; cell viability; proliferation; migration; apoptosis

1. Introduction

Cancer is the second leading cause of mortality worldwide, and more effective therapies to control these severe diseases are urgently needed. A distinctive feature of cancer is the uncontrolled proliferation and spread of tumor cells and the loss of apoptosis. Compounds that block or suppress the proliferation of tumor cells by inducing apoptosis are considered to have potential as anticancer drugs [1]. The interest in algae as one of the major natural sources of novel bioactive compounds with health-promoting immunostimulating and anticancer properties has intensified in recent years. In general, microalgae are rich in a spectrum of compounds including, high-quality proteins (phycobiliproteins, enzymes and oligopeptides), polysaccharides (agar, carrageenan, alginates, fucoidan, etc.), long-chain polyunsaturated fatty acids (especially ω-3 and ω-6 fatty acids), pigments (carotenoids: β-carotene, lutein, astaxanthin, fucoxanthin, etc. and phycocyanin), sterols (sitosterol, fucosterol, etc.), polyphenols, vitamins B12, C, and E, biogenic elements (Ca, P, Na, K, etc.), dietary fiber, etc. [2–4].

Among the high-value compounds from microalgae, EPS are very promising. Polysaccharides are natural biopolymers, composed of monosaccharides (hexoses and pentoses) covalently linked by glycosidic bonds in linear or branched chains with a great variety of molecular weights, monosaccharide compositions, and structural conformations. Based on their function, polysaccharides can be divided into three categories: (i) structural polysaccharides that build cell walls, (ii) storage (reserve) polysaccharides that accumulate inside the cell, and (iii) matrix (protective) polysaccharides released into the environment. The latter are subdivided into two different classes—capsular, which remain attached to the cell wall, and free, which are entirely released into the environment and are described as extracellular polysaccharides [5,6]. The best producers of exopolysaccharides were found in different species of microalgae from *Cyanophyta* and *Rhodophyta*, as well as in some types from *Chlorophyta* and *Dinophyta* [7,8]. The polysaccharide content, composition, and structure are highly variable depending on numerous influencing factors, such as algal species and strain, the area of cultivation, seasonal, physiological, and environmental variations, cultivation parameters, and culture age. Variations can even occur between samples prepared in the same way from different batches of a given species of algae. The type and conditions of extraction also have a very decisive influence on the polysaccharide content [9–11].

The microalgae polysaccharides attract scientific attention due to their diverse biological activities, including the anticoagulant, antithrombotic, immunomodulatory, antiviral, antibacterial, hypoglycemic, antimutagenic, radioprotective, anti-oxidative, antiulcer, anticancer, and anti-inflammatory effects, and find wide application in the pharmaceutical, environmental, cosmetics, and food industries (including functional foods, feed, nutritional supplements, colorants, and drinks) [6–8,11–16].

Numerous studies have indicated that polysaccharides from microalgae sources exhibit antitumor efficacy by inducing apoptosis, inhibiting proliferation and angiogenesis, and modulating the immune response in different cancer models [7,15,17–21].

At present, there are no reports about the pharmacological action of the extracellular polysaccharides from *Coelastarella* species. As a part of our effort to explore the therapeutic potential of the local microalgae strains, we undertook a study on the anticancer activity of the metabolites isolated from the green microalga *Coelastrella* sp. BGV. Our previous studies have shown that aqueous and oil extracts and fatty acids from this strain inhibited cell proliferation and induced apoptotic changes in HeLa tumor cells [22–24]. In this study, we isolated extracellular polysaccharides (EPS) from the green microalga *Coelastrella* sp. BGV, investigated its chemical characteristics, and assessed the antitumor and proapoptotic effects on HeLa human cervical cancer cells. The results obtained provide new data regarding the mechanism of action of EPS against cervical cancer and demonstrate the potential for developing EPS as an agent for cervical cancer prevention and/or therapy. However, more extensive studies are required to better understand the biological mechanisms underlying the antitumor effect of *Coelastrella* EPS and to validate its potential for applications in cancer therapy.

2. Materials and Methods

2.1. Materials and Chemicals

Coelastrella sp. BGV was obtained from the Algae Culture Collection of the Institute of Plant Physiology and Genetics at the Bulgarian Academy of Sciences.

Monosaccharides (L-rhamnose, D-arabinose, D-xylose, D-mannose, D-glucose, D-galactose, and D-fructose) were purchased from the Sigma-Aldrich Chemical Company (St. Louis, MO, US). Dulbecco's Modified Eagle Medium (DMEM), fetal bovine serum, antibiotic solution (penicillin–streptomycin), phosphate-buffered solution (PBS) and trypsin–EDTA solution (2.5 g/L trypsin and 0.2 g/L EDTA), 3-[4,5-dimethylthiazol-2-yl]-2,3-diphenyl tetrazolium bromide (MTT), Acridine Orange (AO), and ethidium bromide (EtBr), were purchased from Merck (Darmstadt, Germany). The Annexin V Apoptosis Detection Kit: sc-4252 AK was the product of Santa Cruz Biotechnology, Inc., Dallas, TX, USA.

2.2. Cell Lines and Culture Conditions

The human cancer cell line HeLa (CCL-2); MCF-7 (HTB-22) and mouse fibroblast cell line BALB/3T3 (CCL-163) were purchased from the American Type Culture Collection (ATCC). The non-tumor human keratinocyte cell line HaCaT was obtained from the CLS Cell Lines Service (Eppelheim, Germany). Cells were maintained in Dulbecco's modified Eagle's medium (DMEM) supplemented with 10% heat-inactivated fetal bovine serum, 2 mM L-glutamine, 50 U/mL penicillin, and 50 mg/mL streptomycin. Both cell lines were cultivated at 37 °C in a humidified atmosphere with 5% CO_2. After achieving 60–80% confluency, the cells were trypsinized with 0.25% trypsin (dissolved in PBS, pH 7.4), counted, and placed at the necessary density for each experiment.

2.3. Algal Strain and Growth Conditions

The green microalga *Coelastrella* sp. strain BGV was isolated from stagnant water in a metal trough near the village of Varvara, Bulgaria (N 42° 10′; E 24° 0–7′) [25]. The strain is maintained in the algal culture collection of the Laboratory of Experimental Algology, at the Institute of Plant Physiology and Genetics at the Bulgarian Academy of Sciences. Algae were cultured as monospecific non-axenic cultures in glass bottles containing 200 mL of autoclaved Šetlik medium modified by Georgiev et al. [26] at 28 °C on a block for intense cultivation. Other experimental conditions included continuous unilateral illumination with cool-white fluorescent lamps at a photon flux density of 132 µmol m^{-2} s^{-1} and a carbon source provided by bubbling 2–3% CO_2 (v/v) in air through the suspensions. The cultures were hand-shaken daily.

2.4. Extraction of Extracellular Polysaccharide

The extracellular polysaccharides from *Coelastrella* sp. BGV were isolated and purified from the cell-free culture liquids using previously described methods [27]. In brief, cultures grown for 20 days under the optimized conditions were subjected to centrifugation at 5000× *g* for 30 min to obtain culture filtrates containing both the released EPS and the culture medium. The resulting supernatant (cell-free culture liquid) was precipitated with cooled 99% ethanol in a ratio of 1:2 (v/v) and pelleted at 5000× *g* for 20 min at room temperature. The precipitate was rewashed three times with 65% ethanol to remove any contaminants (lipophilic substances, carotenoid and chlorophyll-related pigments, and other low molecular weight compounds), and dried at 37 °C. The precipitated materials were dissolved in sterile double distilled water (1%, w/v) on a magnetic stirrer and then extensively dialyzed against distilled water using a cellulose membrane dialysis tubing (Sigma, St. Louis, MO, USA) and finally, were freeze-dried and lyophilized. The EPS was preserved at 4 °C. The obtained crude polysaccharide was used for chemical analysis and bioassays.

2.5. Characterization of Extracellular Polysaccharide (EPS)

2.5.1. Chemical Composition Analysis

The total amount of carbohydrates in EPS was estimated using the phenol–sulfuric acid method of Dubois et al. [28], in which glucose was used as a standard. The protein content of the polysaccharide sample was determined using the dye-binding method of Bradford using bovine serum albumin as a standard [29]. The total uronic acid content of the EPS was analyzed colorimetrically with 3-hydroxybiphenyl by the method of Blumenkrantz and Asboe-Hansen [30], using D-galacturonic acid (D-GalA) as a standard (5.0–100.0 μg/mL) (Sigma-Aldrich Chemical Co., St. Louis, MO, USA). The acetyl content was determined photometrically using the hydroxamic acid reaction method of McComb and McCready [31], using β-D-glucose-pentaacetate (24–120 μg/mL) as a standard. The degree of esterification was measured as well. The polysaccharide sample was saponified (0.5 M NaOH, 1 h) and after neutralization (1 M HCl), the amount of methanol released was determined using a combined enzyme-colorimetric method, using 4-amino-5-hydrazino-1,2,4-triazole-3-thiol (Purpald®) as a chromogen according to the previously reported method [32]. The qualitative estimation of rare sugars was performed according to the periodate-thiobarbituric acid colorimetric method of Karkhanis et al. [33] as described exhaustively by Ognyanov et al. [34].

2.5.2. Determination of Molecular Weight

The determination of the average molecular weight of the EPS was performed using an Agilent 1220 high-performance size-exclusion chromatography-refraction index detector (HPSEC-RID) chromatography system, using pullulan standards with different molecular weights (0.59×10^4–78.8×10^4), a mobile phase of 150 mM NaH_2PO_4 (pH 7.0), and Agilent Bio SEC-3 column (300 A, 4.6 × 300 mm, 3 μm). The sample solution was diluted to a concentration of 1 mg/mL and filtered through a 0.45 μm membrane filter before analysis. Ten microliters of the sample were injected for analysis, and the retention time was recorded.

2.5.3. Determination of Monosaccharide Composition

The monosaccharide composition of the EPS was determined using an HPLC-UV chromatographic system Agilent 1220 (Agilent Technologies, Waldbronn, Germany) employing the method of Honda et al. [35], with a modification by Yang et al. [36]. For this purpose, the EPS (1–5 mg) was hydrolyzed with 2.0 mL of 4M trifluoroacetic acid (TFA), in a sealed tube for 8 h at 110 °C. The released monosaccharides were derivatized with 1-phenyl-3-methyl-5-pyrazolone (PMP) to UV-absorbent products. Separation was performed using an Agilent TC-C18 column (5 μm, 4.6 × 250 mm) with a mobile phase 50 mM phosphate buffer (Na_2HPO_4-NaH_2PO_4, pH 6.9), with added acetonitrile, in gradient elution mode. Identification and quantification were based on response factors relative to standards subjected to the same hydrolytic procedure.

2.5.4. FT-IR Spectroscopy

The Fourier transform infrared (FT-IR) spectra of EPS and its esterified derivatives were recorded at the absorbance mode by a Bruker IR-FT Spectrophotometer in a KBr tablet and analyzed in the wavelength range 500–4000 cm^{-1}.

2.6. Anticancer Activity of Extracellular Polysaccharide/s

2.6.1. Cell Viability Assay

The antiproliferative activity of EPS on human cervical carcinoma cells HeLa, mammary adenocarcinoma MCF-7, human keratinocyte HaCaT and mouse fibroblast BALB/3T3 cells was measured using 3-(4,5-dimethylthiazol-2-yl)-2,5-diphenyltetrazolium bromide (MTT) assay as previously described [37]. The assay detects the reduction of MTT by mitochondrial dehydrogenases to a blue formazan product, which reflects the normal function of mitochondria and cell viability. Briefly, the cells in exponential growth were plated at a final concentration of 1×10^4 cells/well in a 96-well plate with 200 µL of growth medium. After overnight incubation, the growth medium was removed from each well and the cells were treated with rising concentrations of EPS (31.25 µg/mL, 62.5 µg/mL, 125 µg/mL, 250 µg/mL, 500 µg/mL, and 1000 µg/mL) and cultured in a humidified atmosphere with 5% CO_2 for 24 and 48 h. Untreated cells were used as a negative control while cells treated with doxorubicin were used as a positive control. At the indicated times (24 and 48 h) the media was replaced with 100 µL of MTT solution (0.5 mg/mL) into each well. After incubation at 37 °C for 3 h, the medium was removed and 50 µL of DMSO/Ethanol (1:1 *v:v*) was added to each well to dissolve the purple crystals of formazan with shaking for 10 min. Absorbance was measured at 570 nm by a microplate reader (TECAN, SunriseTM, Grödig/Salzburg, Austria). The absorbance value of the control group (without treatment) was considered to be 100%. Relative cell viability was presented as a percentage relative to the control group based on the following formula: Cell viability = [OD of drug-treated sample/OD of non-treated sample] × 100. The 50% inhibitory concentration (IC_{50}) value was determined as the concentration that caused 50% inhibition of cell proliferation. All experiments were performed in triplicate.

2.6.2. Cell Migration Assay

The ability of EPS to inhibit the tumor cells' migration was analyzed by performing a wound-healing scratch assay on HeLa cervical carcinoma cells. Cells were plated in 24-well plates at a density of 2.5×10^5 cells/mL in DMEM containing 10% FBS, and they were cultured in a CO_2 incubator at 37 °C, in an atmosphere with 95% humidity and 5% CO_2, until a monolayer formed. A vertical cut was then created in each well of the plate using a sterile pipette tip with a 10 µL volume. The wells were washed twice with PBS to remove cell debris and were treated with EPS at a concentration of 250 µg/mL. Cell monolayers of untreated HeLa cells with the same vertical scratches served as a negative control of the experiments. The plates were cultured for 72 h in a CO_2 incubator, and images of the scratched area were taken at regular time intervals (0, 24, 48, and 72 h) using an Olympus inverted light microscope with a digital camera to quantify the area of cell migration. The wound area in the control and treated cell cultures was measured at each time point using the ImageJ software package, Version 1.42.

2.6.3. Fluorescence Microscopy

AO/EtBr Staining

Cell morphology changes after treatment with EPS were studied by staining the cells with a combination of the fluorescent DNA-binding dyes acridine orange (AO) and ethidium bromide (EtBr). For this purpose, cancer cells (1×10^5 cells/well) were seeded on a cover slip placed on the bottom of each well in a 24-well plate and incubated overnight to form a monolayer on its surface. Then the cells were exposed for 24 h to the EPS at a concentration of 500 µg/mL, equal to half the maximal inhibitory concentration (IC_{50}) established by the MTT assay. After an additional 24 h of incubation, the cells were stained with 10 µL of aqueous AO/EtBr solution (10 µL /mL of AO in PBS; 10 µL/mL of EtBr in PBS) for 5 min. Tumor cells cultured only in the medium were used as a negative control, and tumor cells cultured in the presence of doxorubicin were used as a positive control. The morphology changes in the AO/EtBr stained cells were observed under a fluorescent microscope (Leica DM 5000B, Wetzlar, Germany).

DAPI Staining

The nuclear morphology of EPS-treated HeLa tumor cells was also investigated by staining with the fluorescent dye 4′, 6 diamino-2phenylindole (DAPI). DAPI has a strong binding affinity for adenine-thymine-rich clusters. The DAPI molecule can pass through an intact cytoplasmic membrane, making it a suitable agent for studying the nuclear morphology of both live and fixed cells. Briefly, HeLa cells were seeded and treated with EPS as described in the previous section. Upon completion of the incubation, the cells were fixed with 3% paraformaldehyde for 10 min, washed three times with PBS, and stained with DAPI solution for 20 min at room temperature in the dark. Samples of treated and untreated (control) tumor cells were coated with Mowiol®, mounted on slides, and observed under a fluorescence microscope (Leica DM 5000B, Wetzlar, Germany).

Annexin V-FITC/PI Staining

Further, we assessed the apoptosis-inducing ability of EPS using an Annexin V-FITC Apoptosis Detection Kit: sc-4252 AK (Santa Cruz Biotechnology, Inc., USA). The translocation of phosphatidylserine from the inner to the outer side of the dual protein-lipid layer of the cell membrane is an early sign of apoptosis. HeLa cells were cultured on glass lamellae and treated with EPS, as described in the previous paragraphs. After that, the culture fluid was removed and the cells were coated with a solution of Annexin V-FITC and propidium iodide (PI), following the manufacturer's instructions. The samples were incubated for 15 min at room temperature, in the dark, and then analyzed on a fluorescence microscope (Leica DM 5000B, Wetzlar, Germany) following a protocol specified by the manufacturer.

2.6.4. Flow Cytometry

The effects of EPS on the cell cycle progression and apoptosis of HeLa cancer cells were analyzed by flow cytometry analysis. HeLa cells were grown to about 80% confluency and were then treated with the EPS at concentrations of 500 μg/mL. Untreated HeLa cells were used as controls. After 24 h of treatment, the medium was aspirated, the cells were washed twice with cold phosphate-buffered saline (PBS), trypsinized with Trypsin-EDTA (Sigma-Aldrich), and centrifuged at 1000 rpm for 10 min. Cell pellets were collected and processed for cell cycle and apoptosis analyses as described below.

Cell Cycle Analysis

The cell pellets of the control and EPS-treated HeLa cell cultures were washed with PBS, resuspended, and fixed with 70% ice-cold ethanol, which was added dropwise while vortexing. Cells were stored at -20°C for at least 12 h. Before analysis, the fixed cells were washed with PBS, treated with RNase A (Roche Diagnostics GmbH, Mannheim, Germany) (20 μg/mL) for half an hour, and stained with propidium iodide (PI; 20 μg/mL). Cell populations at different stages of the cell cycle were analyzed by flow cytometer (Becton Dickinson, Mountain view, CA, USA). From each sample, 10,000 events were recorded, and the percentage of cells in different cell cycle phases (G1, S, and G2-M) was determined using FlowJo ™ v10.8 software (BD Biosciences, San Jose, CA, USA). Data are presented as the mean ± standard error of the mean of three replicates.

Annexin V/PI Analysis of Cancer Cell Apoptosis

Cells were stained using an Annexin V-FITC Apoptosis Detection Kit: sc-4252 AK (Santa Cruz Biotechnology, Inc. USA) according to the manufacturer's protocol. After incubation for 15 min at room temperature, 10,000 cells from each sample were analyzed with a flow cytometer (BD FACSCalibur™) using the FlowJo software (BD Biosciences, San Jose, CA, USA).

2.6.5. Immunocytochemical Analysis

The potential alterations in the expression and intracellular localization of the proliferation marker protein Ki67 and the apoptosis-related proteins p53 and bcl2 were investigated by immunocytochemical analysis of control untreated and EPS-treated HeLa cells. Cells were seeded on clean, sterilized cover slides with a density of 1×10^5 cells/well in 24-well plates. After culturing for 24 h, a negative control (untreated cells), a positive control (cells treated with 2.25 μg/mL Dox), and cells treated with EPS at a concentration of 500 μg/mL were incubated for 24 h under the same conditions. The cover glasses were then washed with PBS, fixed with ice-cold methanol for 10 min, washed three times with PBS, and incubated overnight at 4C with p53 (Monoclonal rabbit Ab-5, clone DO-7, Thermo Scientific, Waltham, MA, USA), Bcl2 (Monoclonal rabbit Ab, clone E17, Zytomed Systems GmbH, Berlin, Germany), and Ki67 (Monoclonal rabbit Ab Clone SP148, Zytomed Systems GmbH, Berlin, Germany) antibodies. Visualization of the antigen-antibody reaction was performed using an immunocytochemical peroxidase reaction with polymer labeling and DAB chromogen (Novolink Polymer detection Systems RE7140-K, Leica Biosystems, Newcastle, UK) according to the manufacturer's recommendations. The procedure was performed at room temperature and the slides were incubated in a humidity chamber. After staining, the preparations were washed several times with distilled water, stained with hematoxylin for 3 min, then dehydrated with an ascending series of alcohols and placed on slides using Bio-Mount DPX synthetic resin (Biognost, Zgreb, Croatia). The prepared immunocytochemical samples were observed with a Leica DM 5000B microscope, Leica Microsystems, Wetzlar, Germany, and documented with a Leica DFC 420 C camera, Wetzlar, Germany and Leica Suite 3.1.0 software.

2.7. Statistical Analysis

All experiments were performed in triplicate (n = 3) and the results were expressed as the mean ± SD (standard deviation). The significance of the differences between the control and experimental groups was analyzed using one-way analysis of the variables (ANOVA) followed by a post-hoc comparison test (Bonferroni) using GraphPAD PRISM software, Version 5 (GraphPad Software Inc., San Diego, CA, USA). A difference was considered statistically significant when the value of $p < 0.05$.

3. Results

3.1. Chemical Characterization of EPS Isolated from Coelastrella sp. BGV

In this study, we isolated and characterized a crude extracellular polysaccharide (EPS) extract from the green microalga Coelastrella sp. BGV, which is endemic to Varvara, Bulgaria. EPS was obtained through ethanol precipitation of a cell-free culture medium. The EPS was washed 3 times with 65% ethanol by centrifugation, dialyzed against distilled water, freeze-dried, and lyophilized. The freeze-dried EPS appeared as a pale yellow pliable fibrous polymer. It was analyzed for carbohydrate and protein content as well as neutral sugar and uronic acid content using colorimetric analyses. The chemical characteristics of EPSs are presented in Table 1. The EPSs contained mainly carbohydrates (36.4%), protein (7.14%), and small amounts of uronic acid (4.5%). The proteins detected in the EPSs were considered to have bonded with the polysaccharide molecules via O-glycosidic or N-glycosidic linkages.

Table 1. Chemical characteristics of exopolysaccharide isolated from *Coelastrella* sp. BGV.

Biochemical Composition	Concentration, *w*/*w*%
Total protein content	7.1
Neutral sugars	
Rhamnose (Rha)	-
Arabinose (Ara)	-
Galactose (Gal)	1.7
Glucose (Glc)	-
Mannose (Man)	-
Xylose (Xyl)	-
Fucose (Fuc)	0.4
Total carbohydrates (Glc equivalent)	36.4
Total uronic acids content	4.5
Degree of methoxylation, mol%	0.74
Acetyl groups content	0.0
Rare sugars test (+ positive, − negative)	+++

The monosaccharide composition of EPS obtained from *Coelastrella* sp. BGV was determined by an Agilent 1220 HPLC-UV chromatography system after hydrolysis of the EPS and derivatization of the released monosaccharides to UV-absorbing products (Figure 1). It was established that EPS from *Coelastrella* sp. BGV is analyzed by employing seven different types of monomer unit standards. Two monosaccharides, including galactose and fucose, were identified, and five others could not be identified (Table 1). Interestingly, EPS tested strongly positive for rare sugars (a pink color was observed), and a positive test result with a 2-thiobarbituric acid reaction suggested the presence of not only 2-keto-3-deoxy-octonate, 3-deoxy-, and 3,6-dideoxy hexoses but also sialic acid and (N-acetyl)hexosamine. It is interesting to note that acetyl groups were not found, which suggests that there were not any acetylated sugar residues. Based on the analyses performed and the origin of the sample, it can be assumed that some of the unidentified monosaccharides are unacetylated galactosamine and/or glucosamine, or that the sample is a proteoglycan. The presence of anhydrous sugars (e.g., 3,6-anhydro-D/L-galactose) cannot be ruled out.

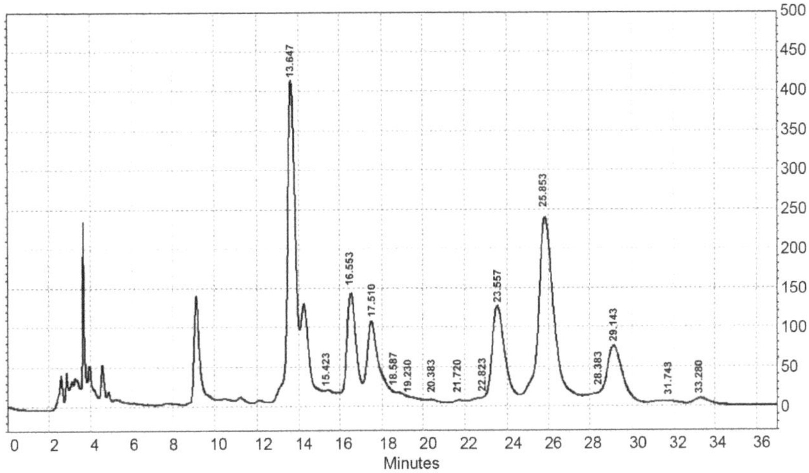

Figure 1. An HPLC-UV chromatogram of PMP (1-phenyl-3-methyl-5-pyrazolone)—monosaccharide derivatives obtained from EPS from *Coelastrella* sp. BGV.

The molecular weight of the EPS obtained from *Coelastrella* sp. BGV was determined using the Agilent 1220 HPSEC-RID chromatography system. The MW of the EPS was calculated by the standard curve of the molecular weight (MW) over the retention time. The elution profile of the EPS is presented in Figure 2.

The molecular weight distribution of EPS showed the presence of three polysaccharide fractions (Figure 2A). The fraction with a molecular weight of 11.5 $\times$ 10^4 Da (marked in the yellow zone of a pronounced peak) made up the largest amount (72.5% of total peak area). In front of it, two fractions (two small peaks) with a higher molecular weight, but in smaller quantities in the sample—72.4 $\times$ 10^4 (11.8%) and 30.7 $\times$ 10^4 (5.7%), respectively, were eluted. The data obtained show that the isolated EPS from *Coelastrella* sp. BGV has a medium molecular weight.

The IR-FT spectrum of the EPS on the IR-FT spectrophotometer in a KBr tablet was taken (Figure 3) and analyzed according to an available database. The individual absorption bands were compared with the presence of well-defined functional groups.

The IR spectrum showed a broad peak at 3400 cm^{-1} that corresponded to the stretching vibration of the hydroxyl groups (–OH), which were the characteristics of polysaccharides. The absorption observed at 3383 cm^{-1} was attributed to the stretching vibration of NH^{3+} (amine group); at 2929 cm^{-1} to the stretching vibration of the methylene (CH_2) group (valence oscillations of the C–H bond of the CH_2 group); at 1650–1550 cm^{-1} for the –NH_2 group of the primary amine and the N–H group of the amide. The peak at 1409 cm^{-1} resulted from the stretching vibrations of the C-N bonds of the amines and amides (in the range of 1400–1418 cm^{-1}). Bands characteristic of polysaccharide sulfate esters were not detected in the spectrum. The two bands noticed at 1542 and 1647 cm^{-1} were assigned to (N–H) and ν(C–N) of the amide II region and the N-linked C=O of the amide I structure vibrations. Bands pointed to the presence of amino sugars and/or protein components. The peak at 1535 cm^{-1} also corresponded to the monosaccharides' C–OH bending vibration. Not found were absorption bands for acetyl groups, which confirmed previous findings made by spectrophotometric analysis. These findings demonstrated that the IR-FT spectrum of EPS from *Coelastrella* sp. BGV is typical of a polysaccharide (or proteoglycan) composed predominantly of neutral sugars.

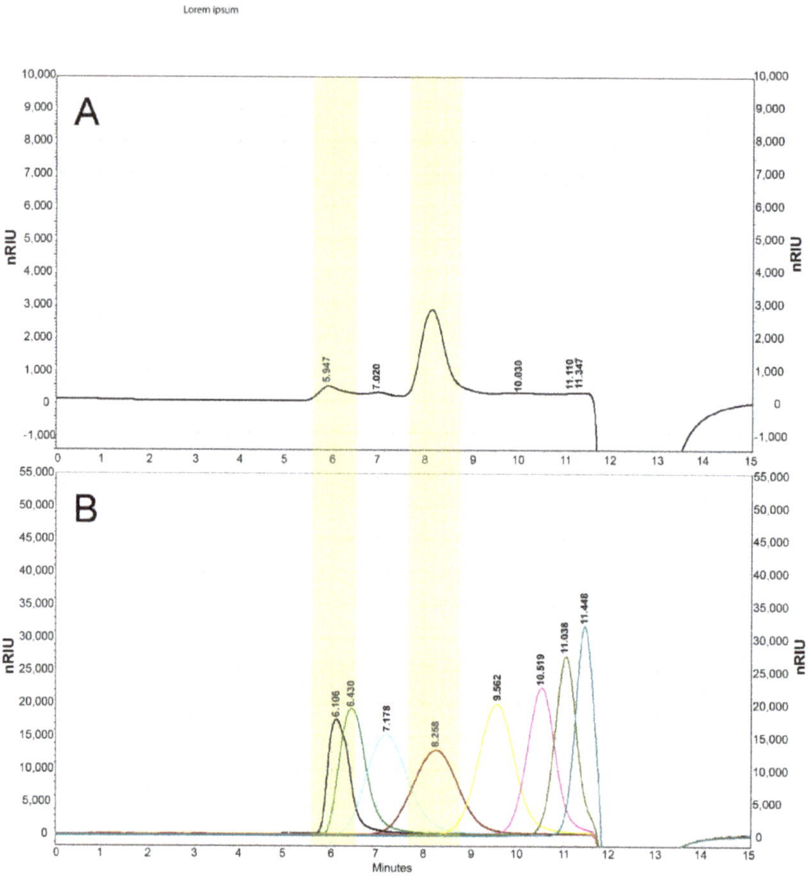

Figure 2. HPSEC elution profile of EPS from *Coelastrella* sp. BGV. (**A**) exopolysaccharide; (**B**) pullulan standards. Molecular weights of the standards used—from left to right: 78.8 × 10^4, 40.4 × 10^4, 21.2 × 10^4, 11.2 × 10^4, 4.73 × 10^4, 2.28 × 10^4, 1.18 × 10^4, 0.59 × 10^4 Da.

3.2. *Anticancer Activity of Extracellular Polysaccharide*

3.2.1. Effects of EPS from *Coelastrella* sp. BGV on Cell Viability

An MTT assay was used to determine the viability of the cancer cell lines HeLa and MCF-7 and the non-cancerous HaCaT and BALB/3T3 cells exposed to increasing concentrations (31.3, 62.5, 125, 250, 500, and 1000 µg/mL) of EPS for 24 and 48 h (Figure 4). The antitumor antibiotic doxorubicin (Dox), widely used in clinical practice for the treatment of human malignancies, was used as a positive control in the experiments. It was established that Dox significantly reduced HeLa cell viability/proliferation, with values between 5%

and 54% at the 24th hour and between 1.0% and 17.0% at the 48th hour of treatment. The observed effect was concentration- and time-dependent. The IC_{50} values determined at the 24th and 48th hour were 2.254 µg/mL and 0.076 µg/mL, respectively.

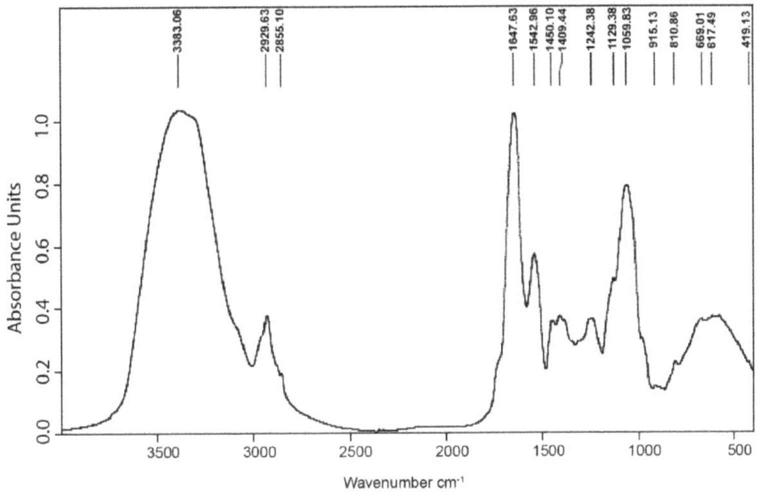

Figure 3. FT-IR absorption spectrum of the EPS from *Coelastrella* sp. BGV over the range of 4000–400 cm^{-1}.

As shown in Figure 4, EPS markedly inhibited the growth of tumor cells in a time- and concentration-dependent manner. It showed a moderate antiproliferative effect on HeLa cells; cell viability was between 45.77 ± 3.93% and 62.35 ± 4.78% at 24h with statistical significance compared to the control. At the high EPS concentrations—500 and 1000 µg/mL—cell viability was lower than that seen for the positive control (doxorubicin-treated HeLa cells). The antiproliferative effect of EPS on mammary carcinoma cells of the MCF-7 line was less pronounced, and the viability of the cells treated with the highest concentration was 71.57%. At the 48th hour, EPS caused a significant decrease in HeLa cell viability as compared to the control. Values were 3 to 10 times lower than those at 24 h and were 22.68 ± 4.296%, 16.04 ± 2.185%, and 11.15 ± 2.690% at EPS concentrations of 31.3 µg/mL, 62.5 µg/mL, and 125 µg/mL, respectively. The highest inhibitions of proliferation reached up to 6.033 ± 0.2418%, 4.878 ± 0.2218%, and 4.833 ± 0.4446% when EPS concentration increased to 250 µg/mL, 500 µg/mL, and 1000 µg/mL. The viability of MCF-7 cells also showed a marked time-dependent decrease, and values ranging between 96.4% and 38.6% were measured at the 48th h. Statistically significant reductions of cell viability compared to the untreated controls were found in all concentrations higher than 31.3 µg/mL.

The control non-cancer cell lines used in the study showed lower sensitivity to the cytotoxic effects of the EPS than the cancer cells. The viability of the human keratinocyte cells HaCa showed a statistically significant increase compared to the untreated control at the lowest tested concentrations of 31.3 µg/mL and 62.5 µg/mL. A decrease in cell viability was established only at the highest tested concentrations of 500 and 1000 µg/mL, with values of 91.17% and 73.96% for the 24th h and 86.77% and 51.75% for the 48th h.

The viability of the EPS-treated mouse fibroblasts BALB/3T3 was not decreased at 24 h and was equal to that of the control. At 48 h, the viability of the EPS-treated fibroblasts was between 76.74 ± 6.195% and 68.54 ± 2.899%. These values were about 10-fold higher than those of the EPS-treated tumor cells.

The inhibitory concentrations of EPS (IC_{50}) were calculated by curve fit analysis of the obtained concentration-response curves for all cell lines tested. The results are presented in Table 2.

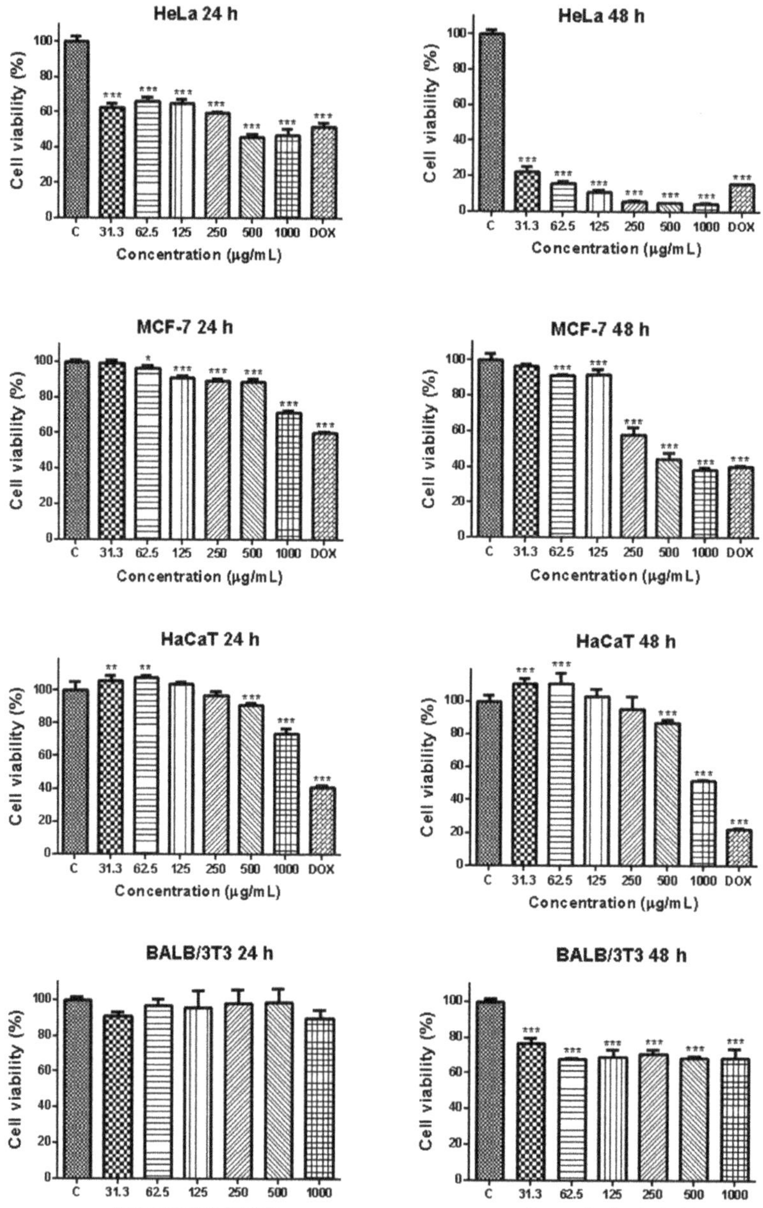

Figure 4. Effect of extracellular polysaccharide from Coelastrella sp. BGV on the viability of HeLa, MCF-7, HaCaT and BALB/3T3 cells assessed by an MTT test at 24 h and 48 h. Untreated cells and cultivated cells treated with the antitumor drug Doxorubicin (Dox; 2.5 µg/mL) were used as negative and positive controls, respectively. The data are expressed as the mean ± SD of five samples from each treatment group. * $p < 0.05$, ** $p < 0.01$, and *** $p < 0.001$ indicate significant differences compared to the negative control.

Table 2. Inhibitory concentrations (IC_{50}; µg/mL) of extracellular polysaccharides isolated from *Coelastrella* sp. BGV, determined by MTT test after 24 h and 48 h treatment of cancer and non-cancer cell lines.

Cell Line	24 h	48 h
HeLa	643.11	<31.3
MCF-7	>1000	486.40
HaCaT	>1000	>1000
BALB/3T3	>1000	>1000

The results presented in Table 2 demonstrate a higher toxicity of EPS (lower IC_{50} values) for the cervical and breast carcinoma cell lines as compared to the non-cancer control cell lines. Based on the MTT results, the HeLa cell line was selected as the most suitable model system for the subsequent analyses of EPS's anticancer potential.

3.2.2. Effects of EPS on HeLa Cancer Cell Migration

The effect of EPS on the migration capacity of cervical carcinoma cells of the HeLa line was examined by a wound-healing assay. The EPS-induced changes in the migration ability of the cancer cells were followed in dynamics during the 72 h period, and measurements of the wound area were performed at regular time intervals (Figure 5).

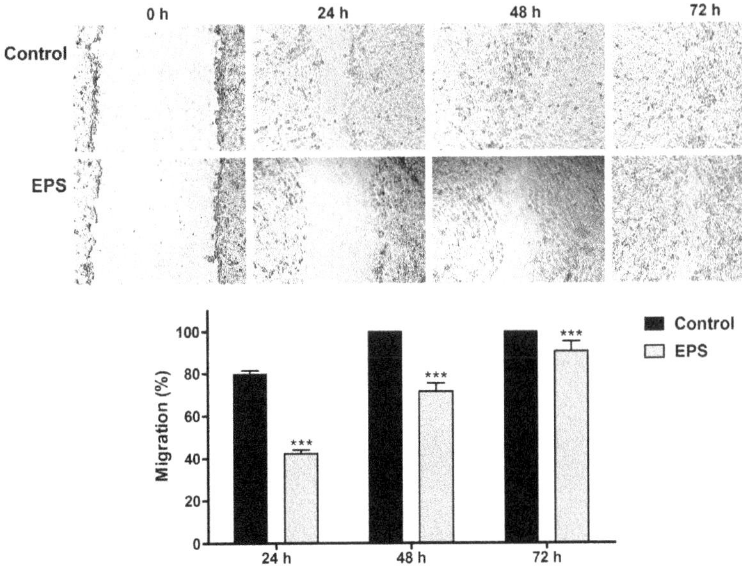

Figure 5. Effect of Coelastrella sp. BGV EPS treatment on the migration of HeLa cervical carcinoma cells evaluated by wound-healing assay. (**Upper panel**) Light microscopy images of untreated cell cultures and cell cultures treated with EPS (250 µg/mL); (**Lower panel**) Quantification of the EPS effect on the migration potential of the cancer cells. Data are presented as Mean ± SD; *** $p < 0.001$ compared to the untreated control.

In the control cell cultures, about 80% reduction of the wound width was measured at 24 h, and complete monolayer healing was observed as early as 48 h. The EPS treatment induced a statistically significant delay in the wound healing as compared to the control, and the mean percentages of cancer cell migration at the three time points measured (24, 48 and 72 h) were 42.3 ± 1.7%, 71.43 ± 3.8% and 90.4 ± 4.7%, respectively.

3.2.3. Fluorescent Microscopy Analysis of EPS-Induced Apoptotic Alterations in HeLa Cancer Cells

To determine whether the growth-inhibitory effect of EPS was related to the induction of apoptosis, HeLa cells were treated with an IC_{50} concentration of EPS for 24 h, and then their morphological changes were analyzed under a fluorescence microscope after double intravital staining with AO and EtBr (Figure 6). Acridine orange is a vital dye that stains both live and dead cells, whereas ethidium bromide stains only the cells that have lost their membrane integrity.

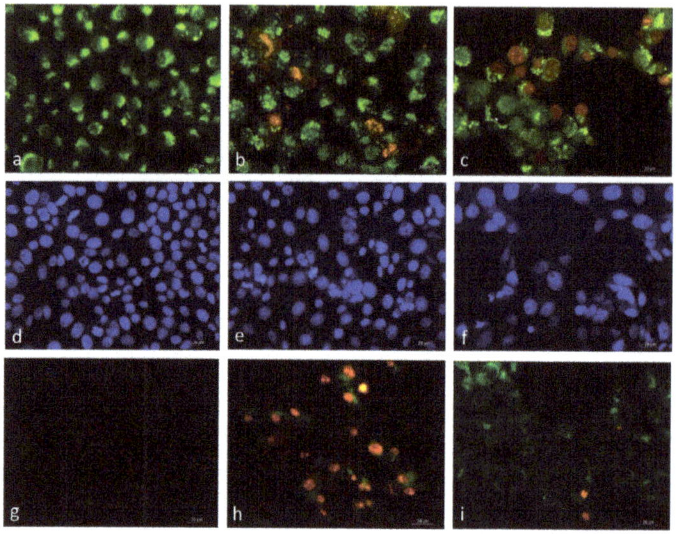

Figure 6. Morphological changes of the HeLa tumor cells cultured in the presence of EPS (500 μg/mL) for 24 h followed by AO/EB (**Upper row**), DAPI (**middle row**), and Annexin V (**Lower row**) staining. Fluorescence micrographs of: (**a**,**d**,**g**)—untreated HeLa cells; (**b**,**e**,**h**)—cells after incubation with 500 μg/mL of EPS; (**c**,**f**,**i**)—cells after incubation with 2.5 μg/mL Dox; Scale bar = 20 μm.

As shown in Figure 6, the HeLa control cells were morphologically normal, with nuclei of similar sizes, regularly shaped, and evenly bright green stain color (Figure 6a). The cells treated by EPS presented the typical morphological characteristics of early and late apoptosis. Wrinkled cells showing chromatin condensation as a bright green area or fragments (early apoptotic) and a significant number of cells with orange to red stained nuclei and condensed or fragmented chromatin (late apoptotic) were observed (Figure 6b). These alterations were accompanied by membrane blebbing and nuclear shrinkage. The nuclear morphology of the cells treated with Dox (Figure 6c) was completely destroyed. Late apoptotic cells with a bright red stained nucleus predominated. The majority of the HeLa cells were detached from the surface of the coverslips and were floating in the medium.

Further confirmation of the EPS-induced apoptosis of tumor cells was obtained by staining with DAPI. The control, untreated HeLa tumor cells had intact nuclei, round to slightly oval in shape and almost uniform in size, with smooth outlines and evenly distributed chromatin. Cell nuclei in different phases of mitosis were observed (Figure 6d). In contrast to the controls, the EPS-treated tumor cells showed significant morphological changes in the nuclei typical of apoptosis, such as nuclear polymorphism, chromatin condensation and margination, nuclear fragmentation, and collapse of the cell into membrane-bound apoptotic bodies (Figure 6e). The reduced number of nuclei with uneven outlines, condensed chromatin, and fragmented nuclei with multiple apoptotic bodies was seen in the samples treated with the anthracycline antitumor antibiotic doxorubicin (Figure 6f). The morphological studies showed that *Coelastrella* EPS was able to induce marked apoptotic morphology in HeLa cells at the cellular and nucleus levels.

The EPS-induced apoptosis of HeLa cells was also studied using Annexin-V staining, which permits the detection of phosphatidylserine exposure on the outer membrane surface of the apoptotic cells [38,39]. The translocation of phosphatidylserine from the inner side of the plasma membrane to the outer layer is one of the earliest steps in the initiation of programmed cell death-apoptosis. In this initial process, chromatin condensation occurs, but the cell membrane still retains its integrity. Annexin is a lipid-binding protein with an affinity for phosphatidylserine. Cells stained only with Annexin V-FITC glow green on the outside of the plasma membrane (early apoptotic). As cells move into late apoptosis, the permeability of the cell membrane is disrupted and DAPI enters the cell and stains the nuclei orange-red (late apoptotic). Late apoptotic cells were both Annexin V-FITC and PI positive. After EPS treatment, HeLa cells in the early and late apoptotic stages were observed under fluorescence microscopy, but those with late apoptosis (Annexin V-FITC and PI positive) predominated (Figure 6h). By contrast, after treatment with Dox, most cells were in the early apoptotic stage (Annexin V-FITC positive) (Figure 6i).

3.2.4. Flow Cytometry Analysis of the Effects of EPS on the Apoptosis and Cell Cycle Progression in HeLa Cancer Cells

Apoptosis Assay

Quantification of the live, early and late apoptotic, and necrotic cells in the HeLa cell cultures treated with 500 μg/mL EPS for 24 h was performed by FACS analysis after Annexin V-FITC/PI fluorescent staining (Figure 7).

The performed Annexin V-FITC/PI flow cytometry demonstrated a statistically significant increase in the early and late apoptotic cells and a decrease of the percentage of live cells in the EPS-treated cell cultures as compared to the untreated control.

Cell Cycle Analysis

The effect of EPS from *Coelastrella* sp. BGV on the cell cycle progression of HeLa carcinoma cells was studied by FACS analysis based on the detection of cellular DNA content after fluorescent staining with PI (Figure 8).

The results of flow cytometry analysis (presented in Figure 8) indicate that the EPS treatment induces a significant increase in the Sub G1 cell population and decreases the percentages of the G1, S, and G2-M cells.

3.2.5. Immunocytochemical Analysis of the EPS-Induced Alterations in the Expression and Intracellular Localization of the p53, bcl2, and Ki67 Proteins

Immunocytochemical analysis of the HeLa cells treated with 500 μg/mL EPS for 24 h was performed to identify the potential alterations in the expression and intracellular localization of the tumor suppressor protein p53, proapoptotic protein bcl2, and proliferation marker protein Ki67. Untreated cells and cells treated with the standard cytostatic Dox were used as negative and positive controls, respectively (Figure 9).

The results of the performed analysis revealed marked alterations in the pattern and intensity of the immunochemical staining of the EPS-treated cancer cells. Nuclear p53 staining was not detected in the control and EPS-treated cells (Figure 9a,b). However, in the cells exposed to EPS, a prominent increase in the cytoplasmic staining intensity was observed (Figure 9b), suggesting the accumulation of p53 protein in the cellular cytoplasm. In contrast, some of the nuclei in the Dox-treated cell cultures were p53 positive (Figure 9c). The intensity of bcl2 cytoplasmic staining of both EPS- and Dox-treated cells (Figure 9e,f) was significantly decreased in comparison to the control (Figure 9d). The effect of the standard cytostatic Dox was more clearly expressed than those of the studied EPS. The immunostaining of the nuclear proliferation marker Ki67 revealed a significant reduction in the number of positive cells as well as a decrease in the staining intensity of the cancer cells after treatment with the studied EPS (Figure 9g,h). A similar but much more pronounced effect was detected in the cells treated with the anticancer drug Dox (Figure 9i).

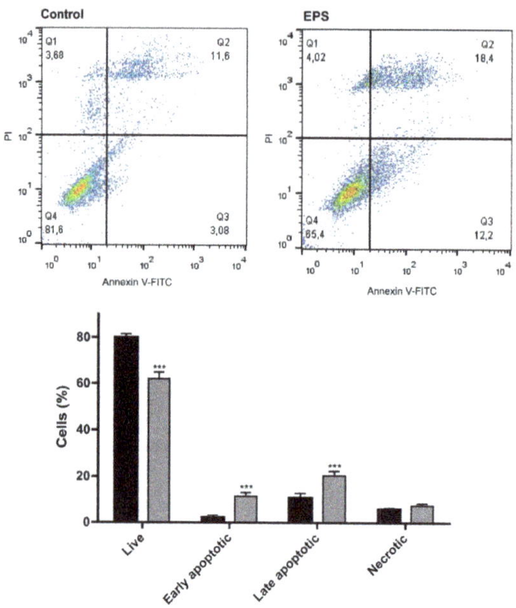

Figure 7. Proapoptotic effect of *Coelastrella* sp. BGV EPS on HeLa cervical carcinoma cells as evaluated by FACS analysis. (**Upper panel**) Representative histogram of control untreated cells and cells treated with 500 µg/mL EPS for 24 h. (**Lower panel**) Bar graph showing the percentages of the live, early and late apoptotic, and necrotic cells. The data are expressed as mean ± SD from three independent experiments; *** $p < 0.001$ indicates significant difference as compared to the negative control.

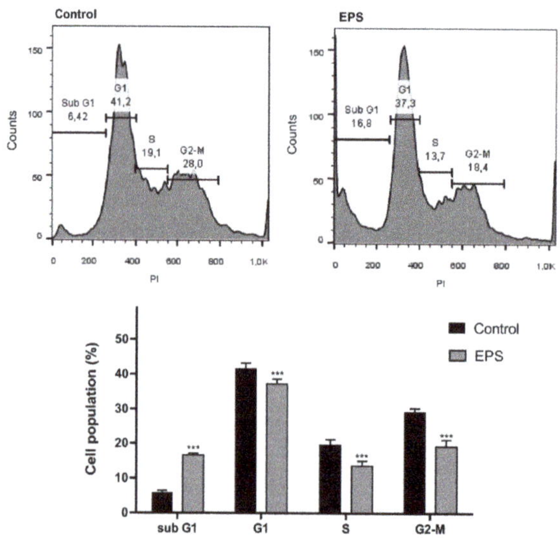

Figure 8. Effect of Coelastrella sp BGV EPS treatment on the cell cycle progression of HeLa cervical carcinoma cells. (**Upper panel**) Representative histogram of control untreated cells and cells treated with 500 µg/mL EPS for 24 h. (**Lower panel**) Bar graph representing the distribution of the cells in the different cell cycle phases. The data are expressed as mean ± SD from three independent experiments; *** $p < 0.001$ indicate significant difference as compared to the negative control.

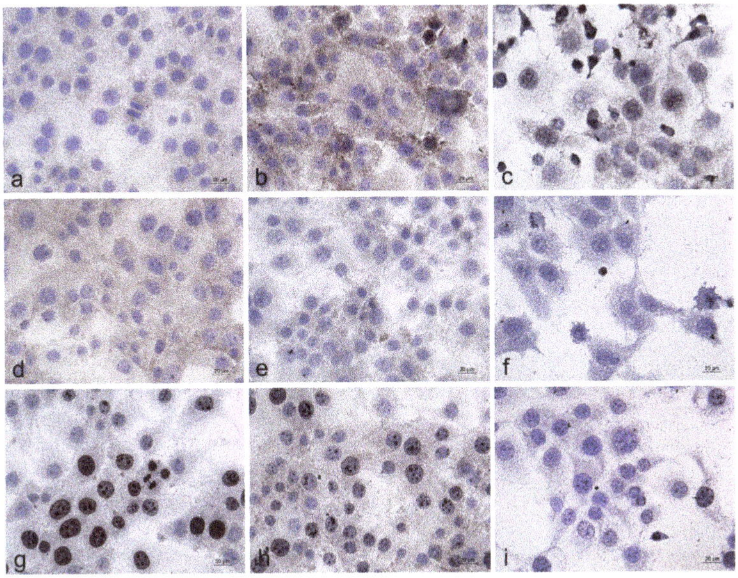

Figure 9. Immunocytochemical analysis of the EPS effects on the expression and intracellular localization of the p53, bcl2, and Ki67 proteins in HeLa carcinoma cells. (**a**,**d**,**g**) untreated control cells; (**b**,**e**,**h**) cells treated with EPS (500 µg/mL); (**c**,**f**,**i**) cells treated with Dox (2.5 µg/mL); (**a**–**c**) p53 immunostaining; (**d**–**f**) bcl2 immunostaining; (**g**–**i**) Ki67 immunostaining.

4. Discussion

Despite the progress in cancer therapy, a number of negative factors such as the increasing incidence of the disease, limited efficacy, multidrug resistance, side effects, and others, stimulate efforts to develop new and effective treatment approaches, as well as to develop new drugs. Nowadays, medicinal substances from natural sources, which offer new and alternative options for cancer treatment, are gaining more and more popularity, compared to synthetic drugs [40]. The inhibition of cancer cell proliferation is a critical effect of anticancer agents. Another major target for cancer therapy is the induction of apoptosis, by which antitumor drugs kill cancer cells [41,42].

As a part of our efforts to explore the therapeutic potential of the local strains of microalgae, we undertook a systematic study on the green microalga *Coelastrella* sp. BGV, which is endemic to Varvara, Bulgaria. In this study, for the first time, we isolated EPS from the Bulgarian strain of green microalga and assessed its antitumor and apoptosis-inducing properties against cervical cancer cells of the HeLa line in vitro. The chemical composition analysis of EPS collected by ethanol precipitation of a cell-free culture medium showed that it was composed mainly of carbohydrates (36.4%) and contained small amounts of proteins (7,14%). The uronic acid content was 4.5%. Moreover, the molecular weight and monosaccharide composition of the isolated exopolysaccharide were also investigated. The presence of three polysaccharide fractions with molecular weights 11.5×10^4 Da, 72.4×10^4 Da, and 30.7×10^4 Da were established by HPSEC-RID chromatography. HPLC-UV chromatography indicated that the isolated extracellular polysaccharides contain seven different types of monomeric units, two of which were identified as galactose and fucose. FT-IR absorption spectra confirmed the existence of various polysaccharide-characteristic substituent groups without establishing the presence of sulfate esters. The results showed that *Coelastrella* EPS is a typical polysaccharide (or proteoglycan) composed mainly of neutral sugars.

The different microalga and cyanobacteria species display significant variability in their ability to produce EPS as well as in the amount, structure, and chemical composition of the secreted EPS. A recent study compared ten species of microalgae that are of commercial interest as a functional food or nutritional supplement, in terms of biomass composition, cell-associated polysaccharides, EPS, and their chemical composition (monosaccharide profile, uronic acid content, and sulfates) [8]. EPSs were identified in only four species of microalgae (*Porphyridium cruentum, Odontella aurita, Arthrospira platensis,* and *Chlorella vulgaris*). The highest content of EPS was found in *P. cruentum*, a red microalga known for its high content of sulfated extracellular polysaccharides [43]. The most abundant monosaccharide in microalgal EPS is glucose, while fructose predominates in cyanobacterial EPS. In the EPS produced by *Rhodophyta*, xylose was found to predominate, followed by galactose, while in *Charophyta*, mainly uronic acids and fucose were detected. Galactose is the most abundant monosaccharide of EPS from *Chlorophyta*. Only a few studies reported EPS production and partial characterization in green alga species, for example *Dunaliella salina, Chlorella vulgaris, Chlorella elipsoidea*, and *Chlorella pyrenoidosa* [44–47]. Chemical composition analysis indicated that these EPSs consisted of different types of monosaccharides and their derivatives. The heteropolysaccharides identified in *Chlorella pyrenoidosa* were found to contain rhamnose, glucosamine, glucose, glucuronic acid, mannose, fucose, galactose, and xylose, and the EPSs from *Spirulina platensis* were composed mainly of glucose monosaccharides and rhamnose and smaller amounts of glucuronic acid, mannose, glucosamine, fucose, and xylose [48]. *Spirulina* sp. LEB 18 heteropolysaccharides were reported to contain glucose, galactose, xylose, glucuronic acid, rhamnose, fucose, arabinose, and galacturonic acid [49]. Polysaccharides isolated from *Chlorella pyrenoidosa* consist of two low molecular weight fractions (69,658 Da and 109,406 Da) that have the same qualitative and different quantitative monosaccharide profile. Both fractions contained rhamnose, mannose, glucose, and galactose and up to 10% unknown monosaccharides [50]. The dominant monosaccharide in one fraction was galactose (46.5%), and in the second rhamnose predominated (37.8%). From the extraction residue of *D. salina*, a crude polysaccharide extract (PD) containing four fractions—PD1, PD2, PD3, and PD4— and the two subfractions PD4a and PD4b were obtained [51]. The results of the monosaccharide analysis showed that PD1 and PD4a are acidic heteropolysaccharides containing glucose and galactose, respectively, and PD4a contains sulfated groups. PD2 and PD3 are glucans, while PD4b is a polysaccharide complex linked to nucleic acids by covalent bonds.

The quantity of the produced extracellular polysaccharides shows significant variations between the different species and strains of green microalga and is substantially impacted by cultivation conditions, the physiological state of the cells, culture age, and the extraction techniques and procedures used. Even EPS obtained from the same algal species by the same methods and conditions but from different lots can be distinguished [6,10,11,47]. The variations in the chemical structure, molecular weights, monosaccharide composition, and chain conformation determine the differences in the biological activities of the microalga-derived EPS.

The anticancer activity of the polysaccharides isolated from different microalga species has been frequently reported in recent years, and the potential mechanisms of action of polysaccharides have been investigated. The EPS derived from the microalga *Thraustochytriidae* sp. GA strain inhibited the proliferation of ovarian, breast, and colon cancer cell lines, altered cell cycle-related protein expression, and displayed immunomodulatory activity by inducing human B cell proliferation and altering T cell cytokine production [15]. The anticancer activities of polysaccharides derived from various species of the *Chlorella* genus in cell culture models have been reported. Polysaccharides from *Chlorella pyrenoidosa* inhibited the growth of A549 human lung cancer cells in vitro, in a dose-dependent manner [50]. Purified EPS from *Chlorella zofingiensis* and *Chlorella vulgaris* exhibited antitumor activities against human colon cancer HCT8 cells in vitro, with IC_{50} values of 1.70 and 3.14 mg/mL, respectively [47]. In another study, similar inhibitory effects of EPSs from *Chlorella pyrenoidosa, Scenedesmus* sp., and *Chlorococcum* sp. on the cell growth, proliferation, and colony formation of the human colon cancer cell lines HCT116 and HCT8 (with better inhibitory effects on HCT8 cells) were reported [52]. Aqueous EPS from *Graesiella* sp. demonstrated a dose-dependent antiproliferative effect on HepG2 (human hepatocellular carcinoma) and Caco-2 (human colon cancer) cell lines, with higher sensitivity reported for Caco2 cells [53].

Moreover, the anticancer efficacy of microalgal EPS has been confirmed by in vivo experiments. The two low molecular weight polysaccharides from *Pavlova viridis* were found to exert strong immunoenhancing activities (significantly increased lymphocyte and macrophage proliferation, and phagocytosis of macrophages), and to inhibit the in vivo growth of implanted S180 tumors in mice after intragastric administration [54]. EPS from *P. cruentum* increased the spreading and phagocytic ability of peritoneal macrophages, stimulated the proliferation of bone marrow cells in a dose-dependent manner, retarded tumor growth, and prolonged the survival time (by 10–16 days) of hamsters implanted with Graffi myeloid tumors [55]. Extracellular polysaccharides from the microalga *Crypthecodinium* sp. SUN suppressed the growth of lung adenocarcinoma tumors in nude mice without affecting their body weight [56].

Despite the numerous studies indicating the cancer-suppressive effects of algal EPSs, currently no data are available regarding the anticancer potential of EPSs isolated from *Coelastrella* species. In this study, we examined the effect of EPS on cell proliferation and the viability of HeLa and MCF-7 human cancer cells and the non-cancer control cell lines HaCaT and BALB/3T3. The cell proliferation of the EPS-treated cells was tested using an MTT assay after 24 and 48 h. The results showed that EPS decreased the proliferation of HeLa at 24 and 48 h in a time- and dose-dependent manner. The results also showed that EPS does not inhibit BALB/3T3 cell proliferation at 24 h, and even increases the proliferation of the human keratinocyte cell line HaCaT at the lower tested concentrations. A significant reduction in the cell viability of HaCaT cells was established only at a concentration of 1000 μg/mL at the 24 h and 500 μg/mL and 1000 μg/mL at the 48 h. The cell viability of BALB/3T3 cells treated for 48 h with EPS was significantly decreased as compared to untreated control. However, it was significantly higher compared to that measured for the tumor cells, thus indicating the EPS's ability to differentially regulate the proliferation of tumor and normal cells. These results are consistent with the previously reported data demonstrating the anticancer potential of algal EPSs.

Several studies have demonstrated that the anticancer effects of microalga-derived EPS stem from their capacity to trigger apoptosis in cancer cells. A novel acid polysaccharide designated as XQZ3, with a molecular weight of 29.13 kDa and mainly composed of galactose and mannose extracted from *Chlorella pyrenoidosa,* led to the induction of mitochondrial dysfunction, autophagy, and apoptosis of cancer cells [57]. The sulfated polysaccharides obtained from *Tribonema* sp. and *Phaeodactylum tricornutum* significantly reduced the proliferation of the liver cancer cell line HepG2 by inducing cell apoptosis without affecting the cell cycle and mitosis of tumor cells, and it showed immune-modulatory activity by stimulating macrophage cytokine production (such as IL-6, IL-10, and TNF-α) [58,59]. EPS from *Gymnodinium* sp. A3 was cytotoxic against various human lymphoid cells, particularly MT-4 cells, and induced apoptosis in the cells, as demonstrated by morphological, flow cytometry, and DNA fragmentation investigations [60]. The same polysaccharide exhibited significant cytotoxicity toward human myeloid leukemia K562 cells by inducing apoptotic cell death through the inhibition of DNA topoisomerases I and II (two nuclear enzymes regulating apoptotic cell death) [61,62]. EPS produced by *Chlorella* sp. inhibited the proliferation and promoted the apoptosis of HeLa cervical cancer cells by activating the MAPK, TNF, and PI3K-Akt signaling pathways [63].

To obtain information about the processes and mechanisms underlying the cancer-suppressive effects of the *Coelastrella* EPS detected in the present study, additional cytomorphological, flow cytometric, and immunocytochemical analyses were performed. Based on the results obtained from the cell viability assays, the HeLa cell line was chosen as a model system for the further analyses because it showed the highest sensitivity to the EPS-induced antiproliferative and cytotoxic effects among the cell lines tested.

The effect of EPS on cancer cell migration was followed in dynamics for 72 h and quantified by the wound-healing assay that analyzes the ability of the cells to fill a gap mechanically created by scratching a cell monolayer. The surface of the wound area measured in the EPS-treated HeLa cells was notably larger and showed a statistically significant difference from those measured in the untreated control at all three tested time intervals, indicating the inhibitory action of EPS on cervical carcinoma cells' migration.

Fluorescence microscopy examination of HeLa cervical cells treated with *Coelastrella* EPS and labeled with the fluorescent dyes AO/EB and DAPI was used to acquire information about the processes that mediate anticancer action and identify the type of cell death. Apoptotic cells are distinguished by the presence of specific cellular and nuclear morphology changes, which allows for their identification using cytomorphological approaches [64]. The observed membrane blebbing, chromatin condensation, nuclear fragmentation, and apoptotic body formation in the treated HeLa cells indicated the ability of the EPS to trigger apoptosis. The proapoptotic activity of the EPS was also confirmed by fluorescent microscopy after staining with Annexin V-FITC/PI. This method allows the detection of the translocation of phosphatidylserine from the inner to the outer membrane surface, which is an apoptosis-specific alteration in the lipid structure of the cytoplasmic membrane occurring at the earliest stage of the apoptotic process. The cytomorphological analysis performed by these three fluorescent methods showed consistent results and allowed the establishment of typical apoptotic alterations in EPS-treated HeLa cervical carcinoma cells.

A fluorescence-activated cell sorting (FACS) analysis of Annexin V-FITC/PI-stained HeLa cells was used to quantify the proapoptotic effects of *Coelastrella* sp. BGV EPS. The results of the investigation revealed a statistically significant increase in both early and late apoptotic cell counts in EPS-treated cell cultures as compared to the untreated control. This finding is in agreement with the results obtained by fluorescent microscopy analysis and provides further confirmation of the detected apoptosis-inducing ability of EPS.

To analyze the effect of EPS from *Coelastrella* sp. BGV on cell cycle progression of HeLa carcinoma cells, a FACS analysis of PI-stained cells was performed to quantify the cell populations in the different phases of the cell cycle based on the differences of their DNA content. The obtained results were consistent with the data of Annexin V-FITC/PI FACS analysis and indicated a significant increase of the cell population that had Sub G1 DNA content, which is an indication of the induction of apoptosis in EPS-treated cancer cells. The percentages of G1, S, and G2-M cell populations in the cell cultures treated with EPS were significantly decreased in comparison with the control, and this effect was most pronounced for the G2-M cells. That is an indication of the ability of EPS to reduce the mitotic activity of the cancer cell.

This finding is consistent with the results of the immunocytochemical analysis of the control untreated and EPS-treated HeLa carcinoma cells, demonstrating a marked decrease in the expression of the nuclear proliferation marker Ki67. Ki-67 is a nuclear protein highly expressed in cycling cells but significantly down-regulated in resting G_0 cells and rapidly degraded upon cell cycle exit [65]. This feature has made Ki-67 a clinically important diagnostic and prognostic marker for grading the primary tumor and metastases and predicting the likelihood of relapses and survival rates [65]. The presented results clearly demonstrate the antiproliferative activity of the studied *Coelastrella* sp. BGV EPS.

The potential involvement of the apoptosis-related proteins p53 and bcl2 in the molecular mechanisms underlying the detected proapoptotic activity was also investigated by immunocytochemical analyses of the control untreated and EPS-treated HeLa carcinoma cells. The cellular protein p53 plays central roles in the regulation of cell cycle progression, DNA repair, and apoptosis [66]. Under normal conditions, the expression levels of p53 are very low. However, the exposure of the cell to internal and external stresses triggers a rapid increase in the intracellular p53 protein levels. Under stress conditions, the p53 protein governs cellular fate decisions and restricts the propagation of damaged cells. Functional loss of the p53 protein has been found in about half of human malignancies, highlighting its key role in cancer suppression. In addition to its known function as a nuclear transcription factor regulating the expression of a number of apoptosis-related genes, more recent studies have discovered that p53 has additional activities in the cytoplasm, where it triggers apoptosis through a transcription-independent mechanism by directly binding and inactivating the anti-apoptotic protein bcl2 [67]. The stress-induced accumulation of p53 in the cytosol is a hallmark of the transcription-independent pathway of p53-mediated apoptosis [68]. The increased intensity of the cytoplasmic p53 staining and the reduced bcl2 staining observed in the EPS-treated HeLa cells suggests that the activation of the cytosolic transcription-independent p53 pathway is a possible mechanism of the EPS-induced apoptosis.

5. Conclusions

The ability to distinguish cancer from non-cancerous cells, suppress tumor cell proliferation, and induce apoptosis in treated tumor cells is an important property of candidate anticancer drugs. The present study provided the first evidence that the EPS isolated from the *Coelastrella* sp. BGV can selectively inhibit the growth of human cancer cell lines in a dose-dependent and time-dependent manner. Moreover, the ability of the *Coelastrella* EPS to inhibit cancer cell proliferation and migration and to induce apoptosis was clearly demonstrated. The presented results reveal that the green microalga *Coelastrella* sp. BGV is a promising source of valuable bioactive compounds and provides a foundation for further investigations of the *Coelastrella* EPS as a potential anticancer drug in other cancer model systems.

Author Contributions: Conceptualization: R.T. and T.T.-Y.; methodology: T.T.-Y., A.G., I.S., V.D., Z.P. and M.O.; software: A.G., I.S. and M.O.; formal analysis: T.T.-Y., I.S., V.D., Z.P. and M.O.; investigation: R.T., A.G., T.T.-Y., M.O., V.D., Z.P. and P.D.; data curation: A.G., T.T.-Y. and I.S.; writing—original draft preparation: T.T.-Y. and R.T.; writing—review and editing: A.G., R.T., M.O. and P.D.; visualization: A.G., I.S. and M.O.; supervision: R.T. and P.D.; project administration: I.S.; funding acquisition: I.S. All authors have read and agreed to the published version of the manuscript.

Funding: This research was partially supported by the Bulgarian Ministry of Education and Science under the National Research Program "Young scientists and postdoctoral students -2" approved by DCM 206/07.04.2022.

Institutional Review Board Statement: Not applicable.

Informed Consent Statement: Not applicable.

Data Availability Statement: All data are comprised in the manuscript.

Conflicts of Interest: The authors declare no conflicts of interest.

References

1. Frankfurt, O.S.; Krishan, A. Apoptosis-based drug screening and detection of selective toxicity to cancer cells. *Anticancer Drugs* **2003**, *14*, 555–561. [CrossRef] [PubMed]
2. Abd El Baky, H.H.; El-Baroty, G.S. Healthy benefit of microalgal bioactive substances. *J. Aquat. Sci.* **2013**, *1*, 11–23.
3. Singh, D.V.; Upadhyay, A.K.; Singh, R.; Singh, D.P.B. Health benefits of bioactive compounds from microalgae. In *Phytomedicine*; Bhat, R.A., Hakeem, K.R., Dervash, M.A., Eds.; Academic Press: Cambridge, MA, USA, 2021; Chapter 10; pp. 291–319.
4. Zhou, L.; Li, K.; Duan, X.; Hill, D.; Barrow, C.; Dunshea, F.; Suleria, H. Bioactive compounds in microalgae and their potential health benefits. *Food Biosci.* **2022**, *49*, 101932. [CrossRef]
5. Gaignard, C.; Laroche, C.; Pierre, G.; Dubessay, P.; Delattre, C.; Gardarin, C.; Michaud, P. Screening of marine microalgae: Investigation of new exopolysaccharide producers. *Algal Res.* **2019**, *44*, 101711. [CrossRef]
6. Tounsi, L.; Hentati, F.; Hlima, H.B.; Barkallah, M.; Smaoui, S.; Fendri, I.; Abdelkafi, S. Microalgae as feedstock for bioactive polysaccharides. *Int. J. Biol. Macromol.* **2022**, *221*, 1238–1250. [CrossRef]
7. Raposo, M.F.D.J.; De Morais, R.M.S.C.; de Morais, A.M.M.B. Health applications of bioactive compounds from marine microalgae. *Life Sci.* **2013**, *93*, 479–486. [CrossRef]
8. Bernaerts, T.M.; Gheysen, L.; Foubert, I.; Hendrickx, M.E.; Van Loey, A.M. The potential of microalgae and their biopolymers as structuring ingredients in food. *Biotechnol. Adv.* **2019**, *37*, 107419. [CrossRef]
9. Mišurcová, L.B. Chemical composition of seaweeds. In *Handbook of Marine Macroalgae, Biotechnology and Applied Phycology*; Kim, S.-K., Ed.; John Wiley & Sons: Hoboken, NJ, USA, 2011; Chapter 7; pp. 171–192.
10. Kumar, K.S.; Kumari, S.; Singh, K.; Kushwaha, P.B. Influence of seasonal variation on chemical composition and nutritional profiles of macro-and microalgae. In *Recent Advances in Micro and Macroalgal Processing: Food and Health Perspectives*; Rajauria, G., Yuan, Y.V., Eds.; John Wiley & Sons, Ltd.: Hoboken, NJ, USA, 2021; Chapter 2; pp. 14–71.

11. Costa Alberto Vieira, J.; Franco Lucas, B.; Gabrielle Pires Alvarenga, A.; Botelho Moreira, J.; Greque de Morais, M. Microalgae polysaccharides: An overview of production, characterization and potential applications. *Polysaccharides* **2021**, *2*, 2673–4176.
12. Kraan, S.B. Algal Polysaccharides, Novel Applications and Outlook. In *Carbohydrates—Comprehensive Studies on Glycobiology and Glycotechnology*; Chang, C., Ed.; IntechOpen: London, UK, 2012; Volume 1, Chapter 2; pp. 490–532.
13. Mišurcová, L.; Orsavová, J.; Ambrožová, J.V.B. Algal Polysaccharides and Health. In *Polysaccharides: Bioactivity and Biotechnology*; Ramawat, K.G., Mérillon, J.-M., Eds.; Springer International Publishing: Cham, Switzerland, 2015; Chapter 4; pp. 109–144.
14. Machu, L.; Misurcova, L.; Vavra Ambrozova, J.; Orsavova, J.; Mlcek, J.; Sochor, J.; Jurikova, T. Phenolic content and antioxidant capacity in algal food products. *Molecules* **2015**, *20*, 1118–1133. [CrossRef]
15. Park, G.T.; Go, R.E.; Lee, H.M.; Lee, G.A.; Kim, C.W.; Seo, J.W.; Hwang, K.A. Potential anti-proliferative and immunomodulatory effects of marine microalgal exopolysaccharide on various human cancer cells and lymphocytes in vitro. *Mar. Biotechnol.* **2017**, *19*, 136–146. [CrossRef]
16. Netanel, L.G.; Ochbaum, G.; Mejubovsky-Mikhelis, M.; Bitton, R.; Arad, S. Physico-chemical characteristics of the sulfated polysaccharides of the red microalgae *Dixoniella grisea* and *Porphyridium aerugineum*. *Int. J. Biol. Macromol.* **2020**, *145*, 1171–1179. [CrossRef]
17. Matsubara, K.; Mori, M.; Matsumoto, H.; Hori, K.; Miyazawa, K. Antiangiogenic properties of a sulfated galactan isolated from a marine green alga, Codium cylindricum. *J. Appl. Phycol.* **2003**, *15*, 87–90. [CrossRef]
18. Raposo, M.F.J.; Morais, A.M.B.; Morais, R.M.S.C. Marine polysaccharides from algae with potential biomedical applications. *Mar. Drugs* **2015**, *13*, 2967–3028. [CrossRef] [PubMed]
19. Yu, Y.; Shen, M.; Song, Q.; Xie, J. Biological activities and pharmaceutical applications of polysaccharide from natural resources: A review. *Carbohydr. Polym.* **2018**, *183*, 91–101. [CrossRef] [PubMed]
20. Yuan, Q.; Li, H.; Wei, Z.; Lv, K.; Gao, C.; Liu, Y.; Zhao, L. Isolation, structures and biological activities of polysaccharides from Chlorella: A review. *Int. J. Biol. Macromol.* **2020**, *163*, 2199–2209. [CrossRef]
21. Gharibzahedi, S.M.T.; Marti-Quijal, F.J.; Barba, F.J.; Altintas, Z. Current emerging trends in antitumor activities of polysaccharides extracted by microwave and ultrasound-assisted methods. *Int. J. Biol. Macromol.* **2022**, *202*, 494–507. [CrossRef] [PubMed]
22. Toshkova-Yotova, T.; Georgieva, A.; Iliev, I.; Alexandrov, S.; Ivanova, A.; Pilarski, P.; Toshkova, R. Antitumor and antimicrobial activity of fatty acids from green microalga *Coelastrella* sp. BGV. *South Afr. J. Bot.* **2022**, *151*, 394–402. [CrossRef]
23. Toshkova-Yotova, T.A.; Georgieva, A.; Pilarski, P.; Toshkova, R. Aqueous extracts, green microalga *Coelastrella* sp. BGV displays antiproliferative, proapoptotic activity in vitro against HeLa tumor cells. *Compt. Rend. Acad. Bulg. Sci.* **2021**, *74*, 696–705.
24. Toshkova-Yotova, T.; Georgieva, A.; Todorova, K.; Pilarski, P.; Toshkova, R. Antitumor properties of vegetable oil extract from green microalga *Coelastrella* sp. *J. Microbiol. Biotechnol. Food Sci.* **2021**, *11*, e2744. [CrossRef]
25. Dimitrova, P.; Marinova, G.; Pilarski, P. Preliminary studies on the growth and biochemical composition of a promising carotenoid producing strain *Coelastrella* sp. *Nat. Math. Sci.* **2016**, *6*, 139–149.
26. Georgiev, D.; Dilov, H.; Avramova, S. Millieu nutritif tamponne et méthode de culture intensive des microal-gues vertes. *Hydrobiology* **1978**, *7*, 14–23.
27. Ivanova, J.G.; Toshkova-Yotova, T.S.; Toshkova, R.A.; Deleva, V.R.; Georgieva, A.K.; Gigova, L.G. Antioxidant and Anticancer Potential of Extracellular Polysaccharide from *Porphyridium aerugineum* (Rhodophyta). *Fermentation* **2024**, *10*, 259. [CrossRef]
28. Dubois, M.; Gilles, K.A.; Hamilton, J.K.; Rebers, P.A.; Smith, F. Colorimetric method for determination of sugars and related substances. *Anal. Chem.* **1956**, *28*, 350–356. [CrossRef]
29. Bradford, M.M. A rapid and sensitive method for the quantitation of microgram quantities of protein utilizing the principle of protein-dye binding. *Anal. Biochem.* **1976**, *72*, 248–254. [CrossRef]
30. Blumenkrantz, N.; Asboe-Hansen, G. New method for quantitative determination of uronic acids. *Anal. Biochem.* **1973**, *54*, 484–489. [CrossRef] [PubMed]
31. McComb, E.A.; McCready, R.M. Determination of acetyl in pectin and in acetylated carbohydrate polymers. *Anal. Chem.* **1957**, *29*, 819–821. [CrossRef]
32. Anthon, G.E.; Barrett, D.M. Combined enzymatic and colorimetric method for determining the uronic acid and methylester content of pectin: Application to tomato products. *Food Chem.* **2008**, *110*, 239–247. [CrossRef]
33. Karkhanis, Y.D.; Zeltner, J.Y.; Jackson, J.J.; Carlo, D.J. A new and improved microassay to determine 2-keto-3-deoxyoctonate in lipopolysaccharide of gram-negative bacteria. *Anal. Biochem.* **1978**, *85*, 595–601. [CrossRef]
34. Ognyanov, M.; Georgiev, Y.; Petkova, N.; Ivanov, I.; Vasileva, I.; Kratchanova, M. Isolation and characterization of pecticpolysaccharide fraction from in vitro suspension culture of *Fumaria officinalis* L. *Int. J. Polym. Sci.* **2018**, *2018*, 570503. [CrossRef]
35. Honda, S.; Akao, E.; Suzuki, S.; Okuda, M.; Kakehi, K.; Nakamura, J. High-performance liquid chromatography of reducing carbohydrates as strongly ultraviolet-absorbing and electrochemically sensitive 1-phenyl-3-methyl5-pyrazolone derivatives. *Anal. Biochem.* **1989**, *180*, 351–357. [CrossRef]
36. Yang, X.; Zhao, Y.; Wang, Q.; Wang, H.; Mei, Q. Analysis of the monosaccharide components in Angelica polysaccharides by high performance liquid chromatography. *Anal. Sci.* **2005**, *21*, 1177–1180. [CrossRef] [PubMed]
37. Mosmann, T. Rapid colorimetric assay for cellular growth and survival: Application to proliferation and cytotoxicity assays. *J. Immunol. Methods* **1983**, *65*, 55–63. [CrossRef] [PubMed]

38. Vermes, I.; Haanen, C.; Steffens-Nakken, H.; Reutelingsperger, C. A novel assay for apoptosis. Flow cytometric detection of phosphatidylserine expression on early apoptotic cells using fluorescein labelled Annexin V. *J. Immunol. Methods* **1995**, *184*, 39–51. [CrossRef] [PubMed]
39. Crowley, L.C.; Marfell, B.J.; Scott, A.P.; Waterhouse, N.J. Quantitation of Apoptosis and Necrosis by Annexin V Binding, Propidium Iodide Uptake, and Flow Cytometry. *Cold Spring Harb. Protoc.* **2016**, *11*, 953–957. [CrossRef]
40. Cheng, F.; Yang, Y.; Zhang, L.; Cao, Y.; Yao, W.; Tang, Y.; Ding, A. A Natural triterpene derivative from Euphorbia kansui inhibits cell proliferation and induces apoptosis against rat intestinal epithelioid cell line in vitro. *Int. J. Mol. Sci.* **2015**, *16*, 18956–18975. [CrossRef]
41. Yin, P.H.; Liu, X.; Qiu, Y.Y.; Cai, J.F.; Qin, J.M.; Zhu, H.R.; Li, Q. Anti-tumor activity and apoptosis-regulation mechanisms of bufalin in various cancers: New hope for cancer patients. *Asian Pac. J. Cancer Prev.* **2012**, *13*, 5339–5343. [CrossRef]
42. Safarzadeh, E.; Sandoghchian Shotorbani, S.; Baradaran, B. Herbal medicine as inducers of apoptosis in cancer treatment. *Adv. Pharm. Bull.* **2014**, *4*, 421–427.
43. Arad, S.M.; Levy-Ontman, O. Red microalgal cell-wall polysaccharides: Biotechnological aspects. *Curr. Opin. Biotechnol.* **2010**, *21*, 358–364. [CrossRef]
44. Yalcin, I.; Hicsasmaz, Z.; Boz, B.; Bozoglu, F. Characterization of the extracellular polysaccharide from fresh-water microalgae *Chlorella* sp. Lebensm. *Wiss. Technol.* **1994**, *27*, 158–165. [CrossRef]
45. Morineau-Thomas, O.; Jaouen, P.; Legentilhomme, P. The role of exopolysaccharides in fouling phenomenon during ultrafiltration of microalgae (*Chlorella* sp. and *Porphyridium purpureum*): Advantage of a swirling decaying flow. *Bioprocess Biosyst. Eng.* **2002**, *25*, 35–42.
46. Xiao, R.; Zheng, Y. Overview of microalgal extracellular polymeric substances (EPS) and their applications. *Biotechnol. Adv.* **2016**, *34*, 1225–1244. [CrossRef] [PubMed]
47. Zhang, J.; Liu, L.; Chen, F. Production and characterization of exopolysaccharides from *Chlorella zofingiensis* and *Chlorella vulgaris* with anti-colorectal cancer activity. *Int. J. Biol. Macromol.* **2019**, *134*, 976–983. [CrossRef] [PubMed]
48. Guo, W.; Zhu, S.; Li, S.; Feng, Y.; Wu, H.; Zeng, M. Microalgae polysaccharides ameliorate obesity in association with modulation of lipid metabolism and gut microbiota in high-fat-diet fed C57BL/6 mice. *Int. J. Biol. Macromol.* **2021**, *182*, 1371–1383. [CrossRef] [PubMed]
49. Deamici, K.M.; Costa, J.A.V.; Santos, L.O. Magnetic fields as triggers of microalga growth: Evaluation of its effect on *Spirulina* sp. *Bioresour. Technol.* **2016**, *220*, 62–67. [CrossRef]
50. Sheng, J.; Yu, F.; Xin, Z.; Zhao, L.; Zhu, X.; Hu, Q. Preparation, identification and their antitumor activities in vitro of polysaccharides from Chlorella pyrenoidosa. *Food Chem.* **2007**, *105*, 533–539. [CrossRef]
51. Dai, J.; Mumper, R.J. Plant Phenolics: Extraction, Analysis and Their Antioxidant and Anticancer Properties. *Molecules* **2010**, *15*, 7313–7352. [CrossRef]
52. Zhang, J.; Liu, L.; Ren, Y.; Chen, F. Characterization of exopolysaccharides produced by microalgae with antitumor activity on human colon cancer cells. *Int. J. Biol. Macromol.* **2019**, *128*, 761–767. [CrossRef]
53. Trabelsi, L.; Chaieb, O.; Mnari, A.; Abid-Essafi, S.; Aleya, L. Partial characterization and antioxidant and antiproliferative activities of the aqueous extracellular polysaccharides from the thermophilic microalgae *Graesiella* sp. *BMC Complement. Altern. Med.* **2016**, *16*, 210. [CrossRef]
54. Sun, L.; Chu, J.; Sun, Z.; Chen, L. Physicochemical properties, immunomodulation and antitumor activities of polysaccharide from Pavlova viridis. *Life Sci.* **2016**, *144*, 156–161. [CrossRef]
55. Gardeva, E.; Toshkova, R.; Minkova, K.; Gigova, L. Cancer protective action of polysaccharide, derived from red microalga Porphyridium cruentum—A biological background. *Biotechnol. Biotechnol. Equip.* **2009**, *23*, 783–787. [CrossRef]
56. Ye, W.; Zhu, J.; Liu, Q.; Zhang, Y.; Yuan, Y.; Guo, S.; Zhang, Z. Characterization and anticancer effects of extracellular polysaccharide from DHA-producing microalga *Crypthecodinium* sp. SUN. *Int. J. Biol. Macromol.* **2023**, *249*, 100–126. [CrossRef] [PubMed]
57. Sun, L.; Ji, M.; Liu, Y.; Zhang, M.; Zheng, C.; Wang, P. XQZ3, a Chlorella pyrenoidosa polysaccharide suppresses cancer progression by restraining mitochondrial bioenergetics via HSP90/AKT signaling pathway. *Int. J. Biol. Macromol.* **2024**, *264*, 130705. [CrossRef] [PubMed]
58. Chen, X.; Song, L.; Wang, H.; Liu, S.; Yu, H.; Wang, X.; Li, P. Partial characterization, the immune modulation and anticancer activities of sulfated polysaccharides from filamentous microalgae *Tribonema* sp. *Molecules* **2019**, *24*, 322. [CrossRef] [PubMed]
59. Yang, S.; Wan, H.; Wang, R.; Hao, D. Sulfated polysaccharides from Phaeodactylum tricornutum: Isolation, structural characteristics, and inhibiting HepG2 growth activity in vitro. *PeerJ* **2019**, *7*, e6409. [CrossRef]
60. Sogawa, K.; Kodama, E.; Matsuda, M.; Shigeta, S.; Okutani, K. Marine microalgal polysaccharide induces apoptosis in human lymphoid cells. *J. Mar. Biotechnol.* **1998**, *6*, 35–38.
61. Sogawa, K.; Yamada, T.; Sumida, T.; Hamakawa, H.; Kuwabara, H.; Matsuda, M.; Muramatsu, Y.; Kose, H.; Matsumoto, K.; Sasaki, Y.; et al. Induction of apoptosis and inhibition of DNA topoisomerase-I in K-562 cells by a marine microalgal polysaccharide. *Life Sci.* **2000**, *66*, 227–231. [CrossRef]
62. Umemura, K.; Yanase, K.; Suzuki, M.; Okutani, K.; Yamori, T.; Andoh, T. Inhibition of DNA topoisomerases I and II, and growth inhibition of human cancer cell lines by a marine microalgal polysaccharide. *Biochem. Pharmacol.* **2003**, *66*, 481–487. [CrossRef]

63. Zhong, R.; Li, J.Q.; Wu, S.W.; He, X.M.; Xuan, J.C.; Long, H.; Liu, H.Q. Transcriptome analysis reveals possible antitumor mechanism of Chlorella exopolysaccharide. *Gene* **2022**, *811*, 127–146. [CrossRef]
64. Elmore, S. Apoptosis: A review of programmed cell death. *Toxicol. Pathol.* **2007**, *35*, 495–516. [CrossRef]
65. Uxa, S.; Castillo-Binder, P.; Kohler, R.; Stangner, K.; Müller, G.A.; Engeland, K. Ki-67 gene expression. *Cell Death Differ.* **2021**, *28*, 3357–3370. [CrossRef]
66. Wei, H.; Qu, L.; Dai, S.; Li, Y.; Wang, H.; Feng, Y.; Chen, X.; Jiang, L.; Guo, M.; Li, J.; et al. Structural insight into the molecular mechanism of p53-mediated mitochondrial apoptosis. *Nat. Commun. Commun.* **2021**, *12*, 2280. [CrossRef] [PubMed]
67. Wang, H.; Guo, M.; Wei, H.; Chen, Y. Targeting p53 pathways: Mechanisms, structures, and advances in therapy. *Signal Transduct. Target. Ther.* **2023**, *8*, 92. [CrossRef] [PubMed]
68. Speidel, D. Transcription-independent p53 apoptosis: An alternative route to death. *Trends Cell Biol. Biol.* **2010**, *20*, 14–24. [CrossRef] [PubMed]

current issues in molecular biology

MDPI

Article

Cacalol Acetate as Anticancer Agent: Antiproliferative, Pro-Apoptotic, Cytostatic, and Anti-Migratory Effects

Gareth Omar Rostro-Alonso [1,†], Alejandro Israel Castillo-Montoya [1,†], Juan Carlos García-Acosta [1], Erick Fernando Aguilar-Llanos [2], Laura Itzel Quintas-Granados [3], Edgar Yebrán Villegas-Vazquez [1], Rosario García-Aguilar [4], Samantha Andrea Porras-Vázquez [1], Lilia Patricia Bustamante-Montes [5], Jesús J. Alvarado-Sansininea [6], Manuel Jiménez-Estrada [6], Lizbeth Cariño-Calvo [7], Manuel González-del Carmen [8], Hernán Cortés [9], Gerardo Leyva-Gómez [10], Gabriela Figueroa-González [1] and Octavio Daniel Reyes-Hernández [1,*]

1 Laboratorio de Farmacogenética, Unidad Multidisciplinaria de Investigación Experimental Zaragoza, Facultad de Estudios Superiores Zaragoza, Universidad Nacional Autónoma de México, Batalla 5 de Mayo s/n Esquina Fuerte de Loreto, Iztapalapa, Mexico City 09230, Mexico; rostroalonsogarethomar@gmail.com (G.O.R.-A.); alex24castillomontoy@gmail.com (A.I.C.-M.); jcarlosga99@gmail.com (J.C.G.-A.); eyebran.villegas@gmail.com (E.Y.V.-V.); andy.porras13@gmail.com (S.A.P.-V.); gabriela.figueroa@zaragoza.unam.mx (G.F.-G.)

2 Laboratorio de Biología Molecular del Cáncer, Unidad Multidisciplinaria de Investigación Experimental Zaragoza, Facultad de Estudios Superiores-Zaragoza, Universidad Nacional Autónoma de México, Iztapalapa, Mexico City 09230, Mexico; fernandoaguilarllanos@gmail.com

3 Colegio de Ciencias y Humanidades, Plantel Cuautepec, Universidad Autónoma de la Ciudad de México, Calle Dr. García Diego 168, Doctores, Cuauhtémoc, Mexico City 06720, Mexico; itzel.quintas@uacm.edu.mx

4 Laboratorio de Citometría de Flujo y Hematología, Diagnóstico Molecular de Leucemias y Terapia Celular (DILETEC), Gustavo A. Madero, Mexico City 06350, Mexico; rgarcia@diletec.com.mx

5 Coordinacion de Investigacion, Centro Universitario Siglo XXI, Edo. de Mex, Mexico City 03100, Mexico; liliapatricia.bustamante@cus21.edu.mx

6 Laboratorio 2–10, Departamento de Productos Naturales, Instituto de Química, Universidad Nacional Autónoma de México, Mexico City 04510, Mexico; javier33@comunidad.unam.mx (J.J.A.-S.); manueljemex@gmail.com (M.J.-E.)

7 Facultad de Ciencias Químicas, Universidad Veracruzana, Orizaba 94340, Mexico; lcarino@uv.mx

8 Facultad de Medicina, Universidad Veracruzana, Ciudad Mendoza 94740, Mexico; manugonzalez@uv.mx

9 Laboratorio de Medicina Genómica, Departamento de Genómica, Instituto Nacional de Rehabilitación Luis Guillermo Ibarra Ibarra, Mexico City 14389, Mexico; hcortes@inr.gob.mx

10 Departamento de Farmacia, Facultad de Química, Universidad Nacional Autónoma de México, Mexico City 04510, Mexico; leyva@quimica.unam.mx

* Correspondence: octavio.reyes@zaragoza.unam.mx; Tel.: +52-1-55-1706-4638

† These authors contributed equally to this work.

Abstract: Cacalol (C), a sesquiterpene isolated from *Psacalium decompositum*, has demonstrated anti-inflammatory and antioxidant activities. Its cytotoxic, antiproliferative, and pro-apoptotic effects have been previously shown in an in vitro breast cancer model. A derivative, cacalol acetate (CA), shows potential in regulating these processes, which has not been previously reported. This study focused on an in vitro cervical cancer model, assessing CA's antiproliferative, pro-apoptotic, cytostatic, and anti-migratory activities using the HeLa cell line. The natural anticancer agent indole-3-carbinol (I3C) was used as a control for comparison. CA demonstrated significant antitumor activities, including inhibiting cell growth, inducing apoptosis, arresting cells in the G2 phase of the cell cycle, and inhibiting cell migration. These effects were notably greater compared to I3C. I3C, while following a similar trend, did not induce Cas-3 expression, suggesting a different apoptotic pathway. Neither CA nor I3C increased p62 and LC3B levels, indicating they do not stimulate autophagy marker expression. Both compounds inhibited HeLa cell migration and induced cell cycle arrest. Despite both holding promise as anticancer agents for cervical cancer, CA's lower cytotoxicity and stronger regulation of tumor phenotypes make it a more promising agent compared to I3C.

Keywords: cacalol; cacalol acetate; antiproliferation; apoptotic effect; cervical cancer cells

1. Introduction

According to the World Health Organization (WHO), cervical cancer (CC) is the fourth most frequently occurring cancer worldwide [1] and is one of the leading causes of cancer death among women [2]. CC is the leading cause of cancer-related deaths among women in Eastern, Western, Middle, and Southern Africa. China and India together account for over one-third of the global cervical cancer burden, with 106,000 cases and 48,000 deaths in China and 97,000 cases and 60,000 deaths in India. Globally, the average age at diagnosis for CC is 53 years, making it one of the top three cancers affecting women under 45 years old [1].

CC remains a significant health burden among young women globally, especially in low- and middle-income countries. Between 2014 and 2017, Paraguay and Venezuela reported the highest cervical cancer mortality rates, while Puerto Rico had the lowest. Overall, most Latin American and Caribbean countries, such as Chile, Colombia, Cuba, El Salvador, Mexico, Nicaragua, Panama, and Peru, showed a decline in cervical cancer mortality during this period. Conversely, Brazil and Paraguay exhibited significant increases [3].

Although CC is a preventable disease, many women present with invasive disease requiring radical surgery (early-stage disease) and/or combined radiation therapy and chemotherapy (locally advanced disease), radiosensitizing nanoparticles [4,5], and immunotherapies [6]; nevertheless, these strategies are not successful interventions. To achieve CC elimination goals, there is a need for new programmatic approaches to introduce emerging technologies and scale up the screening and treatment of cervical precancer. Implementation research, which is underutilized, plays a crucial role in facilitating the widespread adoption of evidence-based interventions [7]. Fortunately, a large amount of information dealing with the clinical aspects of cancer chemotherapy has been generated, including the finding and application of natural-origin drugs.

Against this background, there are two principal requirements of research on antitumor chemotherapy that achieves an efficient antitumoral agent and satisfies a broad population spectrum: to find a more efficient natural antitumoral agent without adverse effects and a more profitable source of this kind of agent. In this way, we previously reported that indole-3-carbinol (I3C), a non-carcinogenic agonist compound of the aryl hydrocarbon receptor (AhR), promotes the activation of AhR and decreases cell proliferation, possibly through UBE2L3 (also known as UBCH7, UbcH7, and E2 Ubiquitin-Conjugating Enzyme L3) mRNA induction, which would result in the ubiquitination of HPV (Human Papilloma Virus) E7 protein [8]. However, it is still unknown whether I3C affects other hallmarks of cancer.

On the other hand, another bioactive molecule is cacalol (C), a phytochemical compound with anti-inflammatory and antioxidant properties [9–11]. It has a strong antiproliferative effect against breast cancer cells, inducing apoptosis by activating a pro-apoptotic pathway. C inhibits tumor growth in vivo by blocking fatty acid synthase (FAS) gene expression through the modulation of the Akt-SREBP pathway [12]. Cacalol exhibits potential anti-FAS activity and induces apoptosis in breast cancer cells, with possible synergistic effects when combined with cyclophosphamide [13]. Furthermore, its derivative compound, cacalol acetate (CA) (see Scheme 1), has shown anti-inflammatory properties [9] and both C and CA demonstrate potential as photoproducers of singlet oxygen and free radical scavengers, making them promising candidates for new therapeutic applications in the treatment of tumors and other diseases [14]. However, their antitumoral activity is not well known yet.

Although there is no evidence of the antitumoral properties of cacalol acetate in CC, this compound has shown potential utility as a chemopreventive and chemotherapeutic agent against cancer biological models. Particularly, in this study, we investigated the antiproliferative, pro-apoptotic, and anti-migratory properties of CA and I3C in a cervical cancer cell line.

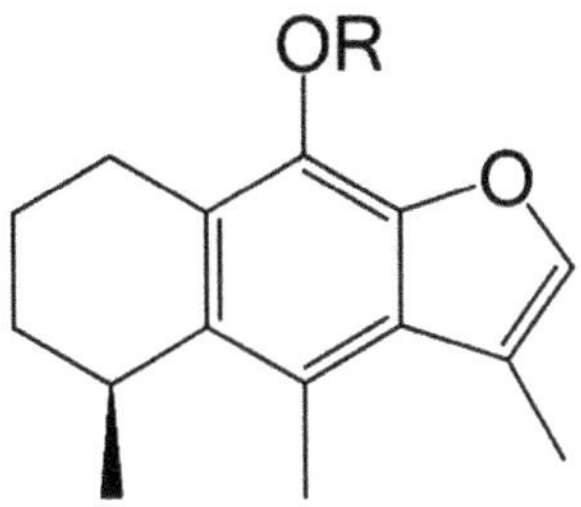

R=H Cacalol

R=$COCH_3$ Cacalol Acetate

Scheme 1. Structure of C and CA. Adapted from Gómez-Vidales and colleagues [14].

2. Materials and Methods

2.1. Cell Cultures

The cervical cancer cell line HeLa (positive to HPV-18) was obtained from the American Type Culture Collection (ATCC, Rockville, MD, USA). For all assays, HeLa cells were cultured in RPMI-1640 media (GIBCO, Carlsbad, CA, USA) and supplemented with 5% newborn calf serum (NCS, GIBCO, USA), L-glutamine, red phenol, and benzylpenicillin. Cultures were maintained in an incubator (Nauire, Plymouth, MN, USA) with a humidified atmosphere at 5% CO_2 and 37 °C. All cell-based assays were performed using culture cells in the exponential growth phase.

2.2. Tested Compounds

CA was solubilized in 100 µL dimethyl sulfoxide (DMSO; Sigma-Aldrich, St. Louis, MO, USA) and 900 µL of RPMI-1640 medium, resulting in a final concentration of 1 µg/µL. I3C (Sigma-Aldrich, St. Louis, MO, USA; purity ≥96%) was solubilized in DMSO and used at a final concentration of 150 µM.

2.3. Cell Proliferation Assays

HeLa cells (6 × 10^3 cell/well) were cultivated in a 96-well tissue culture plate (Corning, New York, NY, USA) with 100 µL of RPMI-1640 medium and growth for 24 h at 37 °C and 5% CO_2. Then, CA was added at several concentrations (from 20 µg/mL to 29 µg/mL) and incubated as mentioned above. I3C was added at a final concentration of 150 µM. As controls, we added 5 µg/mL of DMSO (vehicle) in a cell culture sample and included one cell culture without treatment (control). In addition, HeLa cells were treated with 1 µM of beta-naphthoflavone (BNF), an agonist synthetic ligand of AhR with anticancer activity against mammary carcinoma cells [15] and cervical cancer cells [16] as a control. After 24 h of incubation with CA, we determined the antiproliferative activity (IC_{50}) by crystal violet staining as previously reported [17,18]. Finally, the cell count was performed spectrophotometrically at 590 nm (Awareness Technology INC, Chromate 4300, Palm City, FL, USA). Data were analyzed in a dose–response curve to estimate the concentration at which 50% of the cell population decreases (IC_{50}).

2.4. Determination of Apoptosis by Evaluation of Active Caspase-3

HeLa cells (6 × 10^3 cell/well) were incubated for 24 h with 102.72 µM of CA and I3C (150 µM). As controls, cells were incubated with 5 µg/mL DMSO (vehicle), 1 mg/mL colchicine (positive apoptotic cell death control), and beta-naphthoflavone (BNF) (1 µM). For the immunodetection of active caspase-3, we followed a reported protocol [18]. Briefly, cells were permeabilized with Triton X-100 (1%) for 20 min, after which the cells were washed with phosphate-buffered saline (PBS) pH 7.3. Then, the cells were incubated with rabbit anti-human active caspase-3 polyclonal antibody (Sigma-Aldrich, St. Louis, MO, USA) diluted in PBS (1:1000) for 18 h at 4 °C. Following this, the cells were washed and incubated with goat anti-rabbit IgG secondary antibody coupled to fluorescein-5-isothiocyanate (FITC) diluted 1:1000 in PBS at room temperature for 2 h. Then, the samples were stained with 4′6-diamidino-2-phenylindole (DAPI) and analyzed under epifluorescence microscopy (Eclipse E600, Nikon, Melville, NY, USA) and phase-contrast microscopy (Eclipse TS2R-FL, Nikon, Japan). We used a DXMI200F digital camera (Nikon, Melville, NY, USA) for recorded images.

2.5. Determination of Autophagic (p62 and LC3B) Biomarkers by Western Blot Analysis

HeLa cells treated with CA (102.72 μM), I3C (150 μM), DMSO (5 μg/mL, vehicle), and BNF (1 μM) and untreated cells (control) were grown for 24 h and were subjected to lysis using RIPA buffer (Santa Cruz Biotechnology, Inc., Dallas, TX, USA, sc-24948) supplemented with 0.1% protease inhibitors (Complete Protease Inhibitor Cocktail, Roche, Kansas City, MO, USA, catalog number 11697498008). The lysates were then incubated at 4 °C for 30 min, followed by centrifugation at 13,000× *g* at 4 °C for 25 min. The soluble protein concentrations in the cell lysates were measured spectrophotometrically at 280 nm using the EPOCH Microplate Spectrophotometer (Bio Tek, Winooski, VT, USA). Equal amounts of protein from each sample were combined with 5X Laemmli sample buffer (10% SDS, 50% glycerol, 0.02% bromophenol blue, and 0.3125 M Tris HCl, pH 6.8), supplemented with β-mercaptoethanol, and boiled for 10 min. Subsequently, 50 μg of protein from each sample was separated on 12% SDS-PAGE gels using a vertical electrophoresis system (Mini Trans-Blot® Cell, Bio-Rad, Hercules, CA, USA, catalog number 1703810). The separated proteins were then transferred onto 0.45 μm polyvinylidene difluoride (PVDF) membranes (Thermo Scientific, Waltham, MA, USA, catalog number 88518) using a Trans-Blot Turbo chamber (Bio-Rad) at 25 V and 1 mA for 30 min. The membranes were subsequently blocked with 5% non-fat milk in TBS (pH 7.0) containing 1% Tween-20 for 2 h at room temperature, followed by incubation with primary antibodies against p62 Rabbit pAb (1:3000 dilution, ABclonal, Woburn, MA, USA), LC3B Rabbit pAb (1:3000 dilution, ABclonal), and β-actin mouse mAb (1:10,000 dilution, ABclonal, catalog number AC004) overnight at 4 °C on a rocking platform. After washing the membranes five times with TBS (pH 7.0) containing 0.1% Tween-20, the membranes were incubated for 1 h at 25 °C with peroxidase-conjugated secondary antibodies anti-rabbit IgG (1:10,000 dilution, Cell Signaling Biotechnology, Danvers, MA, USA, catalog number 7074s) or anti-mouse IgG (1:10,000 dilution, Cell Signaling Biotechnology, catalog number 7076s) for β-actin detection. Finally, the membranes were washed with TBS (pH 7.0) containing 0.1% Tween-20 and developed using chemiluminescence with Clarity MaxTM Western ECL (Bio-Rad, catalog number 1705062) following the manufacturer's instructions. Image analysis was performed using the C-DiGit Blot (LI-COR, Lincoln, NE, USA). All experiments were conducted in triplicate. β-actin was consistently detected as a loading control and used for normalizing the densitometry of the target proteins with ImageJ bundled with Java 8 software. Data normalization was carried out by dividing the densitometry data of the target protein by that of the loading control protein (β-actin).

2.6. Determination of Cell Migration

To assess cell migration, a wound healing assay was conducted under sterile conditions. In 96-well plates, adhesive tape (0.5 mm width) was carefully positioned, and a mark with a 2-mm division was applied at the center of each well to demarcate the area for subsequent photographic analysis. Following this, HeLa cells were seeded at a density of 3×10^4 cells per well in 100 μL of RPMI medium supplemented with 10% neonatal serum and incubated for 24 h at 37 °C with 5% CO_2. After the initial incubation period, 10 μM cytarabine (ara-C) was added and cells were further incubated for 2 h under the same conditions. The adhesive tape was then carefully removed to create a wound. The samples were gently washed with PBS (pH 7.0), and HeLa cells were treated with CA (102.72 μM), I3C (150 μM), DMSO

(5 μg/mL, vehicle), and BNF (1 μM). Negative controls (untreated cells) and cells treated with 105 mM TGF-β were included in each experimental set. Cell migration was observed at various time points (0, 24, 48, and 72 h) and documented using a Canon camera. Each experiment was conducted in triplicate, with three biological replicates and technical triplicates for each measurement. The thickness of the wound was analyzed using bioinformatics tools (ImageJ bundled with Java 8) by assessing images captured at different time points within the designated area and quantifying the migration rate of the cells.

2.7. Determination of Cell Cycle Arrest

Cells (3×10^5) were seeded in a 6-well plate and incubated for 24 h at 37 °C with 5% CO_2. Subsequently, the cells were divided into untreated and treated groups. Treatment involved the addition of 20 μL of colchicine (1 mg/mL, as a positive control), 102.72 μM of CA, 150 μM of I3C, 5 μg/mL DMSO (vehicle), and 1 μM of BNF. The cells were then incubated for an additional 24 h at 37 °C with 5% CO_2. Following the incubation period, the cells were trypsinized and collected by centrifugation at 212× *g* for 3 min at room temperature. The collected cells were fixed in ice-cold methanol (500 μL) with PBS (pH 7.0) (500 μL) at 4 °C for 1 h. After fixation, the cells were washed three times with PBS (pH 7.0) (1 mL each wash) and centrifuged as described above. Next, the cells were treated with 30 μL of RNase A (100 U/mL) and incubated for 30 min at 37 °C. After another round of centrifugation, the cells were resuspended in 500 μL of PBS containing 5 μL of propidium iodide (20 μg/mL) and analyzed using the Beckman-Coulter CytoFlex cytometer (Beckman Coulter, Brea, CA, USA). The concentration of colchicine chosen for treatment was based on reported values known to arrest the cell cycle at the G2 phase. Each measurement was conducted with three biological replicates and technical duplicates.

2.8. Statistical Analysis

All data were reported in terms of means and standard errors (SEs). Statistical analyses were performed by variance differences (ANOVA), followed by Holm–Sidak test and Student's *t*-test, using GraphPad Prism 9.0.2.

3. Results

3.1. Cytotoxicity Activity of Phytochemical Compounds on HeLa Cells

First, we determined cellular cytotoxicity by measuring lactate dehydrogenase (LDH), an enzyme that catalyzes the conversion of lactate to pyruvate and is released from cells after membrane dissolution by a toxic stimulus. We did not find cytotoxic activity on HeLa cells from CA or I3C at concentrations of 102.72 μM or 150 μM, respectively, compared to the untreated control or vehicle (Figure 1).

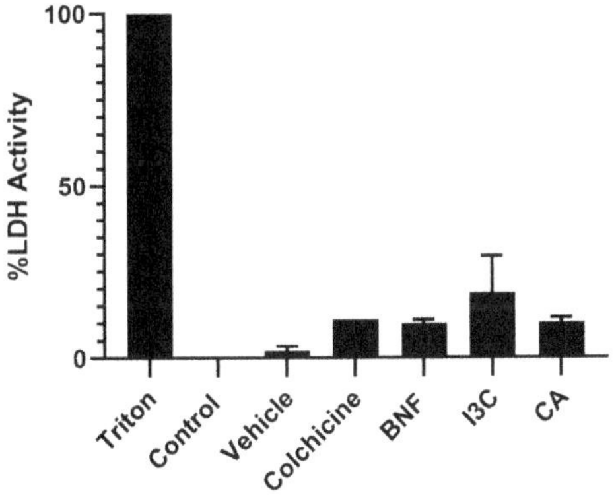

Figure 1. Cytotoxicity effect of CA and I3C on HeLa cells. HeLa cells treated with CA (102.72 μM), I3C (150 μM), DMSO (5 μg/mL, vehicle), BNF (1 μM), and Triton X-100 (positive control) and untreated

cells (control) were analyzed by LDH assay. Bars indicate the percentage of LDH activity in the presence of tested compounds. Experimental data show the means ± standard errors (SEs) of three independent assays performed in triplicate. Statistically significant differences were calculated according to ANOVA test followed by Tukey's test ($p < 0.05$ vs. control).

3.2. *Antiproliferative Activity of CA and I3C in HeLa Cells*

The antiproliferative effect of CA and I3C on HeLa cells was determined. Antiproliferative activity was measured by a decrease in cell growth 24 h after compound administration. Both compounds had the ability to impair HeLa cell proliferation (Figure 2). A concentration of 150 μM of I3C resulted in 66% ± 8.6% of cell growth. In contrast, CA (102.72 μM) resulted in 43% ± 8.5% of cell growth. Taken together, these results suggest that CA has greater antiproliferative activity for HeLa cells than I3C.

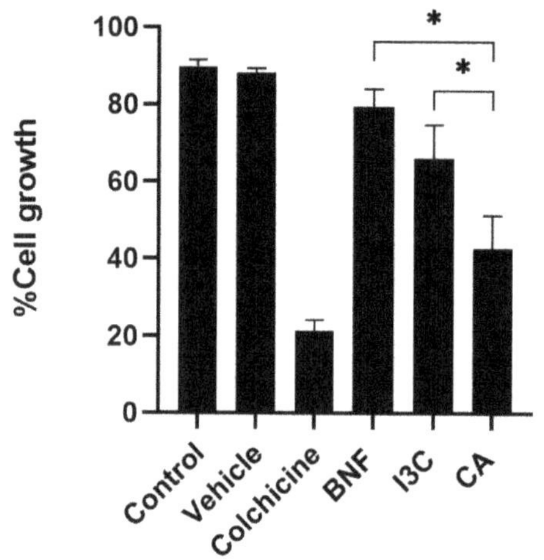

Figure 2. Effect of CA and I3C on cell growth. HeLa cells treated with CA (102.72 μM), I3C (150 μM), DMSO (5 μg/mL, vehicle), BNF (1 μM), or colchicine (25.03 μM) and untreated cells (control) were analyzed by crystal violet staining. Bars indicate the cell growth percentage in the presence of tested compounds. Experimental data show the means ± standard error (SE) of three independent antiproliferative assays performed in triplicate. All groups showed a statistically significant difference when compared with the control and vehicle groups ($p < 0.001$, Holm–Sidak test), as well as when compared with colchicine ($p < 0.002$, Holm–Sidak test). We also observed a statistically significant difference when comparing CA with BNF or I3C (* $p < 0.001$, Holm–Sidak test).

3.3. *Caspase-3-Induced-Apoptosis in HeLa Cells by CA and I3C*

The apoptotic pathway and its initiation may rely on the liberation of cytochrome c and caspase-9 activation, resulting in caspase-3 cleavage [19]. To determine the correlation between Cas-3-induced-apoptosis by CA or I3C, we treated HeLa cells with those compounds (Figure 3). We observed that CA induces the expression of Cas-3, suggesting that CA induces apoptosis via Cas-3. Moreover, after I3C and BNF treatments, the expression of Cas-3 was not increased, suggesting that Cas-3-induced-apoptosis was not triggered by I3C or BNF. The positive control (colchicine) induces Cas-3 expression, thereby activating the Cas-3-induced-apoptosis.

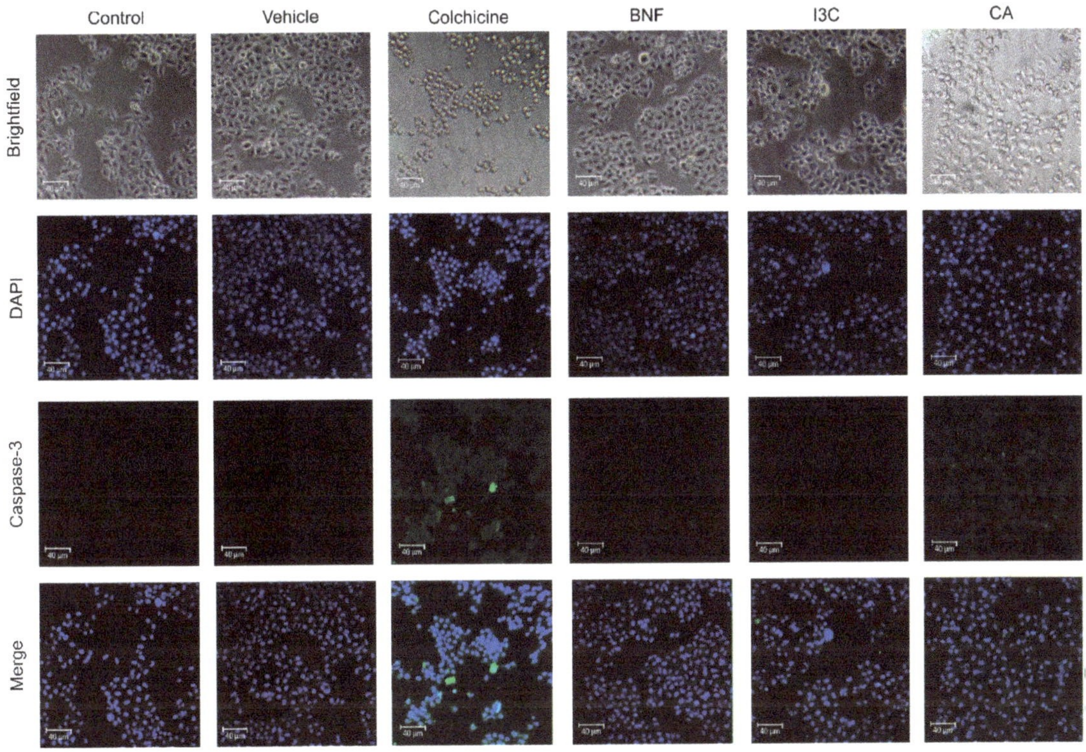

Figure 3. Confocal microscopy of pro-apoptotic Cas-3 protein in HeLa cells. HeLa cells treated with CA (102.72 μM), I3C (150 μM), DMSO (5 μg/mL, vehicle), BNF (1 μM), and colchicine (25.03 μM) or untreated cells (control) were used for immunodetection of caspase-3 (green fluorescence) with DAPI-counterstained nuclei (blue fluorescence).

3.4. Determination of Autophagy Induced by CA and I3C Treatments in HeLa Cells

Autophagy biomarkers such as LC3B and p62 were detected by immunoblotting (Figure 4a) and the expression levels of LC3B and p62 were normalized using the expression of β-actin as a loading control (Figure 4b). In all treatments, the expression levels of LC3B or p62 were not statistically significantly different. Neither CA, I3C, nor BFN induced changes in the expression of LC3B or p62, suggesting that these compounds did not induce autophagy.

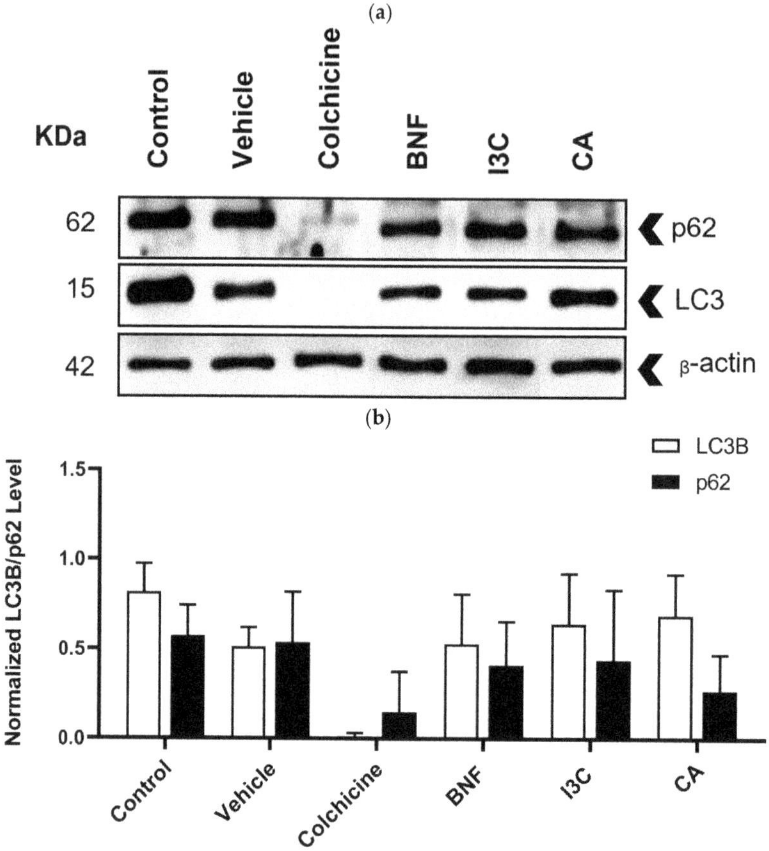

Figure 4. Western blot analysis to determine LC3B and p62 proteins in HeLa cells. (**a**) HeLa cells treated with CA (102.72 μM), I3C (150 μM), DMSO (5 μg/mL, vehicle), BNF (1 μM), colchicine (25.03 μM) and untreated cells (control) were used to detect p62 (62 kDa), LC3B (15 kDa), and β-actin (42 kDa). (**b**) Protein expression levels of p62 and LC3B were normalized using β-actin expression (loading control). Bars indicate the mean levels of protein expression ± standard error (SE) of three independent antiproliferative assays performed in triplicate.

3.5. *Effect of CA and I3C on Cell Cycle Arrest of HeLa Cells*

To explore the impact of CA and I3C on cell cycle progression, we examined the distribution of HeLa cells treated with both compounds (Figure 5a). Approximately 28% of HeLa cells treated with CA remained in the G2 phase. In contrast, 18% of cells treated with I3C remained in this phase. Therefore, CA has a stronger effect on arresting the cell cycle of HeLa cells in phase 2 than I3C. Additionally, HeLa cells treated with I3C predominantly remained in the S phase (48%), while 58% of cells treated with BNF remained in the G1 phase. Approximately 95% of cells treated with colchicine (positive control) remained in the G2 phase (Figure 5b).

(**a**)

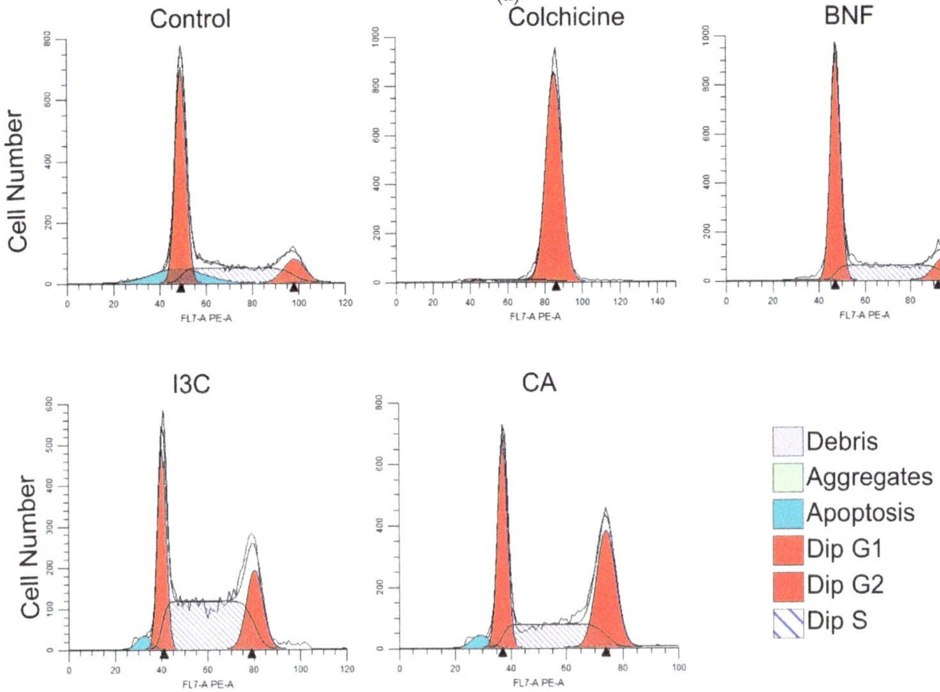

(**b**)

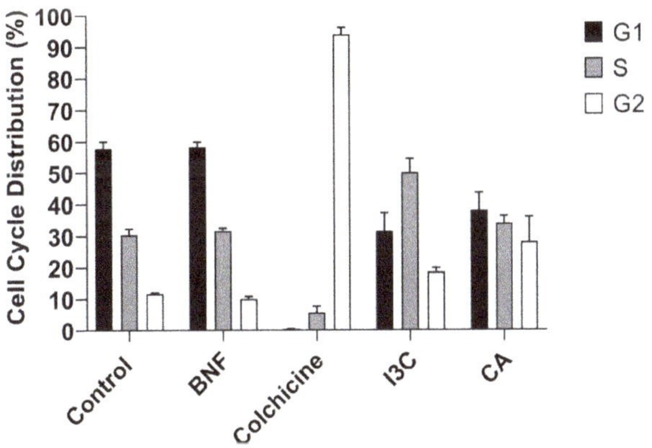

Figure 5. Effect of CA and I3C on cell cycle arrest of HeLa cells. (**a**) Flow cytometry graphs depicting the cell cycle distribution of HeLa cells treated with CA (102.72 µM), I3C (150 µM), BNF (1 µM), and colchicine (25.03 µM). (**b**) The percentages of cells in the G1, S, and G2 phases of the cell cycle for treated HeLa cells.

3.6. Effect of CA and I3C on Cell Migration of HeLa Cells

Wound assays were conducted to assess whether CA or I3C could influence cell migration in HeLa cells (Figure 6a,b). At 72 h, the cell migration of HeLa cells was significantly enhanced following TGF-β treatment (positive control) compared to untreated cells [negative control, C(-)] and vehicle. Conversely, the presence of CA significantly reduced cell migration by 58% in HeLa cells at 72 h ($p > 0.05$) compared to the positive control. On the other hand, in HeLa cells, relative migration decreased by 40% after 72 h of treatment with 150 μM I3C compared to the positive control. Additionally, BNF reduced HeLa cell migration by 75%, while the negative control and vehicle reduced cell migration by approximately 30% compared to the positive control. These results suggested that CA (102.72 μM) reduced HeLa cell migration 1.45-fold more than I3C did. Therefore, CA has a greater effect on reducing the cell migration of HeLa cells compared to I3C.

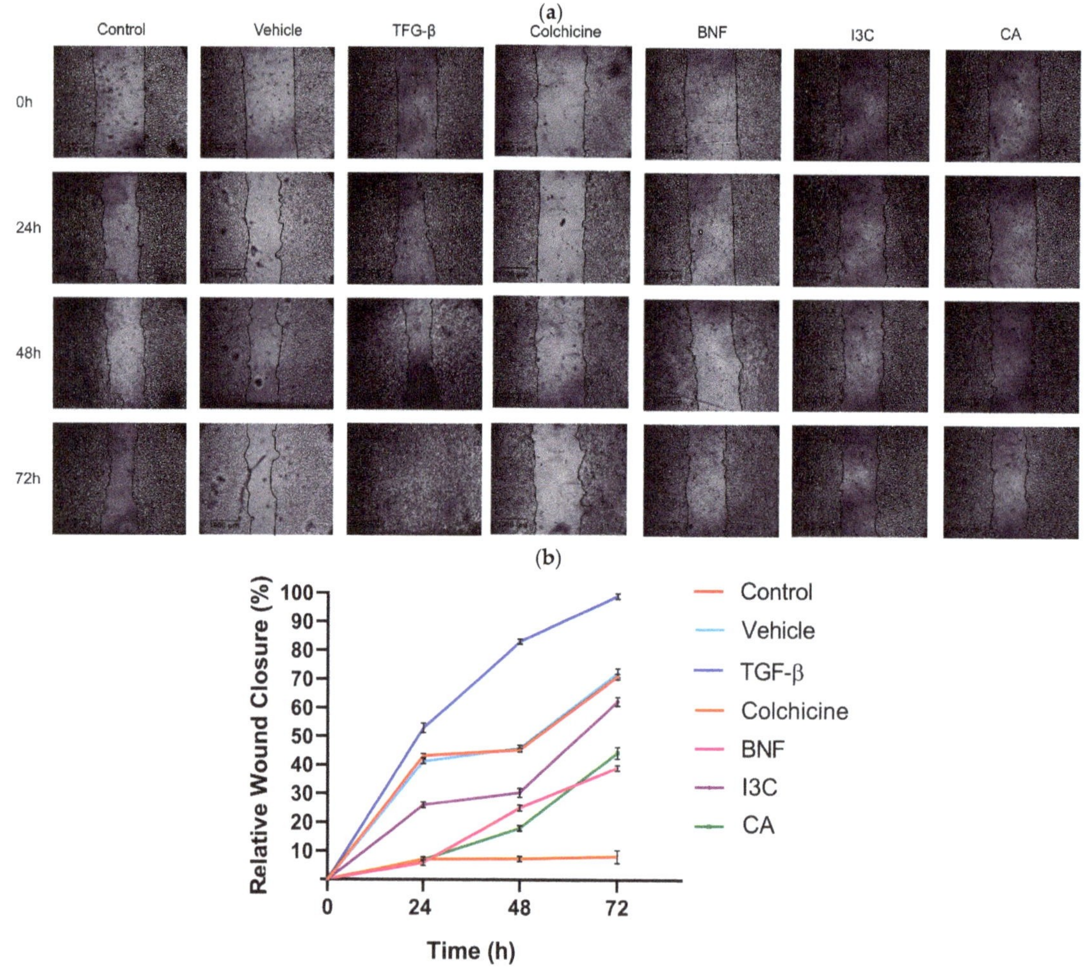

Figure 6. Effect of CA and I3C on cell migration of HeLa cells. (**a**) HeLa cells were subjected to treatment with CA (102.72 μM), I3C (150 μM), DMSO (5 μg/mL, vehicle), BNF (1 μM), TGF-β (105 mM), and colchicine (25.03 μM) and compared to untreated cells (control). Microscopic images were captured at various time intervals, including 0 h, 24 h, 48 h, and 72 h, to visualize the wound closure. The migrating cell edges were delineated by lines. (**b**) Relative wound closure percentage was calculated for all experimental conditions. The lines represent the mean of three independent measurements, with the standard deviation indicated on each bar. Statistical analysis was conducted to compare the experimental conditions with the negative control ($p < 0.05$).

4. Discussion

Sesquiterpenes present in several plant species induce apoptosis in cancer cells through different mechanisms [20]. It has been reported that C has shown anticancer properties inducing apoptosis in several cancer cells, particularly in breast cancer cells.

Our data showed that CA had no cytotoxic effects on HeLa cells and that this compound exhibited antiproliferative activity in a dose-dependent manner. The IC_{50} value of cacalol acetate for HeLa cells was 102.72 μM, whereas for I3C, it was 150 μM, suggesting the strong potential of CA as an anticancer agent through cell growth inhibition. In breast cancer cells (MCF7 and MDA-MD231) and in a xenograft mouse model, cacalol inhibits cell growth without toxic effects and significantly suppresses tumor growth when administered intraperitoneally or orally, suggesting its potential as a preventive and therapeutic agent against cancer [12]. Cacalol and its derivative, CA, have antioxidant activity due to their ability to act as potent free radical scavengers, contributing to their anticancer properties by reducing oxidative stress in cancer cells [14]. Moreover, this phytochemical compound inhibits the lipid peroxidation induced by free radicals [10].

HeLa cells treated with CA showed increased levels in the expression of caspase-3. In contrast, when cells were treated with I3C, the expression of this apoptotic biomarker was not observed, suggesting that CA induces apoptotic cell death via Cas-3, whereas I3C does not. These results are consistent with our previous report, in which we measured apoptosis in I3C-treated HeLa cells by cytometry and did not observe increased levels of apoptosis [8]. Our evidence suggested that the induction of apoptosis by CA is independent of Ahr. However, the molecular mechanism of CA is still unknown. Previous reports suggest that cacalol has an anti-breast cancer effect by inhibiting fatty acid synthase (FAS) at transcriptional and post-transcriptional levels and modulating the Akt-SREBP (sterol regulatory element-binding protein) pathways. In this way, cacalol blocks P13K/Akt signaling resulting in an inhibition of SREBP1, which is the main transcriptional regulator of FAS [12]. Therefore, cacalol induces apoptosis in breast cancer cells by modulating the Akt-SREBP-FAS signaling pathway, leading to the activation of pro-apoptotic proteins DAPK2 and caspase 3 [12]. Furthermore, cacalol inhibits the FAS gene, essential in fatty acid biosynthesis and energy homeostasis, causing apoptosis through its antioxidant activity [13]. Intrinsic apoptosis is a cell death centered in the mitochondrion [21]. The activation of Bax and Bak (BCL-2 family members) results in mitochondrial outer membrane permeabilization (MOMP) and the releasing of pro-apoptotic proteins and cytochrome *c* from the inter-membrane mitochondrial space into the cytosol, where cytochrome *c* binds to Apaf-1, forming an apoptosome and activating caspase-9, which cleaves and activates caspase-3 and -7 [22–26]. Therefore, CA induces apoptotic cell death through promoting more cervical cancer cells expressing caspase-3. The biomarker of late stage of apoptosis (caspase-3) was not significantly upregulated in HeLa cells treated with CA treatment. Previous reports indicated that the treatment of tumor cells with cacalol promote the expression of DAPK2 and caspase-3 [12]. Our results agree, showing that CA induces the expression of caspase-3, suggesting that the acetylation of cacalol might enhance the apoptotic induction mechanism of this compound. Although some evidence suggests that cacalol induces apoptosis through the mechanisms described above, the acetylated molecule (CA) might trigger apoptosis through a different pathway, which we have elucidated.

Furthermore, cacalol has synergistic activity that enhances the apoptotic effect of chemotherapeutic drugs such as taxol and cyclophosphamide, helping to overcome chemoresistance [12]. It is still unclear if CA might have synergistic activity.

In addition, neither CA nor I3C induce autophagic cell death. CA arrests the cell cycle at G2 phase, while I3C also arrests the cell cycle at this phase, albeit to a lesser extent. CA could inhibit cell migration and has a relatively low cytotoxicity, as it does not affect HeLa cell morphology as does BNF (1uM). It is worth mentioning that CA does not cause a morphological cytotoxic effect associated with its ability to inhibit cell migration (Figure 7).

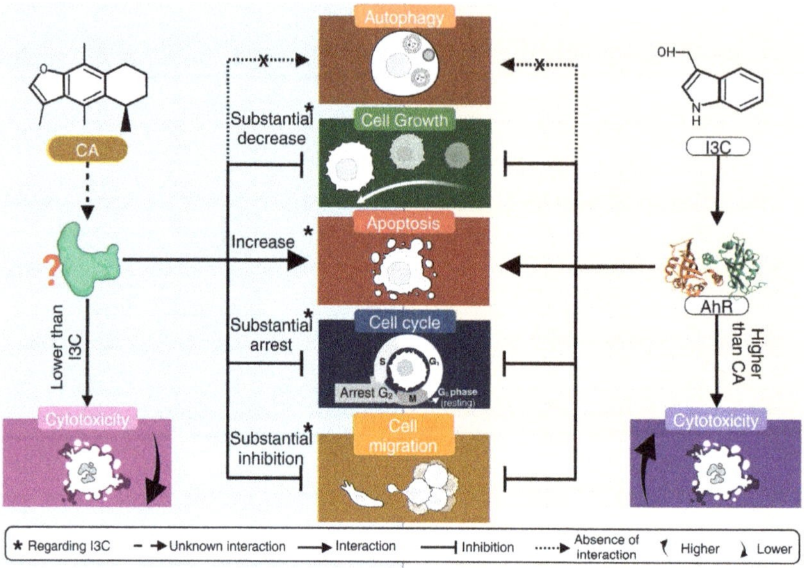

Figure 7. Summary of the anticancer activity of CA and I3C on HeLa cells. CA induces a substantial decrease in cell growth in comparison to I3C and substantially inhibits cell migration in comparison to I3C. CA induces apoptosis and arrests the cell cycle at a higher rate than I3C. CA and I3C do not induce autophagy.

5. Conclusions

CA had a lower cytotoxic effect on HeLa cells than I3C. CA and I3C inhibited cell growth, but CA is more effective in inhibiting cell proliferation than I3C. I3C did not affect the expression of Cas-3, suggesting that this compound did not induce apoptosis via Cas-3. In contrast, CA upregulated the expression of Cas-3, suggesting that CA induces apoptosis via Cas-3. CA and I3C did not induce the expression of p62 and LC3B levels, suggesting that these phytochemical compounds not induce autophagic cell death. CA arrests the cell cycle and inhibits the cell migration of HeLa cells at a higher rate than I3C. Although CA and I3C are promising anticancer agents for the treatment of cervical cancer, the low cytotoxicity of CA compared to I3C and the fact that CA induces apoptosis via Cas-3 and cell cycle arrest and inhibits cell proliferation and migration at a higher rate than I3C make CA a more promising agent than I3C.

Author Contributions: Conceptualization, G.F.-G. and O.D.R.-H.; methodology, G.O.R.-A., A.I.C.-M., J.C.G.-A., E.F.A.-L., R.G.-A., and E.Y.V.-V.; validation, R.G.-A., E.Y.V.-V., H.C., M.G.-d.C., and G.L.-G.; formal analysis, L.I.Q.-G. and O.D.R.-H.; investigation, S.A.P.-V., L.P.B.-M., J.J.A.-S., M.J.-E., and O.D.R.-H.; resources, M.J.-E., G.F.-G., and O.D.R.-H.; data curation, L.I.Q.-G. and O.D.R.-H.; writing—original draft preparation, L.I.Q.-G. and O.D.R.-H.; writing—review and editing, L.C.-C., M.G.-d.C., L.I.Q.-G., G.F.-G., and O.D.R.-H.; visualization, G.L.-G., H.C. and O.D.R.-H.; supervision G.F.-G. and O.D.R.-H.; project administration, G.F.-G. and O.D.R.-H.; funding acquisition, O.D.R.-H. All authors have read and agreed to the published version of the manuscript.

Funding: This research was funded by PAPIIT (projects IA208422 and IA206724 awarded to G.F.-G. and projects IN222321 and IN221824 awarded to O.D.R.-H.). E.Y.V.-V. is a recipient of a postdoctoral fellowship from Dirección General de Asuntos del Personal Académico (DGAPA) from Universidad Nacional Autónoma de Mexico (UNAM).

Institutional Review Board Statement: Not applicable.

Informed Consent Statement: Not applicable.

Data Availability Statement: The original contributions presented in this study are included in the article; further inquiries can be directed to the corresponding author.

Acknowledgments: The authors would like to thank Nieves Herrera-Mundo for technical support. We especially dedicate this work to Leonardo Gabriel Reyes Figueroa for pushing us forward... shine on you crazy diamond!

Conflicts of Interest: The authors declare no conflicts of interest.

References

1. Arbyn, M.; Weiderpass, E.; Bruni, L.; de Sanjosé, S.; Saraiya, M.; Ferlay, J.; Bray, F. Estimates of incidence and mortality of cervical cancer in 2018: A worldwide analysis. *Lancet Glob. Health* **2020**, *8*, e191–e203. [CrossRef]
2. Small, W., Jr.; Bacon, M.A.; Bajaj, A.; Chuang, L.T.; Fisher, B.J.; Harkenrider, M.M.; Jhingran, A.; Kitchener, H.C.; Mileshkin, L.R.; Viswanathan, A.N. Cervical cancer: A global health crisis. *Cancer* **2017**, *123*, 2404–2412. [CrossRef] [PubMed]
3. Torres-Roman, J.S.; Ronceros-Cardenas, L.; Valcarcel, B.; Bazalar-Palacios, J.; Ybaseta-Medina, J.; Carioli, G.; La Vecchia, C.; Alvarez, C.S. Cervical cancer mortality among young women in Latin America and the Caribbean: Trend analysis from 1997 to 2030. *BMC Public Health* **2022**, *22*, 113. [CrossRef] [PubMed]
4. Lopez, M.S.; Baker, E.S.; Maza, M.; Fontes-Cintra, G.; Lopez, A.; Carvajal, J.M.; Nozar, F.; Fiol, V.; Schmeler, K.M. Cervical cancer prevention and treatment in Latin America. *J. Surg. Oncol.* **2017**, *115*, 615–618. [CrossRef]
5. Mayadev, J.S.; Ke, G.; Mahantshetty, U.; Pereira, M.D.; Tarnawski, R.; Toita, T. Global challenges of radiotherapy for the treatment of locally advanced cervical cancer. *Int. J. Gynecol. Cancer* **2022**, *32*, 436–445. [CrossRef]
6. Monk, B.J.; Enomoto, T.; Kast, W.M.; McCormack, M.; Tan, D.S.; Wu, X.; González-Martín, A. Integration of immunotherapy into treatment of cervical cancer: Recent data and ongoing trials. *Cancer Treat. Rev.* **2022**, *106*, 102385. [CrossRef]
7. Broutet, N.; Jeronimo, J.; Kumar, S.; Almonte, M.; Murillo, R.; Huy, N.V.Q.; Denny, L.; Kapambwe, S.; Bhatla, N.; Sebitloane, M. Implementation research to accelerate scale-up of national screen and treat strategies towards the elimination of cervical cancer. *Prev. Med.* **2022**, *155*, 106906. [CrossRef]
8. Arellano-Gutiérrez, C.V.; Quintas-Granados, L.I.; Cortés, H.; González del Carmen, M.; Leyva-Gómez, G.; Bustamante-Montes, L.P.; Rodríguez-Morales, M.; López-Reyes, I.; Padilla-Mendoza, J.R.; Rodríguez-Páez, L. Indole-3-Carbinol, a phytochemical aryl hydrocarbon receptor-ligand, induces the mRNA overexpression of UBE2L3 and cell proliferation arrest. *Curr. Issues Mol. Biol.* **2022**, *44*, 2054–2068. [CrossRef]
9. Jimenez-Estrada, M.; Chilpa, R.R.; Apan, T.R.; Lledias, F.; Hansberg, W.; Arrieta, D.; Aguilar, F.A. Anti-inflammatory activity of cacalol and cacalone sesquiterpenes isolated from *Psacalium decompositum*. *J. Ethnopharmacol.* **2006**, *105*, 34–38. [CrossRef] [PubMed]
10. Shindo, K.; Kimura, M.; Iga, M. Potent antioxidative activity of cacalol, a sesquiterpene contained in *Cacalia delphiniifolia* Sleb et Zucc. *Biosci. Biotechnol. Biochem.* **2004**, *68*, 1393–1394. [CrossRef]
11. Mora-Ramiro, B.; Jiménez-Estrada, M.; Zentella-Dehesa, A.; Ventura-Gallegos, J.; Gomez-Quiroz, L.; Rosiles-Alanis, W.; Alarcón-Aguilar, F.; Almanza-Pérez, J. Cacalol acetate, a sesquiterpene from *Psacalium decompositum*, exerts an anti-inflammatory effect through LPS/NF-KB signaling in Raw 264.7 macrophages. *J. Nat. Prod.* **2020**, *83*, 2447–2455. [CrossRef] [PubMed]
12. Liu, W.; Furuta, E.; Shindo, K.; Watabe, M.; Xing, F.; Pandey, P.R.; Okuda, H.; Pai, S.K.; Murphy, L.L.; Cao, D. Cacalol, a natural sesquiterpene, induces apoptosis in breast cancer cells by modulating Akt-SREBP-FAS signaling pathway. *Breast Cancer Res. Treat.* **2011**, *128*, 57–68. [CrossRef] [PubMed]
13. Liu, W.; Furuta, E.; Watabe, M.; Shindo, K.; Iiizumi, M.; Pai, S.; Watabe, K. Inhibition of Fatty acid synthase and induction of apoptosis in human breast cancer cells by *Cacalia deliphiniifolia*. *Cancer Res.* **2008**, *68*, 629.
14. Gómez-Vidales, V.; Granados-Oliveros, G.; Nieto-Camacho, A.; Reyes-Solís, M.; Jiménez-Estrada, M. Cacalol and cacalol acetate as photoproducers of singlet oxygen and as free radical scavengers, evaluated by EPR spectroscopy and TBARS. *RSC Adv.* **2014**, *4*, 1371–1377. [CrossRef]
15. Wang, C.; Xu, C.-X.; Bu, Y.; Bottum, K.M.; Tischkau, S.A. Beta-naphthoflavone (DB06732) mediates estrogen receptor-positive breast cancer cell cycle arrest through AhR-dependent regulation of PI3K/AKT and MAPK/ERK signaling. *Carcinogenesis* **2014**, *35*, 703–713. [CrossRef]
16. Zidi, I.; Balaguer, P. Potential anti-cervical carcinoma drugs with agonist and antagonist AhR/PXR activities. *Med. Res. Arch.* **2016**, *4*, 1–16.
17. Kueng, W.; Silber, E.; Eppenberger, U. Quantification of cells cultured on 96-well plates. *Anal. Biochem.* **1989**, *182*, 16–19. [CrossRef]
18. Hernández-Vázquez, J.M.V.; López-Muñoz, H.; Escobar-Sánchez, M.L.; Flores-Guzmán, F.; Weiss-Steider, B.; Hilario-Martínez, J.C.; Sandoval-Ramírez, J.; Fernández-Herrera, M.A.; Sánchez, L.S. Apoptotic, necrotic, and antiproliferative activity of diosgenin and diosgenin glycosides on cervical cancer cells. *Eur. J. Pharmacol.* **2020**, *871*, 172942. [CrossRef]
19. Eldeeb, M.A.; Fahlman, R.P.; Esmaili, M.; Ragheb, M.A. Regulating apoptosis by degradation: The N-end rule-mediated regulation of apoptotic proteolytic fragments in mammalian cells. *Int. J. Mol. Sci.* **2018**, *19*, 3414. [CrossRef]
20. Ebrahimi, S.M.; Jafari, S.M. A Review of Potential Anti-Cancer Effect of Sesquiterpene Lactones in Breast Cancer. *Jorjani Biomed. J.* **2022**, *10*, 47–59.

21. Brentnall, M.; Rodriguez-Menocal, L.; De Guevara, R.L.; Cepero, E.; Boise, L.H. Caspase-9, caspase-3 and caspase-7 have distinct roles during intrinsic apoptosis. *BMC Cell Biol.* **2013**, *14*, 32. [CrossRef]
22. Wei, M.C.; Lindsten, T.; Mootha, V.K.; Weiler, S.; Gross, A.; Ashiya, M.; Thompson, C.B.; Korsmeyer, S.J. tBID, a membrane-targeted death ligand, oligomerizes BAK to release cytochrome c. *Genes Dev.* **2000**, *14*, 2060–2071. [CrossRef]
23. Eskes, R.; Desagher, S.; Antonsson, B.; Martinou, J.-C. Bid induces the oligomerization and insertion of Bax into the outer mitochondrial membrane. *Mol. Cell. Biol.* **2000**, *20*, 929–935. [CrossRef]
24. Wei, M.C.; Zong, W.-X.; Cheng, E.H.-Y.; Lindsten, T.; Panoutsakopoulou, V.; Ross, A.J.; Roth, K.A.; MacGregor, G.R.; Thompson, C.B.; Korsmeyer, S.J. Proapoptotic BAX and BAK: A requisite gateway to mitochondrial dysfunction and death. *Science* **2001**, *292*, 727–730. [CrossRef] [PubMed]
25. Li, P.; Nijhawan, D.; Budihardjo, I.; Srinivasula, S.M.; Ahmad, M.; Alnemri, E.S.; Wang, X. Cytochrome c and dATP-dependent formation of Apaf-1/caspase-9 complex initiates an apoptotic protease cascade. *Cell* **1997**, *91*, 479–489. [CrossRef] [PubMed]
26. Srinivasula, S.M.; Ahmad, M.; Fernandes-Alnemri, T.; Alnemri, E.S. Autoactivation of procaspase-9 by Apaf-1-mediated oligomerization. *Mol. Cell* **1998**, *1*, 949–957. [CrossRef] [PubMed]

current issues in molecular biology

Article

Inflammation Factors and Genistein Supplementation in Cancer—Preliminary Research

Karolina Banyś [1], Małgorzata Jelińska [1], Małgorzata Wrzosek [2], Dorota Skrajnowska [1], Robert Wrzesień [3], Wojciech Bielecki [4] and Barbara Bobrowska-Korczak [1,]*

1 Department of Toxicology and Food Science, Faculty of Pharmacy, Medical University of Warsaw, Poland, Banacha 1, 02-097 Warsaw, Poland
2 Department of Biochemistry and Pharmacogenomics, Faculty of Pharmacy, Medical University of Warsaw, Poland, Banacha 1, 02-097 Warsaw, Poland
3 Central Laboratory of Experimental Animals, Medical University of Warsaw, Poland, Banacha 1, 02-097 Warsaw, Poland
4 Department of Pathology and Veterinary Diagnostics, Institute of Veterinary Medicine, Warsaw University of Live Sciences, Nowoursynowska 159c Street, 02-787 Warsaw, Poland
* Correspondence: barbara.bobrowska@wum.edu.pl

Abstract: The purpose of this study was to evaluate the effect of genistein in nano, micro, and macro forms on the intensity of the DMBA-induced tumor process in rats and to understand the mechanisms of this action. The effect of genistein supplementation on the content of selected eicosanoids (HETEs, HODE, and HEPE) in the serum of rats was evaluated. The levels and expression of genes encoding various pro-inflammatory cytokines (IL-1, IL-6) and MMP-9 in the blood of rats were also investigated. The biological material for the study was blood obtained from female rats of the Sprague Dawley strain (n = 32). The animals were randomly divided into four groups: animals without supplementation, and animals supplemented at a dose of 0.2 mg/kg b.w. (0.1 mg/mL) with macro, micro (587 $\pm$ 83 nm), or nano (92 $\pm$ 41 nm) genistein. To induce mammary neoplasia (adenocarcinoma), rats were given 7,12-dimethyl-1,2-benz[a]anthracene (DMBA). The content of selected eicosanoids was determined by liquid chromatography with UV detection. An immunoenzymatic method was used to determine the content of cytokines and MMP-9. The expression of the *IL-6, IL-1beta,* and *MMP-9* genes was determined with quantitative real-time PCR (qRT-PCR) using TaqMan probes. Based on the study, it was shown that supplementation of animals with genistein in macro, micro, and nano forms increased the intensity of the tumor process in rats. It was shown that the content of 12-HEPE, HODE, and 12-HETE in the serum of genistein-supplemented rats was statistically significantly lower with respect to the content of the aforementioned markers in the serum of rats receiving only a standard diet, devoid of supplementation. It was found that animals supplemented with nano-, micro-, and macrogenistein had higher levels of metalloproteinase-9, MMP-9, compared to animals without supplementation. There was a significant increase in MMP-9 gene expression in the blood of macrogenistein-supplemented animals, relative to the other groups of rats. On the basis of the study, it was shown that supplementation of animals with nano-, micro-, and macrogenistein had an effect on the development of the tumor process. Dietary supplementation with genistein significantly decreased the level of selected eicosanoids, which may have significant impacts on cancer development and progression.

Keywords: genistein; cancer; nanoparticles

1. Introduction

In the search for compounds with anticancer effects, research into the use of genistein is receiving considerable attention. Genistein is included in the group of isoflavones. The main dietary source of genistein is soybeans and soy products. It is also found in alfalfa and lima sprouts, broccoli, cauliflower, and barley, among others [1,2]. It is worth noting that a number of preparations containing soy extracts and/or genistein itself are available in pharmacies. Numerous studies have shown that genistein can exhibit anticancer effects by, among other things, inducing apoptosis, affecting the cell cycle, inhibiting angiogenesis, and antiproliferative activity [3]. On the other hand, there are data supporting the pro-cancerous effects of genistein, especially in hormone-dependent cancer types [4–8]. One of the best-known properties of genistein is its estrogenic activity. Phytoestrogens have a chemical structure similar to 17β-estradiol and show the ability to bind to the estrogen receptor. Therefore, they can stimulate the process of carcinogenesis and increase the risk of breast cancer. Estrogens can exert carcinogenic effects through estrogen-receptor-dependent mechanisms, but also through the action of genotoxic products of estrogen metabolism [9]. The effect of genistein in the context of cancer therapy probably depends on the use of a specific dose, the physiological state of the test organism, and diet. We still do not know to whom, and in what doses, genistein should be administered to achieve the desired health effect, the mechanism of its action at the stage of initiation and progression of the cancer process is still unknown. It is also important to answer the question of whether it is safe for women to use supplements containing genistein in the context of cancer risk. Another important aspect is the answer to the question of how genistein in micro and nano forms might work. The studies on nanosized forms of phenolic compounds have become particularly important these days. The nano form changes their bioavailability. Bioavailability is defined in three basic steps: absorption, penetration into systemic circulation, and use in the cells. Reduction of materials at the nanoscale can lead to the development of new physical, chemical, and biological activities compared to the macro compounds [10]. It should be noted that there is still a lack of research in the literature in the field presented [10].

Therefore, the purpose of this study was to evaluate the effect of genistein in nano, micro, and macro forms on the intensity of DMBA-induced tumorigenesis. The effect of genistein supplementation on the content of selected eicosanoids (5-, 12-, and 15-hydroxyeicosatetraenoic acids (HETEs), 12-hydroxyeicosapentaenoic acid (HEPE), and the sum of hydroxyoctadecadienoic acids (HODE)) and levels and expression of genes encoding various pro-inflammatory cytokines (interleukin-1 (IL-1), interleukin-6 (IL-6)) and metalloproteinase-9 (MMP-9) in the blood of rats were also investigated. Despite numerous studies, the influence of genistein on these issues in the early stages of carcinogenesis is still not entirely clear.

2. Materials and Methods

2.1. Laboratory Animals

The biological material for the study was blood obtained from female rats of the Sprague Dawley strain (n = 32). Approval for the study was obtained from the Bioethics Committee at the Warsaw Medical University—document number 645/2018. During the experiment, the animals were housed under controlled conditions and provided with constant access to water and feed. They were fed Labofeed H standard diet (Labofeed H, Żurawia 19, 89-240 Kcynia, Poland). The room temperature was kept at 22 °C, and a 12-h day–night cycle was maintained.

The experiment lasted 100 days. After a 10-day period of adaptation to the experimental conditions, the animals were randomly divided into 4 groups:

Group 1—control group, rats without supplementation, which, in order to maintain the experimental conditions, received 0.4 mL of water via an intragastric probe.

Group 2—animals supplemented with macrogenistein, suspended in 0.4 mL of water, administered via an intragastric probe, at a dose of 0.2 mg/kg b.w.

Group 3—animals supplemented with microgenistein, in the form of particles of 587 ± 83 nm, suspended in 0.4 mL of water, administered via an intragastric probe, at a dose of 0.2 mg/kg b.w.

Group 4—animals supplemented with nanogenistein, in the form of 92 ± 41 nm particles suspended in 0.4 mL of water, administered via an intragastric probe at a dose of 0.2 mg/kg b.w.

The procedure for preparing and evaluating the sizes of the nano- and micro-particles of genistein was presented in the work of Banyś et al. [11]. The dose of genistein used was based on the value of its average daily dietary intake by humans with extrapolation to the body weight of rats [12]. Rats were supplemented from 40 days of age until 20 weeks of age.

2.2. Tumor Formation

To induce mammary tumorigenesis (adenocarcinoma), rats were twice administered 7,12-dimethyl-1,2-benz[a]anthracene (DMBA) (from Sigma-Aldrich, St. Louis, MO, USA) dissolved in rapeseed oil by intragastric probe. The first dose—80 mg/kg b.w.—was administered at day 60 of each animal's life, and the next dose—40 mg/kg b.w.—at day 90 of each animal's life. Examining the development and expansion of tumor nodules was carried out through manual examination. The rats were sacrificed at 150 days old, and an assessment was made regarding the quantity of tumors per rat as well as the weight of each tumor.

2.3. Histopathology

The tumors were placed in a buffered formalin solution, dehydrated, sealed in paraffin and cut into 4 μm thick sections. Hematoxylin and eosin staining of tissue and cell sections was applied. Evaluation of the stained sections was conducted using a BX43 Olympus research microscope (Olympus Europa SE & Co., Hamburg, Germany). Mitoses were quantified in slides sourced from randomly chosen tumors, examining 15 fields of view under a 40× objective magnification.

2.4. Determination of 5-, 12-, and 15-Hydroxyeicosatetraenoic Acids (5-, 12-, and 15-HETE), 12-Hydroxyeicosapentaenoic Acid (12-HEPE), and Hydroxyoctadecadienoic Acids (HODE) in Rat Serum

Serum was obtained from fresh blood (collected when the animals were killed) by centrifugation in a centrifuge at 3000 rpm at 4 °C. The biological material was stored in a low-temperature refrigerator at −70 °C until proper analyses were performed.

The contents of 5-, 12-, and 15-hydroxyeicosatetraenoic acids (5-, 12-, and 15-HETE), 12-hydroxyeicosapentaenoic acid, and hydroxyoctadecadienoic acids (HODE) in the serum of rats supplemented with nano-, micro-, and macrogenistein were determined using high-performance liquid chromatography with UV detection (HPLC/UV) based on the methodology developed by Frohberg et al. [13].

Bakerbond C18 500 mg/3 mL columns (from SPE, J.T. Baker, The Netherlands) were used to extract the 5,12,15-HETE, 12-HEPE, and HODE acids. The column bed was preconditioned with methanol, followed by water at 10 mL per column. A volume of 0.5 mL of 10% methanol was added to the serum sample (0.4 mL) and then applied to the column. After washing with 2 mL of water and 2 mL of 10% methanol, the test compounds were eluted with pure methanol (100%) (3 × 0.5 mL). The samples were evaporated to dryness under a stream of nitrogen at 37 °C and dissolved in 100 μL of ethanol. Before being applied to the chromatography column, each sample was cleaned using a 0.22 μm pore-size filter (Ultrafree-MC, Durapore PVDF, 0.22 μm, from Millipore, Burlington, MA, USA). The content of fatty acid metabolites was determined using a liquid chromatograph with an LC-20AD-type pump, SPD-10AV UV/VIS, detector and CT0-10AS oven (from Shimadzu Corporation, Kyoto, Japan). The tested compounds were separated on a 2.6 μm, 100 mm × 4.6 mm C18 Kinetex-type chromatography column (from Phenomenex, Torrance, CA, USA). The analysis was carried out using the following phase systems: A—methanol: acetic acid (100:0.01); and B—0.01% acetic acid. The composition of the mobile phase (A:B) changed over time as follows: 70:30 at 11 min; 73:27 at 18 min; 90:10 at 25 min, 70:30 at 5 min. The flow rate was 0.8 mL/min, and the column temperature was 35 °C. A 4 μL sample was applied to the chromatography column. The content of fatty acid metabolites was determined at 235 nm. Analysis of the tested compounds was carried out using standard solutions of HODE, 12-HEPE, 5-, 12-, 15-HETE (from Cayman Chemicals, Ann Arbor, MI, USA).

2.5. Determination of the Contents of Interleukin-1, Interleukin-6, and Metalloproteinase-9 in the Serum of Rats

The contents of interleukin-1, interleukin-6, and metalloproteinase-9 in the serum of rats supplemented with nano-, micro-, and macrogenistein were determined using ELISA. Commercially available assays were used for the study: Rat Interleukin-6 (IL-6) ELISA Kit (catalog number: orb219833) and Rat Interleukin-1 (IL-1) ELISA kit (catalog number: 219820) from Biorbyt (Biorbyt® Ltd., 5, Orwell Furlong, Cowley Road, Cambridge, Cambridgeshire, CB4 0WY, UK); and Rat Matrix Metalloproteinase-9 ELISA Kit (catalog number: E0553r) from Wuhan Eiaab Science Co., Ltd. (Wuhan Eiaab Science Co., Ltd., Beneficiary, A1710 Guangguguoji, East Lake Hi-Tech Development Zone, Wuhan 430079, China). In performing the test, the test procedure was followed in accordance with the manufacturer's instructions. A spectrophotometer from Bio-Tek Instruments (JNC, Highland Park, Box 998, Winooski, VT 05404-0998, USA) was used for the determination of IL-6, IL-1, and MMP-9.

2.6. Determination of Gene Expression Activity of Interleukin-1, Interleukin-6, and Metalloproteinase-9 in Rat Blood

The expression of *IL-6*, *IL-1beta* and *MMP-9* genes was determined with quantitative real-time PCR (qRT-PCR) using TaqMan probes. RNA was extracted using a Total RNA Mini kit (A&A Biotechnology, Gdynia, Poland) according to the manufacturer's instruction. The RNA concentration and the purity were evaluated with a micro-volume UV–vis spectrophotometer (Quawell Q3000, Quawell Technology Inc., San Jose, CA, USA). RNA was reverse transcribed to cDNA with a High-Capacity RNA-to-cDNA Kit (Applied Biosystems, Waltham, MA, USA). TaqMan™ Gene Expression Master Mix was used in the research (catalogue no.: 4369016; Thermo Fisher Scientific, Inc., Waltham, MA, USA).

The TaqMan Gene Expression Assays (Thermo Fisher Scientific, Inc., Waltham, MA, USA) were performed with the use of a ViiA™7 Real-Time PCR system (Applied Biosystems; Thermo Fisher Scientific, Inc.) under the following thermocycling conditions: 48 °C for 15 min, 95 °C for 10 min; and 40 cycles of 95 °C for 15 s and 60 °C for 1 min. The TaqMan Probes used for qRT-PCR are presented in Table 1. The data were normalized to the reference genes (*GAPDH* and *ACTB*, Table 1) and the relative expression level of each target gene compared to the control group was expressed as $2^{-\Delta\Delta Ct}$. All qRT-PCR experiments were run in triplicate, and the mean value was used for the determination of mRNA levels [14].

Table 1. TaqMan probes used for qRT-PCR in determination of the gene expression of selected angiogenic factors.

Gene Name	Gene Symbol	Assay ID
Matrix metallopeptidase-9	*MMP-9*	Rn00579162_m1
Interleukin-1 beta	*IL-1b*	Rn00580432_m1
Interleukin-6	*IL-6*	Rn01410330_m1
Glyceraldehyde-3-phosphate dehydrogenase	*GAPDH*	Rn01775763_g1
Actin beta	*ACTB*	Rn00667869_m1

2.7. Statistical Analysis of the Obtained Research Results

Statistical analyses were performed using the statistical package PQStat, version 1.8.2.212.

The results of the study were compared using analysis of variance (ANOVA) and Tukey's post hoc test. A test probability of $p < 0.05$ was considered significant, and a test probability of $p < 0.01$ was considered highly significant.

3. Results

3.1. Effects of Nano-, Micro-, and Macrogenistein on the Development and Progression of DMBA-Induced Tumorigenesis in Rats

The study showed that the incidence of tumors was 100% in all study groups except for the microgenistein-supplemented animals (88%) (Table 2). The first palpable tumors appeared in the group of nanogenistein-supplemented animals as early as 14 weeks of age. For the unsupplemented animals, the first tumors in the group appeared at week 16 (2 weeks later for nanogenistein-supplemented animals), and for the micro- and macrogenistein-supplemented animals at week 17 (3 weeks later for nanogenistein-supplemented animals). The numbers of tumors (assessed at week 20) per individual varied according to the supplementation used, and were for micro: 0–3; nano: 2–5; macro: 1–6, and for the control group: 2–9. Interestingly, the weight of tumors was significantly higher for rats supplemented with microgenistein (mean ± SD: 1.99 ± 1.75; range: 0.11–6.11) and nanogenistein (mean ± SD: 1.59 ± 2.64; range: 0.06–9.50), relative to animals without supplementation (mean ± SD: 0.93 ± 1.34; range: 0.10–7.80).

Table 2. Cancer induction in 7,12-dimethylbenz[a]anthracene-treated rats in relation to supplementation [11].

Supplementation	Rat's Number	Tumor Weight (g) (Mean ± SD) (Week 20)	Number of Tumors per Rat (Week 20)	Incidence of Tumors per Rat in Time (Weeks of Rats Life)
Standard	1	0.90 ± 0.78 (0.1–2.7)	9	17
	2	1.84 ± 3.35 (0.1–7.8)	5	16
	3	0.43 ± 0.30 (0.1–0.8)	4	19
	4	0.45 ± 0.40 (0.1–1.1)	6	18
	5	1.02 ± 1.03 (0.1–2.6)	6	16
	6	0.60 ± 0.00 (0.6)	2	19
	7	1.36 ± 0.92 (0.3–1.96)	3	17
	8	0.61 ± 0.20 (0.47–0.75)	2	17
	mean ± SD	0.93 ± 1.34 (0.10–7.80) [a]		
Macrogenistein	1	2.35 ± 1.96 (0.9–5.14)	4	17
	2	0.52 ± 0.47 (0.14–1.38)	6	17
	3	0.70 ± 0.52 (0.33–1.29)	3	19
	4	1.83 ± 2.48 (0.13–6.39)	6	18
	5	1.74 ± 1.79 (0.24–4.07)	4	17
	6	0.34	1	19
	7	1.58 ± 1.14 (0.29–2.42)	3	17
	8	1.13 ± 1.28 (0.25–3.03)	4	17
	mean ± SD	1.27 ± 1.52 (0.14–6.39)		
Microgenistein	1	0.89 ± 0.40 (0.6–1.17)	2	20
	2	-	-	-
	3	6.11	1	18
	4	1.38 ± 0.69 (0.89–1.86)	2	20
	5	3.31	1	17
	6	2.77 ± 1.81 (0.69–3.89)	3	18
	7	1.45 ± 1.40 (0.19–2.96)	3	18
	8	0.66 ± 0.78 (0.11–1.21)	2	19
	mean ± SD	1.99 ± 1.75 (0.11–6.11) [a]		
Microgenistein	1	0.89 ± 0.40 (0.6–1.17)	2	20
	2	-	-	-
	3	6.11	1	18
	4	1.38 ± 0.69 (0.89–1.86)	2	20
	5	3.31	1	17
	6	2.77 ± 1.81 (0.69–3.89)	3	18
	7	1.45 ± 1.40 (0.19–2.96)	3	18
	8	0.66 ± 0.78 (0.11–1.21)	2	19
	mean ± SD	1.99 ± 1.75 (0.11–6.11) [a]		

Table 2. *Cont.*

Supplementation	Rat's Number	Tumor Weight (g) (Mean ± SD) (Week 20)	Number of Tumors per Rat (Week 20)	Incidence of Tumors per Rat in Time (Weeks of Rats Life)
Nanogenistein	1	1.01 ± 1.02 (0.1–2.43)	4	19
	2	4.58 ± 2.12 (3.08–6.08)	2	17
	3	0.28 ± 0.20 (0.09–0.48)	3	19
	4	0.20 ± 0.07 (0.1–0.26)	4	20
	5	1.92 ± 3.74 (0.11–8.61)	5	14
	6	1.57 ± 1.94 (0.06–4.41)	4	18
	7	5.03 ± 6.32 (0.56–9.50)	2	18
	8	0.30 ± 0.16 (0.18–0.41)	2	20
	mean ± SD	1.59 ± 2.64 (0.06–9.50)		

SD—standard deviation; [a]—statistically significant differences between groups ($p < 0.01$).

Histopathological examination showed that all tumors examined had features of breast cancer—adenocarcinoma (Figure 1, Table 3). A grade II adenocarcinoma was found in animals without supplementation and in animals supplemented with macrogenistein. In tumor samples obtained from microgenistein-supplemented and nanogenistein-supplemented animals, the histopathological examination image indicated grade III malignancy. The groups of animals that were supplemented with genistein showed an increase in the intensity of tumor cell proliferation, as evidenced by the number of mitoses in the field of view of the microscope (at 40× objective magnification), with respect to animals without supplementation (Table 3). The mean numbers of mitoses in genistein-supplemented animals was statistically significantly higher compared to the control animals (mean ± SD: 1.79 ± 1.25), and were mean ± SD: 7.33 ± 1.57 (microgenistein), mean value ± SD: 5.82 ± 1.57 (nanogenistein), and 4.46 ± 2.38 (macrogenistein) [11].

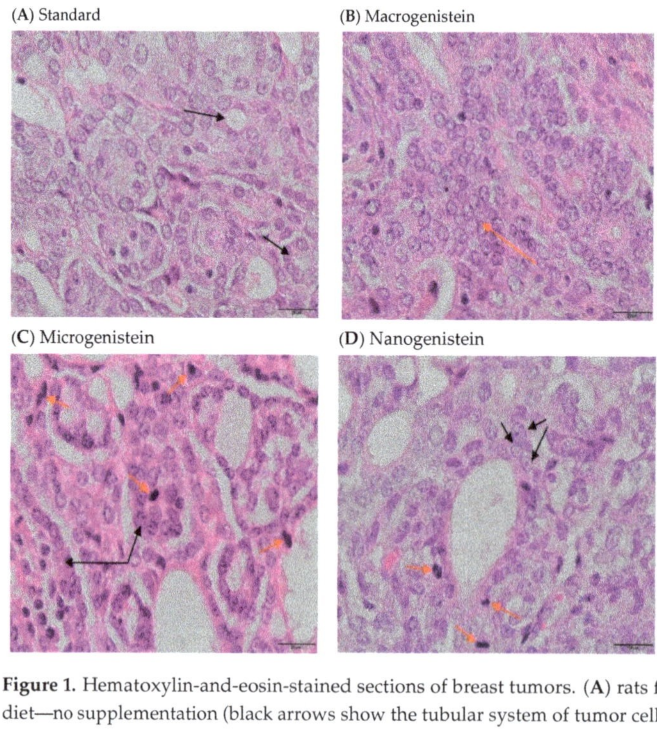

Figure 1. Hematoxylin-and-eosin-stained sections of breast tumors. (**A**) rats fed with a standard diet—no supplementation (black arrows show the tubular system of tumor cells); (**B**) rats fed with

nanogenistein (red arrow indicates infiltrating tumor cell); (**C**) rats fed with a diet supplemented with microgenistein (red arrows indicate mitosis and black bands indicate tumor cells); (**D**) rats fed with a diet supplemented with macrogenistein (red arrows show mitosis and black arrows show cancer cells forming vesicles) [11].

Table 3. Histopathological examination of rats' tumors.

Supplementation	Tumor Grade	The Mean Number of Mitoses in the Field of View Area *
Standard	Adenocarcinoma grade 2	$1.79 \pm 1.25^{a,b,c}$
Macrogenistein	Adenocarcinoma grade 2	$4.46 \pm 2.38^{a,d}$
Microgenistein	Adenocarcinoma grade 3	$7.33 \pm 1.57^{b,d}$
Nanogenistein	Adenocarcinoma grade 3	5.82 ± 1.57^{c}

Data are expressed as mean ± SD (standard deviation). Values sharing letters ([a]: standard, [b]: macrogenistein, [c]: microgenistein, [d]: nanogenistein) indicate statistically significant differences between groups ($p < 0.01$). * Mitoses were counted in slides from randomly selected tumors in 15 fields of view with a 40× objective magnification.

3.2. The Effect of Nano-, Micro-, and Macrogenistein Supplementation on the Body Weight of the Test Animals and the Weight of Their Organs

The data on the kinetics of the changes (7–20 weeks of age of animals) in body weight (g) of animals treated with DMBA and supplemented with genistein in macro, micro, and nano forms and animals without supplementation are shown in Figure 2.

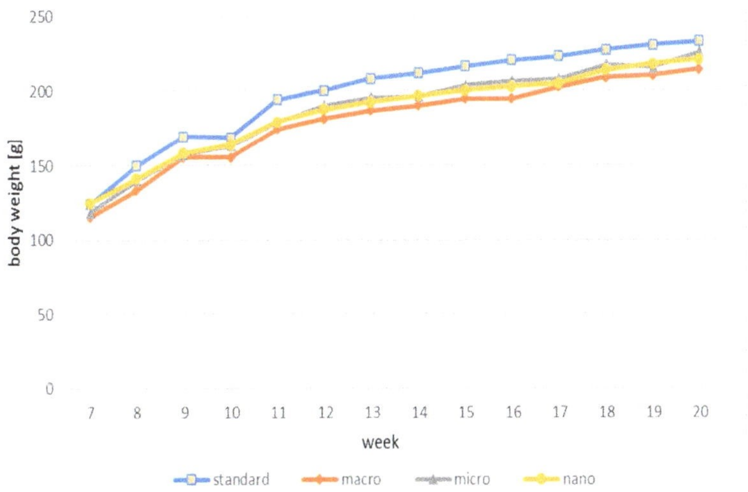

Figure 2. Kinetics of changes (weeks 7–20) in body weight (g) of experimental animals. Standard: animals receiving a standard diet only (no supplementation); macro: animals supplemented with macrogenistein; micro: animals supplemented with microgenistein; nano: animals supplemented with nanogenistein; g: grams; differences not statistically significant ($\alpha = 0.05$).

The results of the statistical analysis of the body weight gain of rats (7–20 week old rats) depending on the supplementation used are shown in Figure 3.

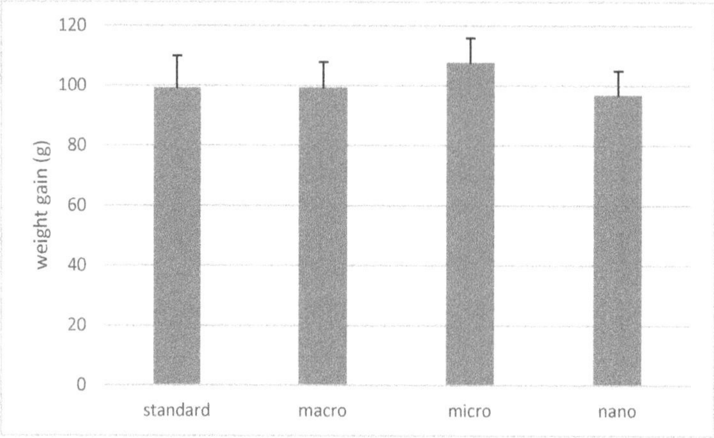

Figure 3. Weight gain of rats (g). Standard: animals without supplementation; macro: animals supplemented with macrogenistein; micro: animals supplemented with microgenistein; nano: animals supplemented with nanogenistein; g: grams; differences not statistically significant ($\alpha = 0.05$).

Based on the results, there were no statistically significant differences in the weight gain of animals (g) over a period of 13 weeks (from 7 to 20 weeks of age) depending on the supplementation used (Figure 3).

The results of a statistical analysis of organ weights (g), liver and spleen of animals supplemented with nano-, micro-, and macrogenistein in relation to animals without supplementation, are shown in Figure 4. The material for the study was obtained at 20 weeks of age of the animals, during their decapitation.

Based on the study, it was shown that the weights of spleens and livers of rats supplemented with macro-, micro-, and nanogenistein were higher with respect to animals without supplementation (control group); however, due to the high values of the standard deviation, these values were not statistically significant (Figure 4).

3.3. Effects of Nano-, Micro-, and Macrogenistein on the Content of Selected Fatty Acid Metabolites in the Serum of Rats Treated with DMBA

The results of 5-, 12-, and 15-hydroxyyeicosatetraenoic acids and hydroxyoctadecadienoic acids in the blood serum of rats treated with DM

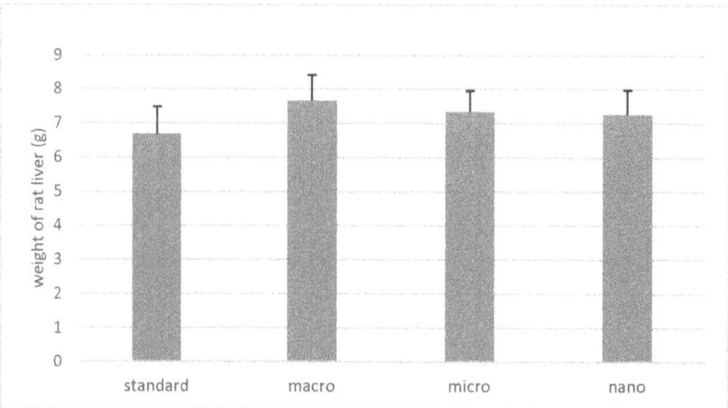

Figure 4. *Cont.*

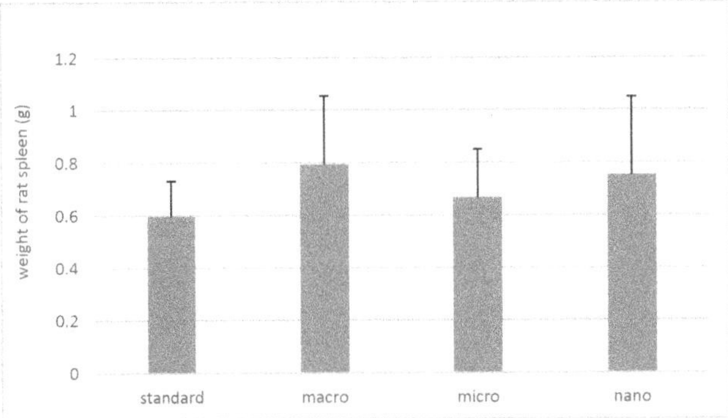

Figure 4. Weight of rats' spleen and liver (g). Standard: rats without supplementation; macro: animals supplemented with macrogenistein; micro: animals supplemented with microgenistein; nano: animals supplemented with nanogenistein; g: grams; differences not statistically significant ($\alpha = 0.05$).

BA and supplemented with nano-, micro-, and macrogenistein are shown in Table 4.

Table 4. The levels of 5-, 12-, and 15-hydroxyeicosatetraenoic acids, 12-hydroxyeicosapentaenoic acid, and the sum of hydroxyoctadecadienoic acids (ng/mL) in the serum of rats treated with a carcinogen and supplemented with macro-, micro-, or nanogenistein.

Eicosanoids	Group				*p*-Value
	Standard	Macro	Micro	Nano	
12-HEPE	458.19 ± 208.09^{b}	69.45 ± 36.42^{a}	61.07 ± 12.68^{a}	60.21 ± 14.18^{a}	0.0013
HODE	226.82 ± 33.67^{b}	110.60 ± 48.13^{a}	130.52 ± 41.90^{a}	116.13 ± 32.58^{a}	0.0001
15-HETE	43.10 ± 7.58^{b}	29.06 ± 6.49^{a}	36.82 ± 14.09^{ab}	36.18 ± 8.68^{ab}	n.s.
12-HETE	6446 ± 1522^{b}	2414 ± 917^{a}	1918 ± 219^{a}	1897 ± 319^{a}	0.0001
5-HETE	10.94 ± 2.81	6.84 ± 3.64	9.29 ± 6.25	15.73 ± 14.17	n.s.

Data are presented as mean values ± standard deviation (SD); standard: animals without supplementation; macro: animals supplemented with macrogenistein; micro: animals supplemented with microgenistein; nano: animals supplemented with nanogenistein; *p*-value: test probability (statistical significance); ^{a,b}—homogeneous groups in rows ($\alpha = 0.05$); n.s.—differences not statistically significant ($\alpha = 0.05$); 12-HEPE—12-hydroxyyeicosapentaenoic acid; HODE—sum of hydroxyoctadecadienoic acids; 15-HETE—15-hydroxyyeicosatetraenoic acid; 12-HETE—12-hydroxyyeicosatetraenoic acid; 5-HETE—5-hydroxyyeicosatetraenoic acid; ng: nanogram; ml: milliliter.

Based on the study, there was a statistically significant lower content of 12-HEPE ($p = 0.001$); HODE ($p = 0.0001$), and 12-HETE ($p = 0.0001$) in the serum of rats supplemented with genistein in the macro, micro, and nano forms, with respect to the content of the markers in the serum of rats without supplementation. There were no statistically significant differences in the content of 5-HETE and 15-HETE acids in the serum of rats depending on the supplementation used (Table 4).

3.4. Effects of Nano-, Micro-, and Macrogenistein on the Contents of Interleukin-1, Interleukin-6, and Metalloproteinase-9 in the Serum of Rats Treated with DMBA

The results of the contents of interleukin-1, interleukin-6, and metalloproteinase-9 in the serum of animals treated with a carcinogenic agent and supplemented with nano-, micro-, or macrogenistein are shown in Table 5.

Based on the results, there were no statistically significant differences in the levels of IL-1, IL-6, and MMP-9 in the serum of genistein-supplemented rats, relative to animals without supplementation.

Table 5. Levels of interleukin-6 (IL-6) (pg/mL), interleukin-1 (IL-1) (pg/mL), and metalloproteinase-9 (MMP-9) (ng/mL) in serum of rats treated with DMBA and supplemented with macro-, micro-, or nanogenistein.

Eicosanoids	Group				p-Value
	Standard	Macro	Micro	Nano	
IL-6	88.47 ± 40.39	109.97 ± 57.64	99.36 ± 43.12	92.01 ± 16.50	n.s.
IL-1	103.64 ± 69.86	86.05 ± 35.07	104.25 ± 32.82	132.43 ± 65.78	n.s.
MMP-9	0.64 ± 0.35	1.67 ± 1.10	1.80 ± 1.05	2.03 ± 2.68	n.s.

Data are presented as mean values ± standard deviation (SD); standard: animals without supplementation; macro: animals supplemented with macrogenistein; micro: animals supplemented with microgenistein; nano: animals supplemented with nanogenistein; *p*-value: test probability (statistical significance); n.s.—differences not statistically significant (α = 0.05); Il-6—interleukin-6; IL-1—interleukin-1; MMP-9—metalloproteinase-9.

3.5. Effects of Nano-, Micro-, and Macrogenistein on Gene Expression of Interleukin-1, Interleukin-6, and Metalloproteinase-9 in the Blood Serum of Rats Treated with DMBA

The results of the gene expression of *IL-1, IL-6,* and *MMP-9* in the blood of animals treated with DMBA and supplemented with nano-, micro-, or macrogenistein are shown in Figure 5.

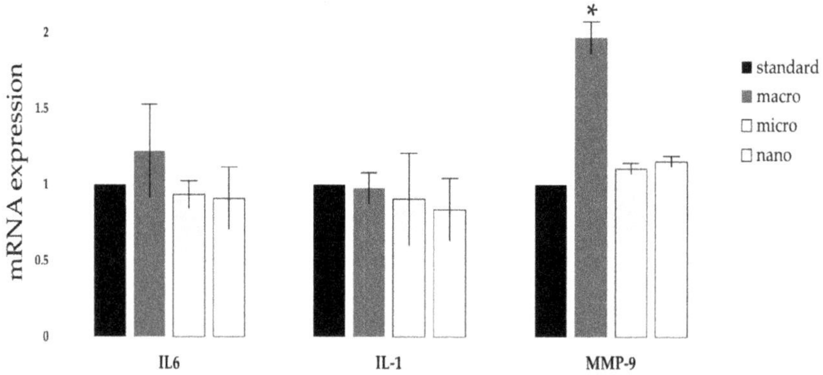

Figure 5. Results of gene expression of interleukin-1, interleukin-6 and metalloproteinase-9 in blood of animals treated with (DMBA) and supplemented with nano-, micro-, or macrogenistein; standard: animals without supplementation; macro: animals supplemented with macrogenistein; micro: animals supplemented with microgenistein; nano: animals supplemented with nanogenistein. The results were expressed as the relative quantification (the fold of standard group). * $p < 0.05$ compared to standard group.

On the basis of the study, we found a significant increase in the expression of the *MMP-9* gene in the blood of rats supplemented with macrogenistein (compared to animals without supplementation or supplemented with micro- or nanogenistein). The expression of the IL-1 gene in the blood of nano- and microgenistein-supplemented rats was shown to be reduced, relative to animals without supplementation; however, this did not reach statistical significance.

4. Discussion

Based on the study, it was shown that supplementation of animals with genistein in macro, micro, and nano forms increased the intensity of the tumor process in rats. Histopathological examination showed that all tumors examined had features of breast cancer—adenocarcinoma. A grade II adenocarcinoma was found in animals without supplementation and in animals supplemented with macrogenistein. In tumor samples obtained from microgenistein-supplemented and nanogenistein-supplemented animals, the histopathological examination image indicated grade III malignancy. The groups of animals that were supplemented with genistein showed an increase in the intensity of tumor cell proliferation, as evidenced by the number of mitoses in the field of view of the microscope (at 40× objective magnification), with respect to animals without supplementation. Macro-, micro-, and nanogenistein caused an increase in the intensity of tumor cell proliferation. Higher proliferative potential is associated with a poor prognosis and indicates rapid proliferation of tumor cells [15]. Ju Y.H. et al. [7] showed that the carcinogenic potential of genistein depended on the dose of genistein. The use of higher concentrations of this compound was associated with breast tumor growth, increased cell proliferation, and pS2 expression. Reducing materials to the nanoscale can sometimes lead to the development of new structural, phytochemical, electronic, and magnetic properties that are not present in larger particles containing the same material. Nanoparticles acquire new physical properties by increasing the surface-to-volume ratio, and having different reactive sites, charge, shape, mobility, and thermal properties. The form of the particles can unambiguously change their properties, and thus, the effect of nanoparticles on biological activity [16]. For this reason, these compounds are used in the diagnosis and treatment of various diseases, allowing earlier detection of pathological changes and more effective treatment of patients [17]. So far, clinical studies and observations indicate that the effect of genistein is inconclusive—some show it to have a protective effect in cancer, while others show it to be carcinogenic. However, given the structure of genistein and its proven potential to enhance the proliferation of some cancer cells, particularly in hormone-dependent cancers, the use of particle size reduction in this study exacerbated cancer. The best known property of genistein is its oestrogenic activity [7,8,18,19]. Genistein is a relatively strong agonist of the oestrogen receptor beta isoform (ERβ). Owing to its structural similarity to oestrogen, genistein shows similar activity to oestrogen [20]. However, the role of genistein in breast cancer can be determined by multiple factors, including age-dependent biological effect, the ratio of alpha and beta oestrogen receptors, gene mutations, individual differences in metabolism, the possibility of action through various metabolic pathways, and inflammation [8,21,22]. Considering that the role of genistein in breast cancer is ambiguous, learning about the mechanisms of action of genistein based on the analysis of selected biomarkers seems to be of great importance in assessing the safety of its use.

Inflammation is one of the factors in the initiation and progression of the cancer process [23,24]. Fatty acids are subject to metabolic processes that produce substances with the character of modulators of immune responses and inflammation, these include, among others, derivatives of hydroxyeicosatetraenoic, hydroxyoctadecadienoic, and hydroxyeicosapentaenoic acids. Arachidonic acid, metabolized by the enzymes 5-, 12-, and 15-lipoxygenase (5-LOX, 12-LOX, 15-LOX), is converted into hydroxyeicosatetraenoic acids: 5-HETE, 12-HETE, and 15-HETE, respectively. HODE are formed by the metabolism of linoleic acid. The oxidation of linoleic acid via 12-LOX and 15-LOX produces 9-hydroxyoctadecadienoic acid (9-HODE) and 13-hydroxyoctadecadienoic acid (13 HODE). With the participation of 12-lipoxygenase, 12-hydroxyeicosapentaenoic acid (12-HEPE) is formed from eicosapentaenoic acid [25,26]. The above-mentioned fatty acid metabolites, even in very low concentrations, are characterized by high biological activity [24–27]. They can play an important role in the development and course of a number of diseases, including atherosclerosis, cardiovascular diseases, allergies, autoimmune diseases, or cancer. The direction of this action depends on the type of compounds formed and the cascade of reactions in which they are involved [25,26]. Based on our study, we found a statistically significantly lower content of 12-HEPE ($p = 0.001$), HODE ($p = 0.0001$), and 12-HETE ($p = 0.0001$) in the blood serum of genistein-supplemented rats, with respect to the content of the aforementioned markers in the serum of rats without supplementation. HEPE acids are considered a possible modulator of the tumor process. Treatment of cancer cells with

HEPE results in inhibition of their growth. 12-HEPE has been found to inhibit the uptake of 3H-thymidine (a marker of cell proliferation and growth) by cancer cells. It has been shown to modulate cell proliferation and apoptosis [28]. 13-HODE acid can affect the development and progression of cancer by regulating cancer cells' motility and their adhesion and migration through capillaries in the endothelium. If cancer cells are unable to adhere to the endothelium and migrate across the barrier, it hinders the stabilization of metastatic foci. It has been shown that tumor cells producing small amounts of 13-HODE are characterized by easier adhesion to the endothelium. In a study by Tavakoli-Yaraki et al. [29], 13-HODE was found to inhibit the growth of both MCF-7- and MDA-MB-231-type cancer cells. It causes cell cycle arrest and induces apoptosis and decreases the level of PPAR-δ receptor expression. Both 15-LOX expression and HODE levels have been shown to be downregulated in cancer cells [30]. Breast cancer patients have significantly reduced levels of 15-LOX in tumor-transformed breast tissues, relative to levels in breast tissues obtained from healthy women [31,32]. It is difficult to explain the decrease in serum levels of 12-HETE in the rats studied, for it is a compound with inhibitory effects on apoptosis, promoting tumor angiogenesis and adhesion of tumor cells to endothelial cells [33]. Perhaps this result is due to the inhibitory effect of genistein on both 15- and 12-lipoxygenase activity [34].

Another objective of the current study was to evaluate the effects of nano-, micro-, and macrogenistein on the content of interleukin-6 (IL-6), interleukin-1 (IL-1), and metalloproteinase-9 (MMP-9) in the serum of DMBA-treated rats. The effect of genistein supplementation on the expression of genes encoding selected compounds in the blood of rats was also evaluated. Interleukins are proteins belonging to the cytokine group [35,36]. Cytokines are responsible for communication between cells. They condition the interaction of cells. At physiological concentrations, interleukins play an important role in cell proliferation, maturation, migration, and adhesion. They have been shown to influence metabolic processes and the neuroendocrine system, thereby taking part in maintaining homeostasis in the body [37]. However, interleukins may also play an important role in tumorigenesis, including initiation of carcinogenesis, angiogenesis, and metastasis [38–40]. Elevated levels of IL-1 interleukins have been shown to occur in the body fluids of cancer patients, relative to healthy individuals [41]. Local or systemic overexpression of the gene encoding IL-6 has been found in cancer patients [40,41]. A study by Kozlowski et al. [40] showed higher serum levels of IL-6 in patients with stage III disease, relative to patients with stage II disease. Elevated serum levels of IL-1 and/or IL-6 in patients are usually associated with poor prognosis and poor survival of breast cancer patients [41,42]. It has been shown that the levels of interleukin family 1 and IL-6 are significantly higher in tumor-lesioned tissue compared to healthy tissue [38]. However, based on this study, there were no statistically significant differences in the content or expression of IL-1 and IL-6 genes in the blood of DMBA-treated rats, depending on the supplementation used. Tang et al. [43] showed that genistein inhibits gene expression and prevents IL-1 formation in UVB-treated keratinocytes. Lee et al. [44] showed that genistein supplementation of diethylnitrosamine (DEN)-treated mice results in decreased IL-6 and TNF gene expression (relative to control animals). The anti-inflammatory effects of genistein have been demonstrated in a number of studies [45]. Interestingly, it was found that animals supplemented with nano-, micro-, and macrogenistein had higher levels of metalloproteinase-9, MMP-9, compared to animals without supplementation. There was a significant increase in MMP-9 gene expression in the blood of macrogenistein-supplemented animals. Extracellular matrix metalloproteinases are a group of metal-dependent proteolytic enzymes belonging to the group of endopeptidases, involved in the degradation of basement membrane proteins and extracellular matrix, which enables tissue remodeling and cell movement, both in the course of physiological processes, inflammation, and cancer. MMP-9 regulates the activity of growth factors, cytokines and especially chemokines [46]. Metalloproteinase-9 plays an important role in tumorigenesis [47]. It is characterized by its ability to degrade type IV collagen, and thus, participates in the mechanism of damage to the vascular basement membrane. This feature determines the process of angiogenesis, local tumor growth, and

38. Wu, T.C.; Xu, K.; Martinek, J.; Banchereau, R.; George, J.; Turner, J.; Kim, K.I.; Zurawski, S.; Wang, X.; Blankenship, D.; et al. IL1 receptor antagonist controls transcriptional signature of inflammation in patients with metastatic breast cancer. *Cancer Res.* **2018**, *1578*, 5243–5258. [CrossRef]
39. Dinarello, C.A. An interleukin-1 signature in breast cancer treated with interleukin-1 receptor blockade: Implications for treating cytokine release syndrome of checkpoint inhibitors. *Cancer Res.* **2018**, *78*, 5200–5202. [CrossRef]
40. Kozłowski, L.; Zakrzewska, I.; Tokajuk, P. Concentration of interleukin-6 (IL-6), interleukin-8 (IL-8) and interleukin-10 (IL-10) in blood serum of breast cancer patients. *Rocz. Akad. Med. W Bialymst.* **2003**, *48*, 82–84.
41. Gelfo, V.; Romaniello, D.; Mazzeschi, M.; Sgarzi, M.; Grilli, G.; Morselli, A.; Manzan, B.; Rihawi, K.; Lauriola, M. Roles of IL-1 in Cancer: From tumor progression to resistance to targeted therapies. *Int. J. Mol. Sci.* **2020**, *21*, 6009. [CrossRef]
42. Shibayama, O.; Yoshiuchi, K.; Inagaki, M.; Matsuoka, Y.; Yoshikawa, E.; Sugawara, Y.; Akechi, T.; Wada, N.; Imoto, S.; Murakami, K.; et al. Association between adjuvant regional radiotherapy and cognitive function in breast cancer patients treated with conservation therapy. *Cancer Med.* **2014**, *3*, 702–709. [CrossRef]
43. Tang, S.C.; Hsiao, Y.P.; Ko, J.L. Genistein protects against ultraviolet B- induced wrinkling and photoinflammation in in vitro and in vivo models. *Genes Nutr.* **2022**, *17*, 4. [CrossRef]
44. Lee, S.R.; Kwon, S.W.; Lee, Y.H.; Kaya, P.; Kim, J.M.; Ahn, C.; Jung, E.M.; Lee, G.S.; An, B.S.; Jeung, E.B.; et al. Dietary intake of genistein suppresses hepatocellular carcinoma through AMPK-mediated apoptosis and anti-inflammation. *BMC Cancer* **2019**, *19*, 6. [CrossRef]
45. Pierzynowska, K.; Podlacha, M.; Brokowska, J.; Gaffke, L.; Mantej, J.; Cyske, Z.; rintz, E.; Osiadły, M.; Bartkowski, M.; Puchalski, M.; et al. Molekularne mechanizmy działania genisteiny w świetle terapii chorób genetycznych i immunologicznych. *Post. Biochem.* **2018**, *64*, 262–275.
46. Kołaczkowska, E. Metaloproteinaza 9 (MMP-9) jako szczególny przedstawiciel metaloproteinaz macierzy zewnątrzkomórkowej: Rola w napływie i apoptozie neutrofili w trakcie reakcji zapalnej. *Post. Biol. Kom* **2010**, *37*, 471–499.
47. Zaręba, I.; Donejko, M.; Rysiak, E. Znaczenie i przydatność diagnostyczna mttaloproteinaz w raku piersi. *J. Oncol.* **2014**, *64*, 491–495.

current issues in molecular biology

MDPI

Review

Anticancer Ribosomally Synthesized and Post-Translationally Modified Peptides from Plants: Structures, Therapeutic Potential, and Future Directions

Hyeon-Jeong Hwang †, Youngsang Nam †, Chanhee Jang, Eun La Kim, Eun Seo Jang, Yeo Jin Lee and Seoung Rak Lee *

College of Pharmacy, Research Institute for Drug Development, Pusan National University, Busan 46241, Republic of Korea
* Correspondence: srlee17@pusan.ac.kr; Tel.: +82-51-510-2803
† These authors contributed equally to this work.

Abstract: Cancer remains a significant medical challenge, necessitating the discovery of novel therapeutic agents. Ribosomally synthesized and post-translationally modified peptides (RiPPs) from plants have emerged as a promising source of anticancer compounds, offering unique structural diversity and potent biological activity. This review identifies and discusses cytotoxic RiPPs across various plant families, focusing on their absolute chemical structures and reported cytotoxic activities against cancer cell lines. Notably, plant-derived RiPPs such as rubipodanin A and mallotumides A–C demonstrated low nanomolar IC_{50} values against multiple cancer cell types, highlighting their therapeutic potential. By integrating traditional ethnobotanical knowledge with modern genomic and bioinformatic approaches, this study underscores the importance of plant RiPPs as a resource for developing innovative cancer treatments. These findings pave the way for further exploration of plant RiPPs, emphasizing their role in addressing the ongoing challenges in oncology and enhancing the repertoire of effective anticancer therapies.

Keywords: phytochemicals; ribosomally synthesized and post-translationally modified peptides; chemical structure; anticancer activity; biosynthesis

1. Introduction

Cancer remains a major global health challenge, ranking as the second leading cause of death worldwide [1–3]. Despite significant advancements in early detection, diagnosis, and treatment, cancer remains a challenging threat to human health due to its inherent complexity [4,5]. The disease is marked by uncontrolled cell proliferation, the capacity to invade surrounding tissues, and, in many cases, the potential to metastasize to distant organs [6,7]. Furthermore, the development of drug resistance poses a significant challenge in cancer therapy [8,9]. Cancer cells can adapt and evolve, ultimately diminishing the efficacy of standard treatments over time. This resistance often results in relapse and disease progression, underscoring the urgent need for new therapeutic compounds [10–13].

Given these challenges, there is an urgent need to discover and develop novel anticancer drugs that are more effective, less toxic, and capable of overcoming drug resistance. Phytochemicals have historically served as a valuable source of therapeutic agents [14–17]. Several drugs currently employed in cancer treatment, such as paclitaxel (Taxol) [18–22] and vinblastine [23], originate from plant sources. This underscores the significant potential of plant-derived compounds in contributing to the next generation of anticancer therapies [24].

Ribosomally synthesized and post-translationally modified peptides (RiPPs) represent a diverse and rapidly growing class of natural products that have garnered significant attention for their effective biological activities and therapeutic potential [25–27]. RiPPs are unique in that they are initially synthesized as precursor peptides by the ribosome, following the standard genetic code, and subsequently undergo extensive post-translational modifications (PTMs) [28,29]. These modifications are catalyzed by specific enzymes and are crucial for converting the linear precursor peptides into biologically active structures. The structural diversity of RiPPs is driven by the wide array of potential PTMs, such as cyclization, methylation, glycosylation, hydroxylation, and the formation of unusual amino acids or cross-links [30,31]. These modifications significantly alter the chemical properties of the peptides, enhancing their stability, specificity, and potency.

Plant-derived RiPPs have emerged as a particularly promising source of new bioactive compounds. Plants have developed a diverse range of chemical defenses to combat herbivores, pathogens, and environmental stressors, many of which are mediated by RiPPs. These peptides frequently exhibit potent bioactivity while remaining minimally toxic to the plants themselves, positioning them as ideal candidates for the development of new therapeutic agents, particularly in oncology [32–37]. Plant-derived RiPPs exhibit a broad spectrum of bioactivities, functioning as potent antimicrobials, insecticides, and vasorelaxants, as well as demonstrating antiviral, immunomodulatory, and notable anticancer properties. For instance, the cyclotide kalata B1, derived from *Oldenlandia affinis*, has demonstrated antimicrobial activity against *Escherichia coli* and *Staphylococcus aureus* [38,39], as well as insecticidal effects by targeting the disruption of insect gut epithelia [40]. Similarly, the orbitide segetalin A, derived from *Vaccaria hispanica*, exhibits vasorelaxant activity, making it beneficial for the treatment of cerebrovascular spasms and hypertension [41]. Another example is the burpitides lyciumin A and lyciumin B, derived from *Lycium chinense*, which have been reported to inhibit angiotensin-converting enzyme (ACE) and renin, highlighting their potential for hypertension management [42]. Additionally, RiPPs can exhibit antiviral activity by interacting with viral proteins through their unique structure, including disulfide bonds and other post-translational modifications, or by inhibiting the entry of viruses into host cells [43,44]. RiPPs also possess immunomodulatory properties that can regulate immune responses. Stimulated by cyclopeptides, RiPPs can enhance the immune system's ability to combat infections or cancer by modulating Caspase 3, which promotes apoptosis in infected or cancerous cells [45]. These examples highlight the diverse ecological and health-related roles of RiPPs, underscoring their potential as valuable resources for the development of bioactive compounds. Thus, RiPPs often demonstrate exceptional bioactivity, including exhibiting antimicrobial, antiviral, and anticancer properties, making them highly promising candidates for drug development [25,26,32].

The study of RiPPs derived from plants is still in its early stages, but it holds great potential. Conventional cancer treatments, such as chemotherapy and radiation, often face significant challenges including drug resistance, off-target effects, and toxic side effects [9]. These limitations underscore the need for novel, targeted therapies. Unlike traditional chemical drugs, some RiPPs exhibit high specificity and potent anticancer activity with unique mechanisms of action, making them attractive candidates for overcoming some of the limitations associated with current therapies [46–48]. RiPPs are naturally derived, structurally diverse peptides that undergo PTMs, enabling them to target multiple cellular pathways, such as inducing apoptosis, inhibiting angiogenesis, and modulating immune responses [49]. Their selective action and ability to be engineered for specific therapeutic purposes position them as an effective alternative to conventional anticancer drugs, offering a targeted approach with potentially fewer side effects [50].

Advances in genomics, bioinformatics, and synthetic biology are accelerating the discovery and characterization of new RiPPs, while improved techniques in structural biology are providing detailed insights into their mechanisms of action. As researchers continue to explore the rich diversity of plant RiPPs, these peptides offer new solutions to some of the most pressing challenges in cancer therapy, including the need for more effective and selective anticancer phytochemicals. In this review, we first offer a comprehensive overview of anticancer plant-derived RiPPs, emphasizing their chemistry, bioactivity, and biosynthesis. This introduction highlights that plant-derived RiPPs are a fascinating and versatile class of natural products, distinguished by their unique biosynthesis and structural complexity. The potential of RiPPs, particularly those derived from plants, represents an exciting frontier in the search for novel anticancer phytochemicals [33,35,48,51–54].

2. Biosynthesis of Plant-Derived RiPPs

Plant-derived peptides exhibit a range of physiological activities, such as antibacterial, anticancer, and antiviral properties, playing key roles in various beneficial biological processes [55–57]. Most known plant-derived peptides to date are produced through a biosynthetic process involving ribosomal synthesis followed by extensive post-translational modifications, classifying them as RiPPs (Figure 1) [58]. These processes allow plant-derived RiPPs to exhibit diverse structures and biological activities, such as anticancer properties, and highlight the significance of the RiPPs in therapeutic applications [59,60].

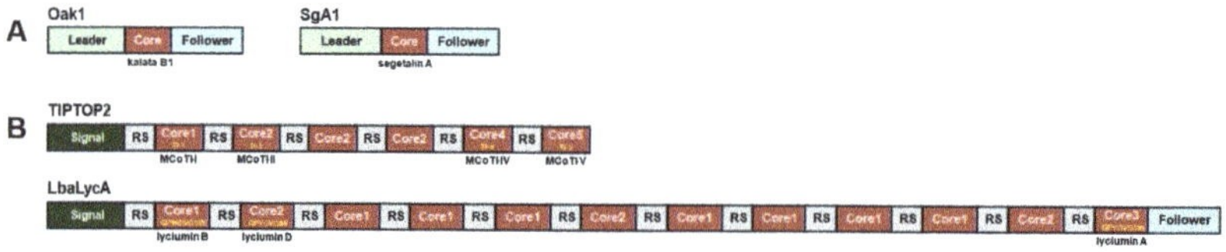

Figure 1. Typical biosynthetic pathway of RiPPs. The RiPP-related gene in DNA is transcribed into mRNA, and the mRNA is subsequently translated by ribosomes, resulting in the formation of a precursor peptide. (**A**) In most cases, precursor peptides are single-core form, containing a leader and core peptide, with the follower peptide being an optional component. (**B**) While less prevalent, some precursor peptides are multi-core form, consisting of two or more core peptides linked by recognition sequences. The precursor peptide undergoes post-translational modification by specific enzymes, which introduce modifications such as cyclization, dehydration, and methylation to the core peptide. Once these modifications are complete, proteases remove the leader and other peptides, converting the modified core peptide into a mature RiPP. At this stage, a variety of mature RiPPs can be produced from the multi-core precursor peptide.

2.1. Ribosomal Synthesis of Precursor Peptides

Plant-derived RiPPs initiate their biosynthesis within the cellular ribosomes as precursor peptides. These precursor peptides are composed of distinct regions, which include the leader peptide, core peptide, and follower peptide, commonly referred to as single-core structures. The leader peptide is typically positioned at the N-terminus of the precursor peptide and ranges in length from approximately 20 to 110 amino acid residues. This peptide region plays a crucial role in the biosynthetic process, functioning primarily as a signal for the activation of various biosynthetic enzymes [61,62]. Furthermore, it aids in the recognition of the core peptide by these enzymes, ensuring the subsequent modifications required for maturation. Central to the precursor peptide is the core peptide, which is the key region responsible for the eventual formation of mature RiPPs through a series of enzymatic modifications. This core peptide undergoes a variety of PTMs that enhance its stability and biological activity, ultimately defining the characteristics of the final RiPPs [63].

At the C-terminus of the precursor peptide lies the follower peptide, which, while not essential for the overall biosynthesis of the RiPPs, plays a supportive role in the modification processes of the core peptide. The follower peptide assists in targeting precise sites for enzymatic modifications, thus influencing the final structure and function of the mature peptide [64]. *O. affinis* has been traditionally used in Africa to aid women during childbirth. From this plant, a single-core precursor peptide, Oak1, is transformed into kalata B1, a member of the cyclotide class of RiPPs (Figure 2) [40]. Similarly, the Chinese herb *Saponaria vaccaria* (Caryophyllaceae), known for its effects in treating amenorrhea, regulating blood flow, and promoting lactation, produces segetalin A, an orbitide-class RiPP, from the precursor peptide SgA1 (Figure 2) [65].

Some precursor peptides of plant-derived RiPPs occur in a multi-core form, containing more than two core peptides. These multi-core precursor peptides possess several distinct recognition sequences that serve to differentiate between the multiple core peptides present within the same precursor. This feature allows them to perform a function analogous to that of follower peptides, effectively guiding the modification processes that ultimately leads to the maturation of the individual core peptides into their respective RiPPs (Figure 1) [66].

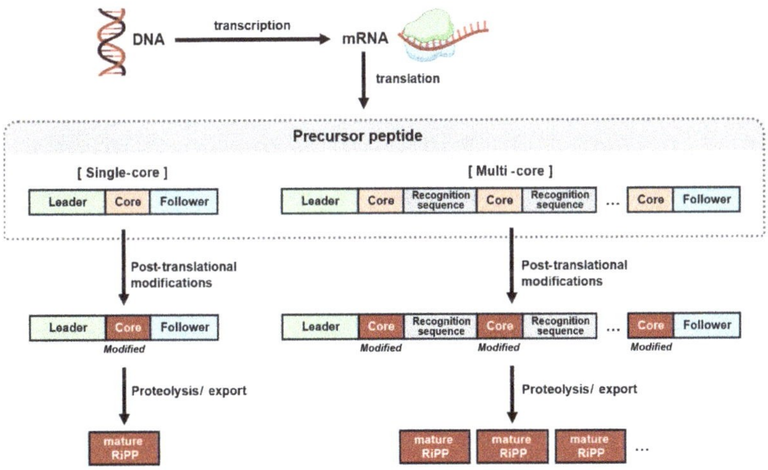

Figure 2. Precursor peptides of several plant-derived RiPPs. Single-core precursor peptides containing one core peptide. The core peptides of Oak1 and SgA1 are subsequently processed into kalata B1 and segetalin A, respectively. Multi-core precursor peptides containing multiple core peptides. TIPTOP2 contains six core peptides, which correspond to four types of core peptides processed into MCoTI-I, MCoTI-II, MCoTI-IV, and MCoTI-V. LbaLycA contains twelve core peptides, composed of three types that will mature into lyciumin A, lyciumin B, and lyciumin D. RS: Recognition sequence.

The multi-core structure of these precursor peptides offers significant advantages over traditional single-core forms, particularly in terms of biosynthetic efficiency. As they possess the capacity to generate multiple plant RiPPs from a single gene cluster, multi-core precursor peptides streamline the production process and enhance the diversity of bioactive compounds that can be obtained from a limited genetic framework. This becomes particularly beneficial in the context of plants with constrained genome sizes, where maximizing the output of bioactive peptides from existing genetic resources is crucial [67]. For instance, the precursor peptide TIPTOP2 (two inhibitor peptide topologies 2), found in the Cucurbitaceae family, contains six core peptides, from which four distinct knottin-class RiPPs—MCoTI (*Momordica cochinchinensis* trypsin inhibitor)-I, MCoTI-II, MCoTI-IV, and MCoTI-V—are produced (Figure 2) [68,69]. Similarly, in the Chinese herb *Lycium barbarum*

(Solanaceae), known for its effectiveness in treating hypertension, the precursor peptide LbaLycA contains twelve linked peptides, but only three core sequences—QPYGVGSW, QPWGVGSW, and QPYGVGIW—leading to the production of the branched cyclic peptides lyciumin A, lyciumin B, and lyciumin D (Figure 2) [70].

2.2. Post-Translational Modifications

The core peptide of plant precursor peptides undergoes a wide range of PTMs, including but not limited to methylation, oxidation/reduction, dehydration, cross-linking between amino acid residues, and macrocyclization [71–73]. These modifications are critical as they enhance both the stability and biological activity of the resulting peptides, contributing to their functional roles in various physiological processes. For instance, methylation influences the charge and hydrophobicity of the peptide [74], while macrocyclization often results in a more stable structure that is less susceptible to enzymatic degradation [75].

The leader peptide plays a pivotal role in facilitating these PTMs, as it enhances the binding affinity between the core peptide and the various enzymes responsible for the modifications [61,76]. Its structural characteristics allow it to interact effectively with these enzymes, thereby ensuring that the core peptide is modified in a precise and efficient manner [77]. Moreover, the leader peptide often functions to maintain the precursor peptide in an inactive state until the modifications of the core peptide are fully completed [78]. This regulation is crucial for ensuring that the peptide remains non-functional until it has undergone the necessary alterations to become biologically active.

Follower peptides and specific recognition sequences also play a significant role in assisting PTM enzymes [48]. They provide crucial information that helps these enzymes accurately target specific sites on the core peptide for modification. For example, in the case of the plant PTM enzyme known as PCY1, it recognizes the core peptide with the assistance of a follower peptide called AYDG. This interaction is vital for catalyzing the macrocyclization of the precursor peptide, leading to the formation of orbitides, structurally characterized by their head-to-tail cyclic peptides with N-to-C amide bonds [79]. A detailed understanding of PTMs not only provides insights into the molecular mechanisms behind peptide maturation, but also opens avenues for exploring the therapeutic potentials of these modified peptides in various biomedical applications.

The maturation of modified precursor peptides into RiPPs is a critical process that occurs through the proteolytic cleavage of the leader peptide and any other accompanying peptide sequences by specific enzymes known as proteases. This proteolytic removal is a finely tuned mechanism that can occur in several distinct ways. One common method is a one-step removal, where a single protease efficiently cleaves the leader peptide in one action, resulting in the immediate release of the mature RiPPs (Figure 3A) [73]. Alternatively, the process may involve a two-step removal, which can be executed either by two separate proteases acting sequentially or by a single protease performing two distinct cleavages at different sites (Figure 3B) [80]. The specificity of protease substrate recognition is a significant aspect of this maturation process, ensuring that the correct peptide sequences are cleaved at the appropriate points. For example, LahT150, a Cys protease, has been reported to remove double Gly-type leader peptides during the proteolysis of lanthipeptide, a microbial RiPP [81,82]. Currently, lantipeptides are classified as RiPPs produced by microorganisms, and the overall context of plant and microbial RiPP bio-synthesis pathways is similar [83].

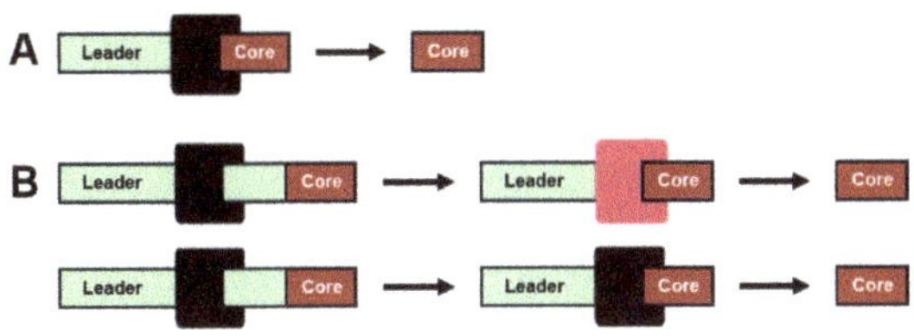

Figure 3. Diagram of proteolysis mechanisms in the biosynthetic pathways of plant RiPPs. (**A**) One-step removal of peptides. In this mechanism, the peptide sequence upstream or downstream of the core peptide is removed in a single step by one enzyme during maturation into the final RiPP product. (**B**) Two-step removal of peptides. In this mechanism, peptide sequences are removed through a multi-step process, either by the sequential activity of different enzymes or by repeated actions of the same enzyme.

2.3. Genetic and Biochemical Regulation of RiPP Biosynthesis

A key characteristic of plant RiPP biosynthesis is that RiPPs contain specific sequences encoding distinct functional domains. These precursor peptides undergo PTMs facilitated by various enzymes, leading to the formation of mature, functional RiPPs. While the exact mechanisms and pathways of biosynthesis differ among plant RiPP classes, much remains to be understood. Nonetheless, cyclotides and orbitides are among the most well-studied classes of plant RiPPs, with their biosynthetic processes being more thoroughly elucidated.

Cyclotides, one of the most recognized classes of plant RiPPs, are head-to-tail macrocyclic peptides characterized by a "cyclic cystine knot" motif, which involves three disulfide bonds [84,85]. These bonds contribute to the remarkable structural stability of cyclotides [86]. The biosynthesis of cyclotides begins with a precursor peptide that typically contains an N-terminal endoplasmic reticulum (ER)-targeting signal sequence, an optional N-terminal leader peptide, one or more core peptide sequences, and a C-terminal follower peptide (Figure 4A). This precursor peptide is first directed to the ER via the signal sequence [87]. In the ER, it undergoes structural stabilization through folding and the formation of disulfide bonds, facilitated by disulfide isomerase [88]. This process establishes the distinct knot structure of the cyclotide, contributing to its stability and function. After stabilization, all peptides upstream of the core peptide are removed by N-terminal processing proteases, such as kalatase A, exposing the N-terminal amino acid (typically glycine) of the core peptide [89]. The final and critical step in cyclotide biosynthesis involves the head-to-tail cyclization of the peptide. This reaction is catalyzed by an asparaginyl endopeptidase (AEP)-like ligase, such as butelase 1 [90,91]. The enzyme catalyzes the formation of a bond between the N-terminal glycine and the C-terminal asparagine (or aspartate), removing the C-terminal peptide and completing the cyclization process. This step is particularly important as it contributes to the unique structural stability and bioactivity of cyclotides, which are known for their resistance to proteolytic degradation and their roles in plant defense [92,93].

Orbitides, another notable class of plant RiPPs, are smaller and simpler head-to-tail macrocyclic peptides that lack disulfide bonds [94]. The precursor peptide of an orbitide typically consists of a leader, one or more core peptides, and a follower peptide (Figure 4B). Its regulation is similar to that of cyclotides, but is less complex due to the absence of disulfide bonds [33,65,95]. The biosynthetic pathway of orbitides varies slightly depending on the type of RiPP. In the biosynthesis of segetalin A in *V. hispanica*, the peptide upstream of the core peptide in the segetalin A precursor peptide is first removed by an unidentified oligopeptidase 1 (OLP1) [79]. The resulting presegetalin A1 then undergoes macrocyclization as the C-terminal peptide is cleaved by peptide cyclase 1 (PCY1).

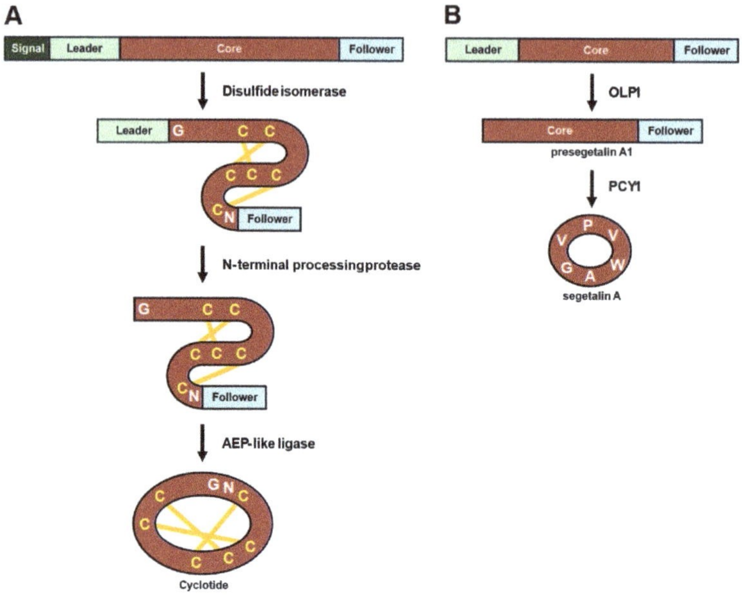

Figure 4. Scheme of biosynthetic pathways for a typical cyclotide (**A**) and the orbitide, segetalin A (**B**). (**A**) Cyclotide biosynthesis. The cyclotide precursor peptide is transported to the ER via an N-terminal signal sequence. Disulfide bonds are first formed by a disulfide isomerase. Subsequently, N-terminal processing proteases remove all peptides upstream of the core peptide, including the leader peptide. Finally, the head-to-tail cyclization of the core peptide is facilitated by an AEP-like ligase, which also removes the downstream peptide sequences, yielding the mature cyclotide. (**B**) Segetalin A biosynthesis. The precursor peptide for segetalin A first undergoes leader peptide removal by OLP1, resulting in presegetalin A1. Subsequently, PCY1 catalyzes macrocylization to produce the mature segetalin A.

Understanding the specific regulatory mechanisms of plant RiPP biosynthesis can offer valuable insights into the production and discovery of promising compounds that may be utilized in the development of new therapeutics [96,97]. However, many aspects of the biosynthesis process remain to be explored, and further research appears necessary to discover new RiPPs.

3. Discovery of Plant-Derived RiPPs

3.1. Ethnobotanical Approaches and Traditional Knowledge

The discovery and identification of plant-derived RiPPs often stems from the foundational knowledge provided by ethnobotanical research, which focuses on the medicinal use of plants in traditional cultures [98]. For centuries, plants have been employed in treating various ailments, including cancer, and this historical context provides valuable insight into identifying species with potential bioactive RiPPs [99–101]. Ethnobotanical data are instrumental in guiding the selection of specific plants for further investigation, particularly those with documented therapeutic properties against cancer [102]. Once promising species are identified, their compounds are isolated and subjected to biological activity screening. This targeted approach, informed by traditional knowledge, enables researchers to prioritize species and extracts with a higher probability of yielding biologically active RiPPs, thereby enhancing the efficiency of discovering therapeutically relevant peptides [103,104].

3.2. High-Throughput Screening and Bioassay-Guided Isolation

High-throughput screening (HTS) and bioassay-guided isolation are essential methodologies in uncovering plant-derived RiPPs with anticancer potential [105]. These techniques enable efficient identification and isolation of bioactive phytochemicals from complex plant extracts, significantly advancing the discovery of new phytochemicals. HTS serves as a powerful tool, allowing researchers to rapidly evaluate the biological activity of large libraries of compounds, including plant extracts, fractions, or purified substances. The value of HTS lies in its ability to simultaneously screen thousands to millions of samples against a specific biological target, such as cancer cell lines, within a relatively short timeframe, making it indispensable in the field of compound discovery [106].

HTS usually relies on automation to efficiently handle the vast number of samples and assays involved. Robotic systems are employed for sample preparation, mixing, and dispensing into microtiter plates, which typically contain 96, 384, or 1536 wells. Each well contains a small volume of plant extract or fraction along with the designated biological target, such as cancer cells or enzymes, for screening. Detection methods in HTS, including fluorescence, luminescence, absorbance, and radioactivity, are selected based on the assay type [107]. For instance, fluorescent markers are frequently used to measure cell viability, where a reduction in fluorescence signifies cytotoxic effects on cancer cells. In cases where specific plants are already known to produce RiPPs from prior phytochemical studies, HTS can be applied to screen various plant extracts or purified fractions for their ability to inhibit cancer cell proliferation, induce apoptosis, or target cancer-specific pathways. By combining HTS with bioassay-guided isolation, researchers can adopt a comprehensive approach to identify novel RiPPs, presenting promising leads for the development of new anticancer therapies [108].

3.3. Genomic and Bioinformatic Approaches

Recent advancements in genomic and bioinformatic technologies have revolutionized the discovery of plant-derived RiPPs [109]. These cutting-edge approaches enable researchers to investigate the genetic information of plants, uncovering the specific genes and pathways involved in RiPP biosynthesis. Through comprehensive analysis of plant genomes and transcriptomes, biosynthetic gene clusters (BGCs) responsible for RiPP production can be identified, with predictions about the structure and function of the specific RiPPs [110,111]. Genome sequencing across various plant species, particularly those used in traditional medicine, has led to the discovery of novel RiPP BGCs that may have remained unidentified through conventional bioassay-guided methods. This genomic approach is especially valuable for finding RiPPs with anticancer potential, as each plant species harbors unique BGCs that produce structurally diverse and biologically potent peptides [112]. Advanced bioinformatics platforms, such as antiSMASH, PRISM, and RiPPER, further enhance this process by predicting and annotating RiPP BGCs, significantly streamlining the discovery of new bioactive peptides [113–115]. Moroidins, a newly characterized class of plant RiPPs, exhibit a unique biosynthetic mechanism involving a copper-dependent BURP domain, KjaBURP, which catalyzes their macrocyclization [35]. Notably, moroidin peptides differ from other BURP-domain-derived RiPPs, as they feature a histidine at the C-terminus instead of a tyrosine or tryptophan, resulting in distinct imidazole-indole cross-links.

Genomic approaches not only help in identifying gene clusters but also provide insights into the regulation and expression of specific RiPP BGCs [116]. Advanced techniques like RNA sequencing allow researchers to examine gene expression profiles across different plant tissues or under varying environmental conditions. By understanding the expression of RiPP BGCs, researchers can optimize experimental conditions for RiPP production in heterologous systems [117]. This knowledge is crucial for scaling up the production of RiPPs, facilitating further biological testing, and advancing their development as potential therapeutics.

4. Anticancer RiPPs from Plants

4.1. Anticancer RiPPs from the Caryophyllaceae Family

The Caryophyllaceae family, commonly referred to as the carnation or pink family, encompasses around 90 genera and over 2000 species of flowering plants. Many species within this family are widely cultivated as ornamental plants, some have also garnered scientific attention for their bioactive properties. Among these, certain species produce RiPPs, which have demonstrated significant therapeutic potential. Notably, these RiPPs have been found to exhibit anticancer properties, with the ability to suppress cancer cell growth and trigger apoptosis. This has positioned plants from the Caryophyllaceae family as valuable natural sources in the discovery for physiologically active phytochemicals, particularly in the development of novel anticancer lead compounds [118–120].

Dianthus superbus L. is a pinkish herbaceous perennial plant growing up to 80 cm in height. It is distributed in Europe, northern Asia, France, and Japan. *D. superbus*, a plant from the Caryophyllaceae family, is commonly utilized in traditional Chinese medicine, particularly as a diuretic and anti-inflammatory agent. It is traditionally employed in the treatment of urinary infections, carbuncles, and carcinoma of the esophagus [121,122]. Phytochemical investigation on the methanolic extract of the dried and powdered whole plants of *D. superbus* led to the isolation of four phytochemicals (Figure 5). The cytotoxic activities of all identified compounds (**1–4**) were evaluated against five cancer cell lines: HepG2 (hepatocellular carcinoma), Hep3B (hepatocellular carcinoma), MCF-7 (breast adenocarcinoma), A549 (lung cancer cell line), and MDA-MB-231 (breast cell line), with doxorubicin serving as the positive control. The IC_{50} values (μg/mL) were used to evaluate the cytotoxic efficacy of all isolated compounds. Among the compounds tested, dianthin E (**1**) exhibited the highest cytotoxicity against the HepG2 cell line, with an IC_{50} value of 2.37 μg/mL, followed by 4-methoxydianthramide B (**4**), which showed moderate activity against 4.08 μg/mL (HepG2) and 16.02 μg/mL (Hep3B). Dianthin C (**2**) displayed weak cytotoxicity against 17.17 μg/mL (HepG2), while dianthin D (**3**) demonstrated no significant cytotoxic effects, as its IC_{50} values were greater than 20 μg/mL for all cell lines tested [123].

Stellaria yunnanensis Franch. is native to the Yunnan and Sichuan regions of China, flourishing in temperate environments. This perennial plant grows in shaded, moist areas, featuring long stems that extend over significant distances. Previous phytochemical investigations from the plant have uncovered several bioactive compounds in its root extracts, including cyclic peptides like yunnanin A, B, and C [124]. These peptides, particularly yunnanin C (**5**), have demonstrated potent cytotoxic activities. Yunnanin C (**5**) showed strong inhibitory effects against murine leukemia cells (P-388), with an IC_{50} value of 2.2 μg/mL (Figure 5). Additionally, it has shown antiproliferative activity against various cancer cell lines, including J774.A1 and WEHI-164, with IC_{50} values ranging from 2.1 to 7.5 μg/mL. Interestingly, synthetic analogs of these peptides, which involve slight modifications, did not exhibit the same level of cytotoxicity, potentially due to conformational changes in proline residues during synthesis [125,126].

Dianthus chinensis L., commonly known as the China pink or rainbow pink, is an herbaceous perennial plant and has been widely distributed to various regions of East Asia, including northern China, Korea, Mongolia, and southeastern Russia. While *D. chinensis* has not been extensively documented for medicinal use, related species in the Dianthus genus have been used in traditional medicine for their potential anti-inflammatory, antioxidant, and antimicrobial properties [127,128]. Phytochemical investigation on *D. chinensis* has led to the discovery of a class of proline-containing cyclic peptides, known as dianthiamides, and commonly referred to as orbitides. The identification and structural elucidation of dianthiamides A–E were achieved by the analysis of nuclear magnetic resonance (NMR) and mass spectrometry (MS) data [129]. Notably, dianthiamide A (**6**) exhibited cytotoxic effects against the A549 human lung cancer cell line, with an IC_{50} value of 47.9 μM, signifying a moderate ability to inhibit the proliferation of these cancer cells (Figure 5) [129].

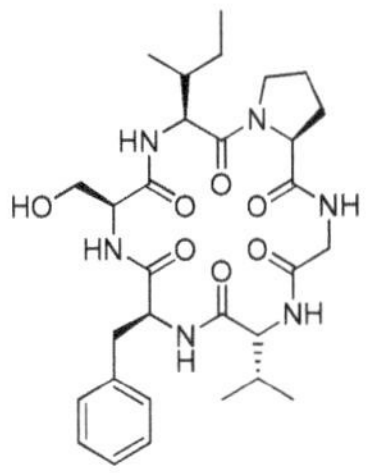

1

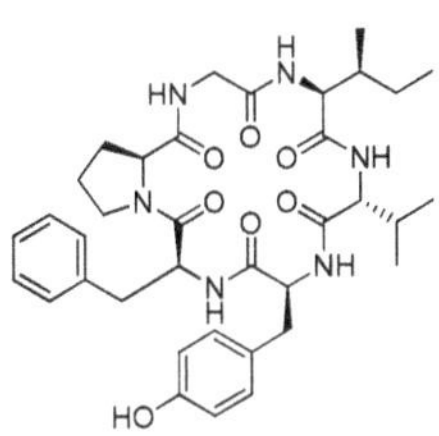

2

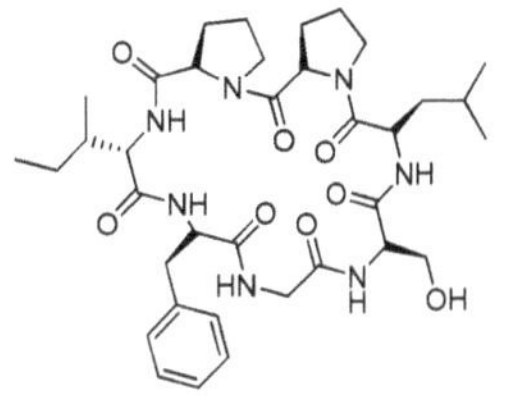

3

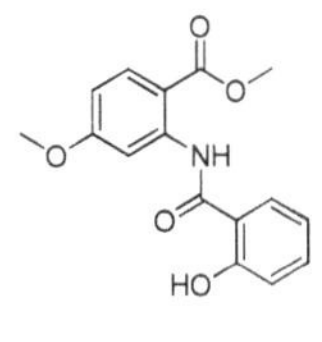

4

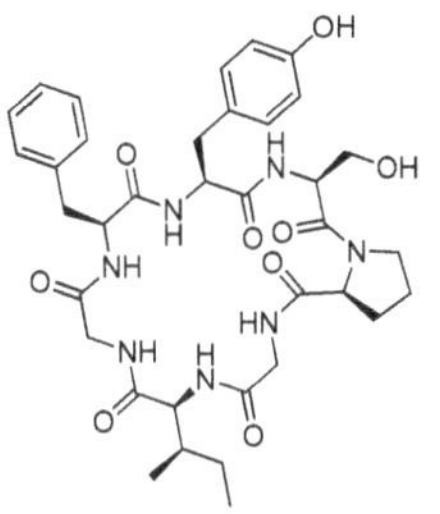

5

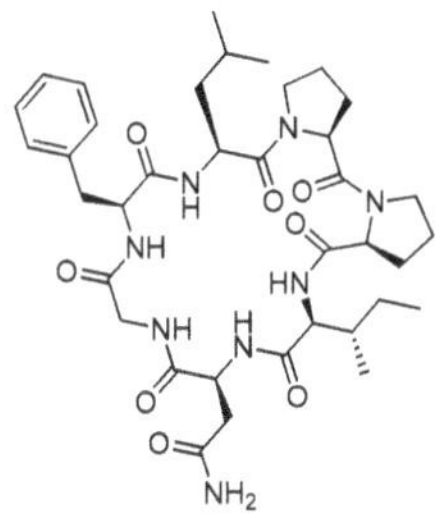

6

Figure 5. Chemical structures of compounds **1–6**.

4.2. *Anticancer RiPPs from the Rubiaceae Family*

Rubia cordifolia L. is a perennial climber native to tropical and subtropical regions of Asia, including India, Nepal, and China. This plant has long been utilized in traditional folk medicine for treating various ailments such as cough, bladder and kidney stones, joint inflammation, uterine hemorrhage, and uteritis [130]. The plant is particularly rich in anthraquinones like alizarin and purpurin, compounds that not only contribute to its dyeing properties but also its medicinal effects [131–134]. Recent studies have shown that methanol extract of the dried root of *R. cordifolia* contains the cyclic hexapeptides RA-XXIII (**7**) and RA-XXIV (**8**) (Figure 6). These compounds have demonstrated notable cytotoxic activity, particularly against leukemia cells. RA-XXIII exhibited an IC_{50} value of 0.16 μg/mL and RA-XXIV showed a value of 0.48 μg/mL against P-388 leukemia cells [135]. Notably, cyclic hexapeptide RA-V has shown potential to modulate cancer-related signaling pathways, particularly targeting pathways like Wnt, Myc, and Notch [136].

Rubia podantha Diels is a perennial shrub native to Europe and North Africa, thriving in various habitats such as grasslands, scrub forests, and rocky areas. The roots and rhizomes of *R. podantha* have been traditionally employed in herbal medicine to address a range of digestive disorders, attributed to the plant's mild laxative properties that facilitate digestion and alleviate constipation [137]. Additionally, phytochemical analyses suggested that extracts from the plant possess significant anti-inflammatory effects, indicating its potential utility in the management of conditions such as arthritis and muscle pain. Compounds **9–14** were isolated from the roots and rhizomes of *R. podantha* (Figure 6). The cytotoxic effect of compounds **9–14** was assessed against cancer cell lines, including MDA-MB-231, SW620 (human colon cancer cell line), and HepG2, with IC_{50} values ranging from 0.015

to 10.27 μM. The cytotoxic effect of compounds **15** and **16** was also assessed against HeLa (cervical cancer cell line), A549, and SGC-7901 (gastric cancer cell line). RA-X (**15**) showed IC_{50} values of 3.80 ± 0.17 μM for SGC-7901, 7.14 ± 0.81 μM for A549, and 7.22 ± 0.76 μM for HeLa. Rubipodanin A (**16**) showed IC_{50} values of 0.0058 ± 0.0016 μM for SGC-7901, 0.017 ± 0.0026 μM for A549, and 0.015 ± 0.0014 μM for HeLa [138,139].

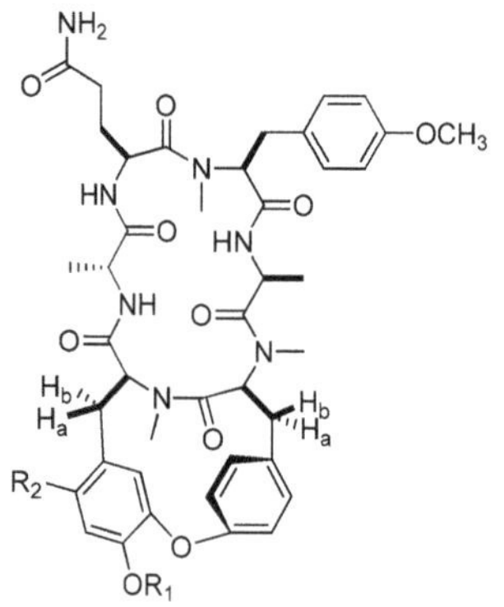

7 $R_1 = CH_3$, $R_2 = H$
8 $R_1 = R_2 = H$

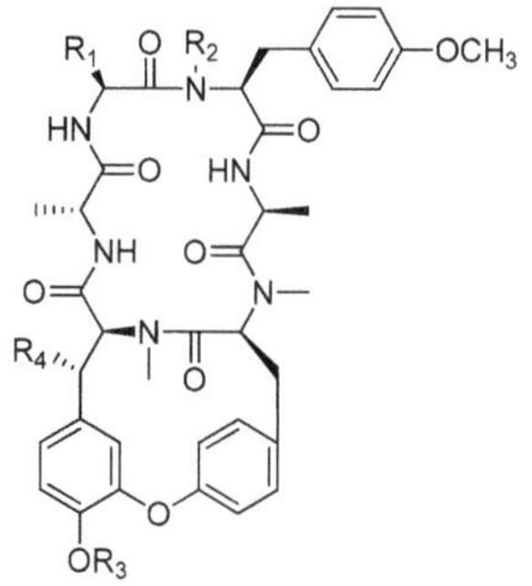

9 $R_1 = CH_3$, $R_2 = CH_3$, $R_3 = H$, $R_4 = H$
10 $R_1 = CH_3$, $R_2 = CH_3$, $R_3 = H$, $R_4 = H$
11 $R_1 = CH_2CH_2COOEt$, $R_2 = CH_3$, $R_3 = H$, $R_4 = H$
12 $R_1 = CH_2CH_2COOCH_3$, $R_2 = CH_3$, $R_3 = CH_3$, $R_4 = H$
13 $R_1 = CH_2CH_2COOCH_3$, $R_2 = CH_3$, $R_3 = H$, $R_4 = H$
14 $R_1 = CH_2COOH$, $R_2 = CH_3$, $R_3 = H$, $R_4 = H$

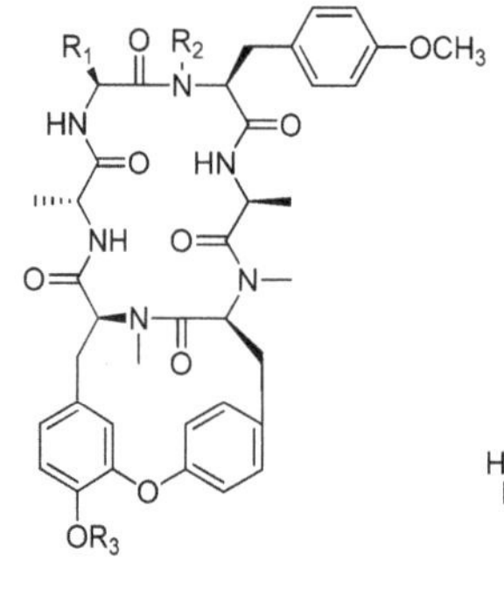

15 $R_1 = CH_3$, $R_2 = CH_3$, $R_3 = H$
16 $R_1 = CH_3$, $R_2 = H$, $R_3 = H$

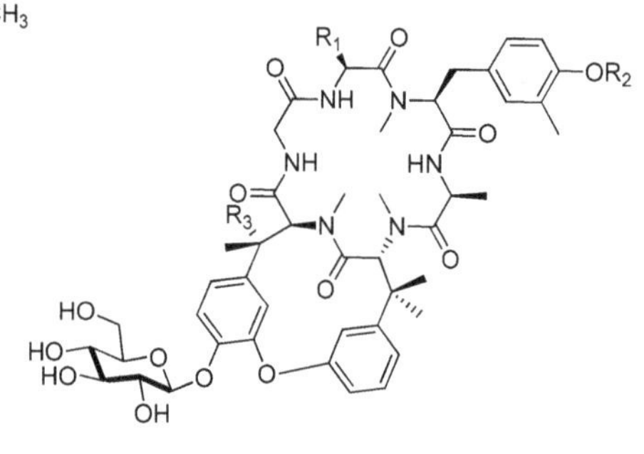

17 $R_1 = CH_2CH_2CONH_2$, $R_2 = CH_3$, $R_3 = H$
18 $R_1 = CH_3$, $R_2 = H$, $R_3 = H$
19 $R_1 = CH_3$, $R_2 = CH_3$, $R_3 = OH$
20 $R_1 = CH_3$, $R_2 = CH_3$, $R_3 = H$
21 $R_1 = CH_2OH$, $R_2 = CH_3$, $R_3 = H$

Figure 6. Chemical structures of cyclic peptides **7–21**.

Rubia yunnanensis Diels. is a perennial herb native to Yunnan province in China. Traditionally, its roots have been employed in Chinese medicine to address various health issues, including tuberculosis, and specifically to aid in treating respiratory conditions. It is also utilized for reliving menoxenia and possesses anti-inflammatory properties beneficial for rheumatism. Furthermore, *R. yunnanensis* is effective in treating contusions and hematemesis, assisting with bruising and blood coughing, which are common in respiratory and gastrointestinal disorders [140–143]. Additionally, it supports blood production in anemia and is used to treat lipomas, benign fatty tumors, in traditional practices. Rubiyunnanins (**17–21**) isolated from the plant exhibit significant bioactivity, including cytotoxic effects against various cancer cell lines and the ability to inhibit nitric oxide (NO) production, which is associated with inflammation (Figure 6). They also suppress the NF-κB signaling pathway, a critical regulator of inflammation, immune responses, and cancer, positioning them as promising candidates for anti-cancer and anti-inflammatory therapies. Among the compounds, compound **10** showed exceptional cytotoxicity, with IC_{50} values as low as 0.01 μM against several cancer cell lines, including HepG2 (human hepatocellular carcinoma) and A549 (non-small cell lung carcinoma). This compound exhibits particularly potent activity in MDA-MB-231 (human breast carcinoma) and B16 (murine melanoma) cell lines, where it achieves IC_{50} values of 0.01 μM and 0.001 μM, respectively, highlighting its broad-spectrum antitumor efficacy. The low IC_{50} values suggest that **17** may interact effectively with critical cellular pathways, potentially leading to apoptosis in cancer cells while sparing normal cells [144].

4.3. Anticancer RiPPs from the Euphorbiaceae Family

Mallotus spodocarpus Airy Shaw. is native to Southeast Asia, particularly Thailand. Traditionally, the roots of the plant are often processed into a fine powder and applied topically to the skin to lighten pigmentation, treat dark spots, and enhance overall skin complexion. In addition to its cosmetic applications, *M. spodocarpus* has been employed in traditional remedies for various ailments, such as wound healing and treating skin conditions [145]. The plant's extract is also believed to possess antioxidant properties, which contribute to its effectiveness in promoting skin health and potentially preventing skin damage. Recent studies have explored the phytochemical composition of *M. spodocarpus*, revealing the presence of various bioactive compounds, including flavonoids and tannins, which may enhance its medicinal properties. Mallotumides A–C (**22**–**24**) were isolated and structurally characterized from the roots of *M. spodocarpus* (Figure 7). These compounds demonstrate potent cytotoxic activity against various cancer cell lines, including KKU-M213 (intrahepatic cholangiocarcinoma), FaDu (squamous cell carcinoma), HT-29 (colon carcinoma), MDA-MB-231 (human breast adenocarcinoma), A549 (lung carcinoma), and SH-SY5Y (neuroblastoma). The cytotoxic effects of mallotumides A–C were notably strong, with IC_{50} values ranging from 0.60 to 4.80 nM across all tested cell lines, highlighting their remarkable potential to inhibit cell proliferation [146].

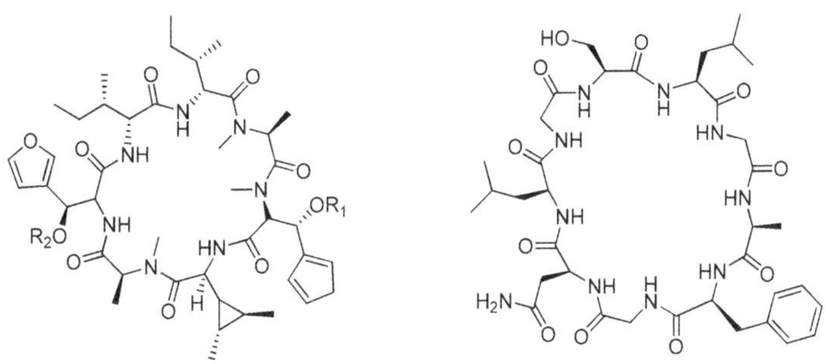

Figure 7. Chemical structures of cyclic peptides **22**–**25**.

Croton urucurana Baillon, native to the tropical and subtropical regions of South America, is commonly found in Argentina, Paraguay, Bolivia, and Brazil. In traditional medicine, *C. urucurana* has been used for its antimicrobial properties, often employed to treat infections due to its effectiveness against various pathogens. The plant's extracts have shown significant antimicrobial activity, supporting its historical use as a remedy for infections [147–149]. Additionally, the leaves and bark of the plant have been utilized for their anti-inflammatory effects. This characteristic makes the plant beneficial in treating conditions such as arthritis and other inflammatory diseases. Its extracts are thought to alleviate inflammation and associated discomfort. In a previous phytochemical study, [1-9-NαC]-crourorb A1 (**25**) was isolated from a 95% ethanol extract of *C. urucurana* (Figure 7). The compound was assessed for its cytotoxic activity against six human cancer cell lines: 786-0 (kidney carcinoma), HT-29 (colon carcinoma), MCF-7 (breast adenocarcinoma), NCI-ADR/RES (ovarian adenocarcinoma with multidrug resistance), Hep-G2 (liver carcinoma), and PC-03 (prostate carcinoma). The GI_{50} values, indicating the concentration required to inhibit 50% of cell growth, were as follows: Hep-G2 (41.31 $\pm$ 2.70 µg/mL), HT-29 (37.28 $\pm$ 0.57 µg/mL), MCF-7 (35.49 $\pm$ 2.59 µg/mL), PC-03 (29.80 $\pm$ 0.34 µg/mL), 786-0 (18.69 $\pm$ 0.82 µg/mL), and NCI-ADR/RES (3.98 $\pm$ 0.20 µg/mL) [150].

4.4. Anticancer RiPPs from the Miscellaneous Families

Celosia cristata L. (Amaranthaceae) is a medicinal herb traditionally employed to treat various ailments, including fatigue, atherosclerosis, leucorrhea, and osteoporosis. This annual plant, originating from tropical regions, is characterized by its herbaceous structure, which lacks a woody stem [151–154]. From the butanol-soluble fraction of a 70% ethanol extract of *C. cristata* seeds, the cytotoxic moroidin (**26**) was purified and structurally characterized (Figure 8). The cytotoxic effects of compound **26** were tested against six cancer cell lines: A549 (lung), H1299 (lung), U87 (human brain), U251 (human brain), HCT116 (human colon), and MCF-7 (breast). The results demonstrated that **26** displayed significant cytotoxicity against A549 lung cancer cells, with an IC_{50} value of 3.2 $\pm$ 0.5 µM. Additionally, it exhibited moderate cytotoxic effects against the H1299 (IC_{50} = 8.3 $\pm$ 0.7 µM), U87 (IC_{50} = 9.6 $\pm$ 1.8 µM), U251 (IC_{50} = 5.2 $\pm$ 0.8 µM), and HCT116 (IC_{50} = 9.9 $\pm$ 1.7 µM) cell lines. However, it was less effective against MCF-7 breast cancer cells [155].

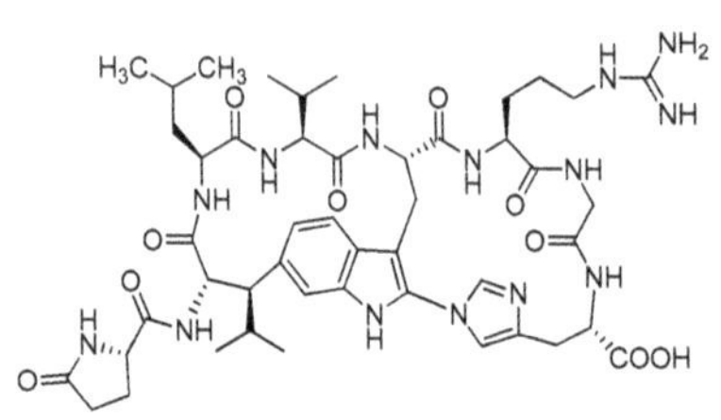

26

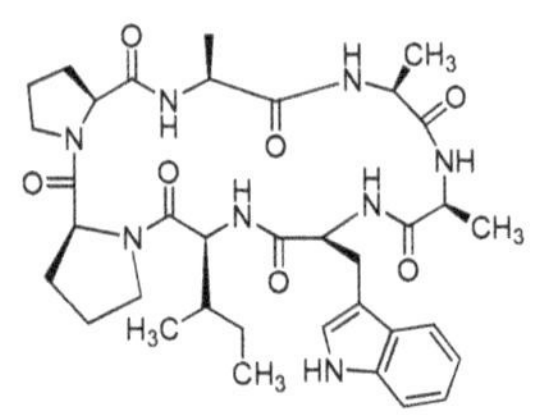

27

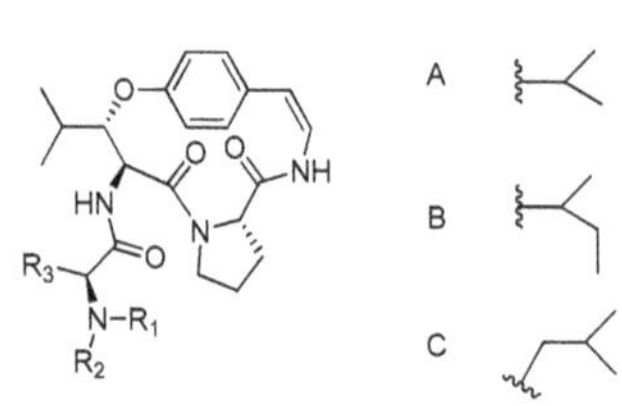

28 $R_1 = R_2 = CH_3$, R_3 = A
29 $R_1 = R_2 = CH_3$, R_3 = B
30 $R_1 = R_2 = CH_3$, R_3 = C

Figure 8. Chemical structures of cyclic peptides **26–30**.

Annona cherimola Miller. (Annonaceae), commonly known as cherimoya, is a species of fruit-bearing tree native to the Andean valleys of Ecuador, Peru, and Colombia that is now also cultivated in various tropical and subtropical regions. In traditional medicine, *A. cherimola* has been used for various purposes. Indigenous peoples in South America have utilized the leaves and bark for their potential therapeutic effects [156,157]. Traditionally, the leaves have been employed to treat digestive issues and respiratory ailments, while the seeds are known for their insecticidal properties. Moreover, the fruit is highly nutritious, rich in vitamins, minerals, and antioxidants, which may contribute to overall health and wellness. Cherimolacylopeptide C (**27**) was isolated from dried and ground seeds of *A. cherimola* (Figure 8). The cytotoxic effect of compound **27** was evaluated against KB cells (oral cancer cell line), with IC_{50} values of 0.072 μM [158].

Heisteria parvifolia Sm. (Olacaceae) is native to the Amazon rainforest, primarily found in countries such as Brazil, Colombia, and Peru. The leaves and bark of the plant have often been employed in folk remedies, believed to possess anti-inflammatory and analgesic properties. Traditionally, preparations made from the plant have been used to treat ailments such as fevers, gastrointestinal issues, and skin conditions. Cycloheisterin B (**28**), cycloheisterin D (**29**), and anorldianine (**30**) were isolated from the chloroform fraction of the leaves of *H. parvifolia* (Figure 8). The anti-proliferative activities of these cyclopeptide alkaloids were evaluated against K562 cells, a human chronic myeloid leukemia cell line. Compounds **28–30** exhibited significant anti-proliferative effects, with cell growth inhibition rates of 46%, 44%, and 43%, respectively, at a concentration of 100 μM [159].

Thymus musilii Velen (Lamiaceae) is a rare plant species primarily found in the Ha'il region of Saudi Arabia and is traditionally used in Mediterranean folk medicine. Local populations utilize the leaves and flowers of *T. musilii* as garnishes, in teas, and for treating various microbial diseases, particularly valuing its antimicrobial and anti-inflammatory properties [160–162]. A tripeptide (**31**) isolated from the methanolic extract of *T. musilii* exhibited significant cytotoxic effects, with IC_{50} values of 107.69 μg/mL against MCF-7, 153.54 μg/mL against HCT-116, and 194.70 μg/mL against A549 cell lines (Figure 9). Additionally, its docking score of −8.983 kcal/mol indicates a strong binding affinity to the MLK4 kinase domain (4UYA), suggesting its potential to disrupt critical cancer signaling pathways such as JNK and ERK [161].

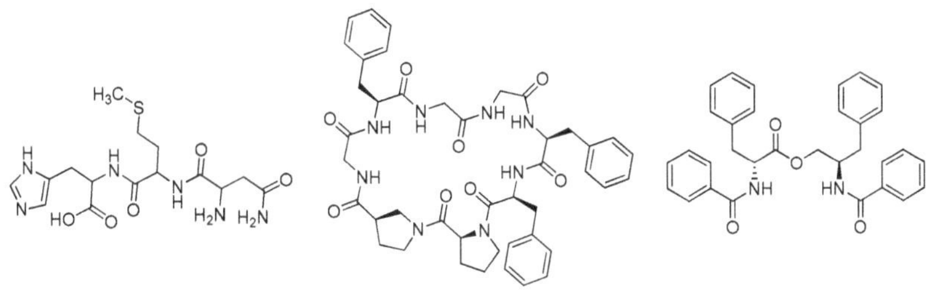

Figure 9. Chemical structures of peptides **31–33**.

Zanthoxylum riedelianum L. (Rutaceae) is widely distributed in South America, particularly found in Brazil and surrounding regions. The barks, leaves, and fruits of *Z. riedelianum* have been utilized for their potential medicinal properties, including anti-inflammatory, analgesic, antifungal, and antimicrobial effects [148,163]. In some cultures, extracts from the plant have been used to treat gastrointestinal disorders, respiratory issues, and skin ailments. Additionally, its antiseptic properties make it valuable for wound healing and in the preparation of traditional remedies against infections. *Z. riedelianum* yields a significant cyclic peptide known as [1-8-NαC]-zanriorb A1 (**32**), which exhibits notable cytotoxic activity against leukemia T cells (Jurkat) with an IC_{50} value of 218 nM (Figure 9) [164].

Colubrina asiatica L. (Rhamnaceae) is a climbing shrub native to Southeast Asia, northern Australia, and the Pacific islands, reaching heights of up to 4 m and commonly found in wetlands and coastal areas. This plant has traditional medicinal applications wherein its leaves and bark are used to treat skin diseases, while the roots are utilized to alleviate fever and thirst [165–167]. A derivative of *N*-benzoyl-D-phenylalanine (**33**) has been found to possess weak cytotoxicity against various cancer cell lines, including HeLa cervical cancer (KB), small cell lung carcinoma (NCI-H187), and human breast cancer (MCF-7). Specifically, compound **33** exhibited notable cytotoxicity against the NCI-H187 cell line, with an IC_{50} value of 19.51 μg/mL, marking it as the only peptide in this study to demonstrate such activity (Figure 9) [168].

5. Apoptotic Mechanisms Induced by Plant-Derived RiPPs in Cancer Cells

Caspases, a family of cysteine proteases, are central to the initiation and execution of apoptosis. Distinct caspases mediate either the intrinsic mitochondrial pathway or the extrinsic death receptor pathway, which converge to break apart cellular components and execute programmed cell death [169,170]. Identifying the specific caspases activated by plant-derived RiPPs is crucial for the identification of their apoptotic mechanisms. By selectively engaging caspase-3, caspase-8, caspase-3/7, or caspase-9, RiPPs effectively disrupt cancer cell survival pathways, providing a mechanistic foundation for their therapeutic potential [171,172]. Furthermore, understanding the link between the chemical structure of RiPPs and their ability to activate caspases is crucial for designing and optimizing RiPP-based anticancer agents (Table 1).

Vigno 5, a cyclotide isolated from *Viola ignobilis*, induced apoptosis in HeLa by activating caspase-3 and caspase-9 [173]. The apoptosis was mediated through the mitochondrial pathway, characterized by the release of cytochrome C, upregulation of Bax, downregulation of Bcl-2, and cleavage of PARP1, ultimately leading to DNA fragmentation. Similarly, orbitides identified from *Linum usitatissimum* L. have been shown to activate caspase-3 and caspase-9 in SGC-7901 via mitochondrial depolarization and Bax/Bcl-2 ratio modulation, resulting in PARP cleavage and apoptosis [174].

[1–9-NαC]-crourorb A1, a orbitide identified from *C. urucurana* latex, activated caspase-3/7 in Huh-7 (human hepatocarcinoma cell line) [175], inducing apoptosis through G2/M cell cycle arrest and a JNK-mediated pathway. This process was accompanied by increased expression of pro-apoptotic proteins, including Bak, Bax, and Puma, highlighting its potential for targeting liver cancer.

Another orbitide, flaxseed-derived linusorbs, also exhibited significant caspase activation in various cancer cells. [1–9-NαC]-linusorb B2 activated caspase-3 and caspase-8 in HepG2 [176] and SGC-7901 [177]. In HepG2, the DR4 death receptor pathway was involved, while in SGC-7901, the Fas/FasL signaling cascade triggered apoptosis, resulting in mitochondrial dysfunction and PARP cleavage. [1–9-NαC]-linusorb B3 demonstrated a broad apoptotic profile across multiple cancer cell lines. In HepG2, it activated caspase-3 and caspase-8 via DR4-mediated apoptosis, involving Bax upregulation, cytochrome C release, and Bcl-2 downregulation [176]. In SGC-7901, it activated caspase-3, caspase-8, and caspase-9, involving dual intrinsic and extrinsic pathways [177]. Furthermore, in C6 (glioblastoma cell line), it induced caspase-3 and caspase-9 activation via mitochondrial-mediated apoptosis, characterized by mitochondrial membrane depolarization and p53 suppression [178].

Moroidin, isolated from the seeds of *C. cristata*, activated caspase-3 and caspase-9 in A549 through the intrinsic mitochondrial pathway [155]. This involved cytochrome C release, Bax upregulation, Bcl-2 downregulation, and PARP cleavage, resulting in apoptotic cell death. Moroidin is categorized as a burpitide, a subclass of RiPPs derived from or associated with the BURP domain, which plays a key role in plant development and responses to environmental stress. [179].

RA-V, a cyclopeptide isolated from *R. cordifolia*, selectively activated caspase-3 in Kras-dependent non-small-cell lung carcinoma (NSCLC) cell lines (H441 and H358) [180]. This apoptotic activity was mediated by TAK1 inhibition, leading to reduced expression of anti-apoptotic proteins such as Bcl-2 and Bcl-XL. RA-V from *R. yunnanensis* also activated caspase-3 and caspase-9 in breast cancer cell lines (MCF-7 and MDA-MB-231) [181], with apoptosis mediated by mitochondrial dysfunction, cytochrome C release, and PARP cleavage. Additionally, RA-XII, another cyclopeptide from *R. yunnanensis*, induced caspase-3, caspase-8, and caspase-9 activation in HepG2 through Bax upregulation, Bcl-2 downregulation, and cytochrome C release, ultimately leading to mitochondrial-mediated apoptosis [182].

Table 1. Types of caspases activated by plant-derived RiPPs for cancer cells.

Compounds	Type	Source (Plant)	Target	Cell Line	Ref.
Vigno 5	Cyclotide	*Viola ignobilis*	Caspase-3, -9	HeLa	[173]
Flaxseed orbitides (extract)	Orbitide	*Linum usitatissimum* L.	Caspase-3, -9	SGC-7901	[174]
[1–9-NαC]-crourorb A1	Orbitide	*Croton urucurana*	Caspase-3/7	Huh-7	[175]
[1–9-NαC]-Linusorb B2	Orbitide	*L. usitatissimum* L.	Caspase-3, -8	HepG2	[176]
			Caspase-3, -8	SGC-7901	[177]
[1–9-NαC]-Linusorb B3	Orbitide	*L. usitatissimum* L.	Caspase-3, -8	HepG2	[176]
			Caspase-3, -8, -9	SGC-7901	[177]
			Caspase-3, -9	C6	[178]
Moroidin	Burpitide	*Celosia cristata*	Caspase-3, -9	A549	[155]
RA-V	Undefined	*Rubia cordifolia*	Caspase-3	H441	[180]
			Caspase-3	H358	[180]
		R. yunnanensis	Caspase-3, -9	MCF-7	[181]
			Caspase-3, -9	MDA-MB-231	[181]
RA-XII	Undefined	*R. yunnanensis*	Caspase-3, -8, -9	HepG2	[182]

6. Challenges in the Development of Plant-Derived RiPPs as Anticancer Agents

6.1. Complexity of RiPP Biosynthesis

A significant challenge in developing plant-derived RiPPs lies in the complexity of their biosynthetic processes. RiPPs are produced from precursor peptides through a series of enzymatic modifications, which can differ greatly across plant species. This variability is due to the diversity of BGCs in different plants, resulting in structural variations in RiPPs. These variations are driven by evolutionary forces that adapt biosynthetic pathways for advantages such as increased pathogen resistance or better ecological interactions. As a result, discovering and characterizing these BGCs is a critical yet difficult task in the search for novel anticancer RiPPs [54].

RiPPs undergo extensive post-translational modifications (PTMs) following their initial ribosomal synthesis, adding complexity to the identification and characterization of plant-derived RiPPs [48]. Although different plants may produce similar precursor peptides, the modifications they undergo can vary significantly, leading to distinct biological activities. Understanding these modifications is essential for harnessing the therapeutic potential of plant-derived RiPPs. Many plant-derived RiPPs possess cyclic structures that enhance their stability and resistance to enzymatic breakdown, contributing to stronger interactions with biological targets. These PTMs, such as methylation, hydroxylation, and phosphorylation, affect the peptide's charge, hydrophobicity, and structure, ultimately influencing its affinity and specificity for binding to cellular receptors or enzymes, and improving its therapeutic efficacy [183,184].

The complexity of RiPP biosynthesis presents both challenges and opportunities for the development of plant-derived RiPPs as anticancer agents [185]. While the diverse PTMs and genetic variability complicate the identification and characterization of their chemical structures, they also provide a rich source of novel compounds with unique structures and mechanisms of action. By leveraging advanced genomic, proteomic, and metabolomic approaches, researchers can unlock the potential of RiPPs, optimizing their biosynthesis for therapeutic applications and ultimately paving the way for the development of new cancer treatments [186].

6.2. *Low Yield and Purification Challenges*

Identification of plant-derived RiPPs as anticancer agents is significantly hindered by the low yield and purification challenges. Many plant-derived RiPPs occur in minute quantities within their natural plant hosts, which poses a considerable challenge for their isolation and identification. RiPPs are classified as secondary metabolites, which are not essential for the primary growth and reproduction of plants. Plants often produce them in response to specific environmental stimuli, such as defense against pathogens, herbivores, or stress [187]. Consequently, RiPP production tends to be inconsistent and varies depending on external factors. This makes it difficult to predict or control the amounts of RiPPs that can be extracted from plants under natural conditions. The BGCs responsible for RiPP biosynthesis in plants are often expressed at low levels or are activated only under specific conditions. As a result, even though a plant may possess the genetic capacity to produce a RiPP, the actual quantities synthesized may be insufficient for practical extraction and subsequent chromatographic isolation. This variability further complicates the production of RiPPs in quantities suitable for pharmaceutical research and development [188].

Plant tissues contain a wide array of biomolecules, including proteins, polysaccharides, lipids, and secondary metabolites, which complicate the isolation of RiPPs [47,186]. These compounds interfere with extraction and purification processes, making it challenging to isolate RiPPs. Moreover, RiPPs are often chemically unstable and susceptible to degradation when exposed to harsh extraction conditions, such as organic solvents, extreme pH, or elevated temperatures [189]. This instability results in the breakdown or modification of RiPPs, leading to diminished yields and loss of biological activity. Purification typically involves multiple chromatography steps, which are labor-intensive and costly [190]. The low yield of RiPPs from plants, combined with the complex purification protocols required, leads to significant losses and further reduces the overall efficiency of RiPP production.

While *D. chinensis* has demonstrated promising anticancer activity due to its RiPP-derived peptides, the yield of these compounds remains a challenge for large-scale production [191]. Additionally, toxicity concerns associated with certain peptides may limit their therapeutic application in clinical settings [192,193]. Similarly, *R. cordifolia* showed potential in traditional medicine, but the complexities involved in extracting and optimizing RiPPs for therapeutic use, alongside issues of limited yields and potential toxicity, need to be carefully addressed for future drug development [194].

Several strategies are being explored to overcome the low yield and extraction challenges associated with plant-derived RiPPs. Among the approaches, heterologous expression systems offer an alternative method for producing RiPPs in higher yields [195]. By transferring the BGCs responsible for RiPP production into microbial hosts, such as bacteria or yeast, researchers bypass the need for direct extraction from plants. These microbial systems can be engineered to overproduce RiPPs in controlled conditions, thereby increasing the yield and simplifying the purification process. Synthetic biology approaches that optimize RiPP BGCs for expression in heterologous hosts are being actively explored to address this challenge [196].

7. Conclusions

The exploration of plant RiPPs represents a significant advancement in the discovery of novel anticancer agents. This innovative field of research merges centuries of traditional ethnobotanical knowledge, derived from the medicinal use of plants, with cutting-edge genomic and bioinformatic technologies. By harnessing insights from ethnobotanical studies, researchers have identified plant species with documented therapeutic properties, thereby guiding the selection of candidates for further phytochemical investigation. This integrated approach markedly enhances the efficiency of discovering biologically active RiPPs that hold great promise for cancer treatment.

In this review, we focus on the discovery of plant RiPPs as valuable candidates for therapeutic applications in cancer treatment. While recent reviews have addressed various aspects of plant RiPPs, our emphasis lies specifically on their chemical structures and cytotoxic activities. The application of high-throughput screening (HTS) and bioassay-guided isolation methodologies has revolutionized the identification of bioactive RiPPs from complex plant extracts. These techniques facilitate the rapid evaluation of a wide array of phytochemicals, including fractions and purified RiPPs, against specific biological targets such as cancer cell lines.

Despite the promising advancements in the field of plant RiPPs as anticancer agents, several challenges impede their effective utilization. One significant hurdle lies in the inherent complexity of RiPP biosynthesis, as these peptides undergo a series of enzymatic modifications that exhibit considerable variability among different plant species. This variability in BGCs often leads to distinct structural variations among RiPPs, each associated with unique biological activities. A comprehensive understanding of these variations is essential for fully harnessing the therapeutic potential of plant RiPPs; however, this complexity complicates the identification and characterization processes. Additionally, the low yields of RiPPs and the challenges associated with their purification further exacerbate the difficulties faced in RiPP discovery. As secondary metabolites, RiPPs are typically found in minute quantities within their natural plant hosts, necessitating the development of sophisticated extraction and purification techniques to isolate these valuable compounds effectively.

To overcome these significant challenges, researchers are actively investigating innovative strategies, including heterologous expression systems and synthetic biology approaches. By transferring the BGCs responsible for RiPP production into microbial hosts such as bacteria or yeast, scientists have been able to achieve higher yields and simplify purification processes, thereby enabling more efficient production of these peptides.

Advances in synthetic biology and heterologous expression systems have significantly enhanced the potential for RiPP-based drug development. Synthetic biology facilitates the design and optimization of biosynthetic pathways, enabling the creation of novel RiPPs with tailored properties. This addresses critical challenges such as low yields and structural complexity. By manipulating BGCs, researchers can design peptides with enhanced bioactivity, stability, and specificity, thereby broadening their therapeutic applications. Moreover, heterologous expression systems, particularly when applied to plant or microbial BGCs, allow for the scalable production of RiPPs that are difficult to obtain from natural sources. These systems enable the expression of complex RiPPs in high yields, overcoming limitations associated with low natural production or host toxicity. This capability opens new avenues for pharmaceutical development, accelerating the testing and commercialization of novel RiPP-based therapeutics. As synthetic biology and heterologous expression technologies continue to evolve, the rapid and cost-effective development of RiPP-based drugs is becoming increasingly feasible. These advancements are driving transformative changes in drug discovery and biotechnology. Additionally, complementary technologies such as HTS, bioassay-guided isolation, and genomic studies play pivotal roles in overcoming existing barriers, enabling the discovery and production of more efficient RiPP-based treatments.

In conclusion, the future of plant RiPPs as anticancer agents is promising yet fraught with challenges. The ongoing collaboration between ethnobotanists, molecular biologists, and chemists is essential to navigate the complexities associated with RiPP biosynthesis and to unlock their full therapeutic potential. By combining traditional knowledge with modern scientific advancements, we may pave the way for innovative cancer treatments that not only harness the rich biodiversity of various natural sources but also contribute to the development of safer and more effective therapeutic options. Ultimately, this synergy can unlock the full potential of plant-derived RiPPs, paving the way for advancements in cancer treatment and contributing to the field of natural product research.

Author Contributions: Conceptualization, S.R.L.; formal analysis, H.-J.H., Y.N. and C.J.; investigation, H.-J.H., Y.N. and C.J.; writing—original draft preparation, H.-J.H., Y.N., C.J. and S.R.L.; writing—review and editing, S.R.L.; visualization, H.-J.H., Y.N., C.J., E.L.K., E.S.J., Y.J.L. and S.R.L.; supervision, S.R.L.; project administration, S.R.L.; funding acquisition, S.R.L. All authors have read and agreed to the published version of the manuscript.

Funding: This work was supported by a 2-Year Research Grant of Pusan National University.

Data Availability Statement: Not applicable.

Conflicts of Interest: The authors declare no conflicts of interest.

References

1. Sivaram, S.; Perkins, S.; He, M.; Ginsburg, E.; Dominguez, G.; Vedham, V.; Katz, F.; Parascandola, M.; Bogler, O.; Gopal, S. Building capacity for global cancer research: Existing opportunities and future directions. *J. Cancer Educ.* **2021**, *36*, 5–24. [CrossRef]
2. de Araújo, C.P. Introduction. In *Palliative Treatment for Advanced Cancer Patients*; Springer: Cham, Switzerland, 2023; pp. 1–7.
3. OECD. *Health at a Glance 2023*; OECD Indicator: Paris, France, 2023.
4. Grizzi, F.; Di Ieva, A.; Russo, C.; Frezza, E.E.; Cobos, E.; Muzzio, P.C.; Chiriva-Internati, M. Cancer initiation and progression: An unsimplifiable complexity. *Theor. Biol. Med. Model.* **2006**, *3*, 37. [CrossRef] [PubMed]
5. Swanton, C.; Bernard, E.; Abbosh, C.; André, F.; Auwerx, J.; Balmain, A.; Bar-Sagi, D.; Bernards, R.; Bullman, S.; DeGregori, J. Embracing cancer complexity: Hallmarks of systemic disease. *Cell* **2024**, *187*, 1589–1616. [CrossRef]
6. Cheema, P.S.; Kumar, G.; Mittal, S.; Parashar, D.; Geethadevi, A.; Jadhav, K.; Tuli, H.S. Metastasis: A major driver of cancer pathogenesis. In *Drug Targets in Cellular Processes of Cancer: From Nonclinical to Preclinical Models*; Springer: Singapore, 2020; pp. 185–211.
7. Fan, T.; Kuang, G.; Long, R.; Han, Y.; Wang, J. The overall process of metastasis: From initiation to a new tumor. *Biochim. Biophys. Acta Rev. Cancer* **2022**, *1877*, 188750. [CrossRef]
8. Vijayakumar, S.; Dhakshanamoorthy, R.; Baskaran, A.; Krishnan, B.S.; Maddaly, R. Drug resistance in human cancers—Mechanisms and implications. *Life Sci.* **2024**, *352*, 122907. [CrossRef]
9. Koirala, M.; DiPaola, M. Overcoming cancer resistance: Strategies and modalities for effective treatment. *Biomedicines* **2024**, *12*, 1801. [CrossRef]
10. Nagaraju, G.P.; Kamal, M.A. Challenges in the discovery of novel therapeutic agents in cancer. *Curr. Drug Metab.* **2019**, *20*, 931–932. [CrossRef] [PubMed]

11. Khan, S.U.; Fatima, K.; Aisha, S.; Malik, F. Unveiling the mechanisms and challenges of cancer drug resistance. *Cell Commun. Signal.* **2024**, *22*, 109. [CrossRef] [PubMed]
12. Das, S.; Dey, M.K.; Devireddy, R.; Gartia, M.R. Biomarkers in cancer detection, diagnosis, and prognosis. *Sensors* **2023**, *24*, 37. [CrossRef] [PubMed]
13. Milner, D.A., Jr.; Lennerz, J.K. Technology and future of multi-cancer early detection. *Life* **2024**, *14*, 833. [CrossRef]
14. Ullah, S.; Khan, T.; Khan, T.; Ali, M.; Jan, A.K.; Shinwari, Z.K.; Khan, A.; Al-Farsi, M.; Waqas, M. Phytochemicals for cancer treatment: An update on plant-derived anti-cancer compounds and their mechanisms of action. *Curr. Top. Med. Chem.* **2024**, *24*, 1–20. [CrossRef] [PubMed]
15. Paudel, S.; Mishra, N.; Agarwal, R. Phytochemicals as immunomodulatory molecules in cancer therapeutics. *Pharmaceuticals* **2023**, *16*, 1652. [CrossRef] [PubMed]
16. Chihomvu, P.; Ganesan, A.; Gibbons, S.; Woollard, K.; Hayes, M.A. Phytochemicals in drug discovery—A confluence of tradition and innovation. *Int. J. Mol. Sci.* **2024**, *25*, 8792. [CrossRef] [PubMed]
17. Maddala, V.K.S.; Asha, S.; Singh, S. Phytopharmaceuticals of medicinal plants for the treatment of common illnesses. In *Phytopharmaceuticals and Biotechnology of Herbal Plants*; CRC Press: Boca Raton, FL, USA, 2022; pp. 201–211.
18. Ahmed Khalil, A.; Rauf, A.; Alhumaydhi, F.A.; Aljohani, A.S.; Javed, M.S.; Khan, M.A.; Khan, I.A.; El-Esawi, M.A.; Bawazeer, S.; Bouyahya, A. Recent developments and anticancer therapeutics of paclitaxel: An update. *Curr. Pharm. Des.* **2022**, *28*, 3363–3373. [PubMed]
19. Junjua, M.; Jafar, S.; Karamat, F.; Ahmed, F. From lab to pharmacy shelves: The story of a plant derived anticancer drug, "Paclitaxel". *J. Bioresour. Manag.* **2015**, *2*, 4.
20. Weaver, B.A. How Taxol/Paclitaxel kills cancer cells. *Mol. Biol. Cell.* **2014**, *25*, 2677–2681. [CrossRef] [PubMed]
21. Liebmann, J.; Cook, J.; Lipschultz, C.; Teague, D.; Fisher, J.; Mitchell, J. Cytotoxic studies of paclitaxel (Taxol®) in human tumour cell lines. *Br. J. Cancer* **1993**, *68*, 1104–1109. [CrossRef] [PubMed]
22. Howat, S.; Park, B.; Oh, I.S.; Jin, Y.-W.; Lee, E.-K.; Loake, G.J. Paclitaxel: Biosynthesis, production and future prospects. *New Biotechnol.* **2014**, *31*, 242–245. [CrossRef] [PubMed]
23. Sarkar, S. Role of paclitaxel and vinblastine in modern cancer therapy. In *Progress in Chemical and Biological Science*; Lincoln University College: Johor, Malaysia, 2023; pp. 15–25.
24. Rahman, M.A.; Hannan, M.A.; Dash, R.; Rahman, M.H.; Islam, R.; Uddin, M.J.; Sohag, A.A.M.; Rahman, M.H.; Rhim, H. Phytochemicals as a complement to cancer chemotherapy: Pharmacological modulation of the autophagy-apoptosis pathway. *Front. Pharmacol.* **2021**, *12*, 639628. [CrossRef]
25. Velásquez, J.E.; Van der Donk, W.A. Genome mining for ribosomally synthesized natural products. *Curr. Opin. Chem. Biol.* **2011**, *15*, 11–21. [CrossRef]
26. Cao, L.; Do, T.; Link, A.J. Mechanisms of action of ribosomally synthesized and posttranslationally modified peptides (RiPPs). *J. Ind. Microbiol. Biotech.* **2021**, *48*, kuab005. [CrossRef] [PubMed]
27. Skinnider, M.A.; Johnston, C.W.; Edgar, R.E.; Dejong, C.A.; Merwin, N.J.; Rees, P.N.; Magarvey, N.A. Genomic charting of ribosomally synthesized natural product chemical space facilitates targeted mining. *Proc. Natl. Acad. Sci. USA* **2016**, *113*, E6343–E6351. [CrossRef]
28. Russell, A.H.; Truman, A.W. Genome mining strategies for ribosomally synthesised and post-translationally modified peptides. *Comput. Struct. Biotechnol. J.* **2020**, *18*, 1838–1851. [CrossRef] [PubMed]
29. Hu, L.; Qiao, Y.; Liu, J.; Zheng, C.; Wang, X.; Sun, P.; Gu, Y.; Liu, W. Characterization of histidine functionalization and its timing in the biosynthesis of ribosomally synthesized and posttranslationally modified thioamitides. *J. Am. Chem. Soc.* **2022**, *144*, 4431–4438. [CrossRef]
30. Funk, M.A.; Van Der Donk, W.A. Ribosomal natural products, tailored to fit. *Acc. Chem. Res.* **2017**, *50*, 1577–1586. [CrossRef]
31. Cao, L.; Beiser, M.; Koos, J.D.; Orlova, M.; Elashal, H.E.; Schroder, H.V.; Link, A.J. Cellulonodin-2 and lihuanodin: Lasso peptides with an aspartimide post-translational modification. *J. Am. Chem. Soc.* **2021**, *143*, 11690–11702. [CrossRef] [PubMed]
32. Papagianni, M. Ribosomally synthesized peptides with antimicrobial properties: Biosynthesis, structure, function, and applications. *Biotechnol. Adv.* **2003**, *21*, 465–499. [CrossRef]
33. Fisher, M.F.; Zhang, J.; Berkowitz, O.; Whelan, J.; Mylne, J.S. Cyclic peptides in seed of *Annona muricata* are ribosomally synthesized. *J. Nat. Prod.* **2020**, *83*, 1167–1173. [CrossRef] [PubMed]
34. Craik, D.J.; Lee, M.-H.; Rehm, F.B.; Tombling, B.; Doffek, B.; Peacock, H. Ribosomally-synthesised cyclic peptides from plants as drug leads and pharmaceutical scaffolds. *Bioorg. Med. Chem.* **2018**, *26*, 2727–2737. [CrossRef] [PubMed]
35. Kersten, R.D.; Mydy, L.S.; Fallon, T.R.; de Waal, F.; Shafiq, K.; Wotring, J.W.; Sexton, J.Z.; Weng, J.-K. Gene-guided discovery and ribosomal biosynthesis of moroidin peptides. *J. Am. Chem. Soc.* **2022**, *144*, 7686–7692. [CrossRef] [PubMed]
36. Grundemann, C.; Koehbach, J.; Huber, R.; Gruber, C.W. Do plant cyclotides have potential as immunosuppressant peptides? *J. Nat. Prod.* **2012**, *75*, 167–174. [CrossRef] [PubMed]

37. Pfeiffer, I.P.; Schroder, M.P.; Mordhorst, S. Opportunities and challenges of RiPP-based therapeutics. *Nat. Prod. Rep.* **2024**, *41*, 990–1019. [CrossRef]
38. Gran, L.; Sletten, K.; Skjeldal, L. Cyclic peptides from *Oldenlandia affinis* DC. Molecular and biological properties. *Chem. Biodivers.* **2008**, *5*, 2014–2022. [CrossRef]
39. Tam, J.P.; Lu, Y.-A.; Yang, J.-L.; Chiu, K.-W. An unusual structural motif of antimicrobial peptides containing end-to-end macrocycle and cystine-knot disulfides. *Proc. Natl. Acad. Sci. USA* **1999**, *96*, 8913–8918. [CrossRef] [PubMed]
40. Jennings, C.; West, J.; Waine, C.; Craik, D.; Anderson, M. Biosynthesis and insecticidal properties of plant cyclotides: The cyclic knotted proteins from *Oldenlandia affinis*. *Proc. Natl. Acad. Sci. USA* **2001**, *98*, 10614–10619. [CrossRef] [PubMed]
41. Morita, H.; Eda, M.; Iizuka, T.; Hirasawa, Y.; Sekiguchi, M.; Yun, Y.S.; Itokawa, H.; Takeya, K. Structure of a new cyclic nonapeptide, segetalin F, and vasorelaxant activity of segetalins from *Vaccaria segetalis*. *Bioorg. Med. Chem. Lett.* **2006**, *16*, 4458–4461. [CrossRef] [PubMed]
42. Yahara, S.; Shigeyama, C.; Ura, T.; Wakamatsu, K.; Yasuhara, T.; Nohara, T. Cyclic peptides, acyclic diterpene glycosides and other compounds from *Lycium chinense* Mill. *Chem. Pharm. Bull.* **1993**, *41*, 703–709. [CrossRef]
43. Vassiliev, P.; Gusev, E.; Komelkova, M.; Kochetkov, A.; Dobrynina, M.; Sarapultsev, A. Computational analysis of CD46 protein interaction with SARS-CoV-2 structural proteins: Elucidating a putative viral entry mechanism into human cells. *Viruses* **2023**, *15*, 2297. [CrossRef]
44. Fu, Y.; Jaarsma, A.H.; Kuipers, O.P. Antiviral activities and applications of ribosomally synthesized and post-translationally modified peptides (RiPPs). *Cell. Mol. Life Sci.* **2021**, *78*, 3921–3940. [CrossRef]
45. Chen, D.; Ermine, K.; Wang, Y.-J.; Chen, X.; Lu, X.; Wang, P.; Beer-Stolz, D.; Yu, J.; Zhang, L. PUMA/RIP3 mediates chemotherapy response via necroptosis and local immune activation in colorectal cancer. *Mol. Cancer Ther.* **2024**, *23*, 354–367. [CrossRef]
46. Raina, K.; Forbes, C.D.; Stronk, R.; Rappi, J.P., Jr.; Eastman, K.J.; Gerritz, S.W.; Yu, X.; Li, H.; Bhardwaj, A.; Forgione, M. Regulated induced proximity targeting chimeras (RIPTACs): A novel heterobifunctional small molecule therapeutic strategy for killing cancer cells selectively. *bioRxiv* **2023**. [CrossRef]
47. Zhong, G.; Wang, Z.J.; Yan, F.; Zhang, Y.; Huo, L. Recent advances in discovery, bioengineering, and bioactivity-evaluation of ribosomally synthesized and post-translationally modified peptides. *ACS Bio Med Chem Au* **2023**, *3*, 1–31. [CrossRef]
48. Han, S.W.; Won, H.S. Advancements in the application of ribosomally synthesized and post-translationally modified peptides (RiPPs). *Biomolecules* **2024**, *14*, 479. [CrossRef] [PubMed]
49. Ongpipattanakul, C.; Desormeaux, E.K.; DiCaprio, A.; Van Der Donk, W.A.; Mitchell, D.A.; Nair, S.K. Mechanism of action of ribosomally synthesized and post-translationally modified peptides. *Chem. Rev.* **2022**, *122*, 14722–14814. [CrossRef]
50. Bauso, L.V.; La Fauci, V.; Munaò, S.; Bonfiglio, D.; Armeli, A.; Maimone, N.; Longo, C.; Calabrese, G. Biological activity of natural and synthetic peptides as anticancer agents. *Int. J. Mol. Sci.* **2024**, *25*, 7264. [CrossRef] [PubMed]
51. Santos-Aberturas, J.; Chandra, G.; Frattaruolo, L.; Lacret, R.; Pham, T.H.; Vior, N.M.; Eyles, T.H.; Truman, A.W. Uncovering the unexplored diversity of thioamidated ribosomal peptides in Actinobacteria using the RiPPER genome mining tool. *Nucleic Acids Res.* **2019**, *47*, 4624–4637. [CrossRef] [PubMed]
52. Moyer, T.B.; Parsley, N.C.; Sadecki, P.W.; Schug, W.J.; Hicks, L.M. Leveraging orthogonal mass spectrometry based strategies for comprehensive sequencing and characterization of ribosomal antimicrobial peptide natural products. *Nat. Prod. Rep.* **2021**, *38*, 489–509. [CrossRef]
53. Frattaruolo, L.; Lacret, R.; Cappello, A.R.; Truman, A.W. A genomics-based approach identifies a thioviridamide-like compound with selective anticancer activity. *ACS Chem. Biol.* **2017**, *12*, 2815–2822. [CrossRef] [PubMed]
54. Chekan, J.R.; Mydy, L.S.; Pasquale, M.A.; Kersten, R.D. Plant peptides-redefining an area of ribosomally synthesized and post-translationally modified peptides. *Nat. Prod. Rep.* **2024**, *41*, 1020–1059. [CrossRef]
55. Ali, A.; Ambrose, S.; Hussain, D.; Hafeez, F.; Asghar, T.; Shah, S.N.A.; Ahsan, M.; Shakir, M.; Ali, A.; Khan, A.M.A. Antimicrobial resistance and antimicrobial activity of plant-based antimicrobial peptides against bacteria: Plant-based antimicrobial peptides. *Lett. Anim. Biol.* **2024**, *4*, 19–27. [CrossRef]
56. Szerszunowicz, I.; Kozicki, S. Plant-Derived Proteins and Peptides as Potential Immunomodulators. *Molecules* **2023**, *29*, 209. [CrossRef]
57. Kadam, D.; Kadam, A.; Koksel, F.; Aluko, R.E. Plant-derived bioactive peptides: A comprehensive review. *Sustain. Food Proteins* **2024**, *2*, 183–214. [CrossRef]
58. Gruber, C.W. Plant-derived peptides: (neglected) natural products for drug discovery. *Planta Med.* **2024**, *90*, 627–630. [CrossRef]
59. Miller, F.S.; Crone, K.K.; Jensen, M.R.; Shaw, S.; Harcombe, W.R.; Elias, M.H.; Freeman, M.F. Conformational rearrangements enable iterative backbone N-methylation in RiPP biosynthesis. *Nat. Commun.* **2021**, *12*, 5355. [CrossRef]
60. Mahanta, N.; Hudson, G.A.; Mitchell, D.A. Radical S-adenosylmethionine enzymes involved in RiPP biosynthesis. *Biochemistry* **2017**, *56*, 5229–5244. [CrossRef] [PubMed]
61. Oman, T.J.; Van Der Donk, W.A. Follow the leader: The use of leader peptides to guide natural product biosynthesis. *Nat. Chem. Biol.* **2010**, *6*, 9–18. [CrossRef] [PubMed]

62. Jin, L.; Wu, X.; Xue, Y.; Jin, Y.; Wang, S.; Chen, Y. Mutagenesis of NosM leader peptide reveals important elements in nosiheptide biosynthesis. *Appl. Environ. Microbiol.* **2017**, *83*, e02880-16. [CrossRef] [PubMed]
63. Walsh, C.T.; Garneau-Tsodikova, S.; Gatto Jr, G.J. Protein posttranslational modifications: The chemistry of proteome diversifications. *Angew. Chem. Int. Ed.* **2005**, *44*, 7342–7372. [CrossRef]
64. Arnison, P.G.; Bibb, M.J.; Bierbaum, G.; Bowers, A.A.; Bugni, T.S.; Bulaj, G.; Camarero, J.A.; Campopiano, D.J.; Challis, G.L.; Clardy, J. Ribosomally synthesized and post-translationally modified peptide natural products: Overview and recommendations for a universal nomenclature. *Nat. Prod. Rep.* **2013**, *30*, 108–160. [CrossRef] [PubMed]
65. Condie, J.A.; Nowak, G.; Reed, D.W.; Balsevich, J.J.; Reaney, M.J.T.; Arnison, P.G.; Covello, P.S. The biosynthesis of Caryophyllaceae-like cyclic peptides in *Saponaria vaccaria* L. from DNA-encoded precursors. *Plant J.* **2011**, *67*, 682–690. [CrossRef] [PubMed]
66. Trabi, M.; Mylne, J.S.; Sando, L.; Craik, D.J. Circular proteins from Melicytus (Violaceae) refine the conserved protein and gene architecture of cyclotides. *Org. Biomol. Chem.* **2009**, *7*, 2378–2388. [CrossRef]
67. Rubin, G.M.; Ding, Y. Recent advances in the biosynthesis of RiPPs from multicore-containing precursor peptides. *J. Ind. Microbiol. Biotechnol.* **2020**, *47*, 659–674. [CrossRef]
68. Jones, P.M.; George, A.M. Computational analysis of the MCoTI-II plant defence knottin reveals a novel intermediate conformation that facilitates trypsin binding. *Sci. Rep.* **2016**, *6*, 23174. [CrossRef] [PubMed]
69. Mylne, J.S.; Chan, L.Y.; Chanson, A.H.; Daly, N.L.; Schaefer, H.; Bailey, T.L.; Nguyencong, P.; Cascales, L.; Craik, D.J. Cyclic peptides arising by evolutionary parallelism via asparaginyl-endopeptidase–mediated biosynthesis. *Plant Cell* **2012**, *24*, 2765–2778. [CrossRef]
70. Kersten, R.D.; Weng, J.-K. Gene-guided discovery and engineering of branched cyclic peptides in plants. *Proc. Natl. Acad. Sci. USA* **2018**, *115*, E10961–E10969. [CrossRef] [PubMed]
71. Rodríguez, V. Insights into post-translational modification enzymes from RiPPs: A toolkit for applications in peptide synthesis. *Biotechnol. Adv.* **2022**, *56*, 107908. [CrossRef] [PubMed]
72. Fu, Y.; Xu, Y.; Ruijne, F.; Kuipers, O.P. Engineering lanthipeptides by introducing a large variety of RiPP modifications to obtain new-to-nature bioactive peptides. *FEMS Microbiol. Rev.* **2023**, *47*, fuad017. [CrossRef] [PubMed]
73. Eslami, S.M.; van der Donk, W.A. Proteases involved in leader peptide removal during RiPP biosynthesis. *ACS Bio Med Chem Au* **2024**, *4*, 20–36. [CrossRef] [PubMed]
74. Mittal, S.; Saluja, D. Protein post-translational modifications: Role in protein structure, function and stability. In *Proteostasis and Chaperone Surveillance*; Singh, L.R., Dar, T.A., Ahmad, P., Eds.; Springer: New Delhi, India, 2015; pp. 25–37.
75. Haim, A.; Neubacher, S.; Grossmann, T.N. Protein macrocyclization for tertiary structure stabilization. *Chembiochem* **2021**, *22*, 2672–2679. [CrossRef] [PubMed]
76. Thibodeaux, G.N.; McClerren, A.L.; Ma, Y.; Gancayco, M.R.; van der Donk, W.A. Synergistic binding of the lader and core peptides by the lantibiotic synthetase HalM2. *ACS Chem. Biol.* **2015**, *10*, 970–977. [CrossRef] [PubMed]
77. Koehnke, J.; Mann, G.; Bent, A.F.; Ludewig, H.; Shirran, S.; Botting, C.; Lebl, T.; Houssen, W.; Jaspars, M.; Naismith, J.H. Structural analysis of leader peptide binding enables leader-free cyanobactin processing. *Nat. Chem. Biol.* **2015**, *11*, 558–563. [CrossRef]
78. Si, T.; Tian, Q.; Min, Y.; Zhang, L.; Sweedler, J.V.; van der Donk, W.A.; Zhao, H. Rapid screening of lanthipeptide analogs via in-colony removal of leader peptides in *Escherichia coli*. *J. Am. Chem. Soc.* **2018**, *140*, 11884–11888. [CrossRef]
79. Chekan, J.R.; Estrada, P.; Covello, P.S.; Nair, S.K. Characterization of the macrocyclase involved in the biosynthesis of RiPP cyclic peptides in plants. *Proc. Natl. Acad. Sci. USA* **2017**, *114*, 6551–6556. [CrossRef] [PubMed]
80. Koehnke, J.; Bent, A.F.; Houssen, W.E.; Mann, G.; Jaspars, M.; Naismith, J.H. The structural biology of patellamide biosynthesis. *Curr. Opin. Struct. Biol.* **2014**, *29*, 112–121. [CrossRef]
81. Ayikpoe, R.S.; Shi, C.; Battiste, A.J.; Eslami, S.M.; Ramesh, S.; Simon, M.A.; Bothwell, I.R.; Lee, H.; Rice, A.J.; Ren, H.; et al. A scalable platform to discover antimicrobials of ribosomal origin. *Nat. Commun.* **2022**, *13*, 6135. [CrossRef] [PubMed]
82. Bothwell, I.R.; Caetano, T.; Sarksian, R.; Mendo, S.; van der Donk, W.A. Structural analysis of Class I lanthipeptides from *Pedobacter lusitanus* NL19 reveals an unusual ring pattern. *ACS Chem. Biol.* **2021**, *16*, 1019–1029. [CrossRef] [PubMed]
83. Lee, H.; van der Donk, W.A. Macrocyclization and backbone modification in RiPP biosynthesis. *Annu. Rev. Biochem.* **2022**, *91*, 269–294. [CrossRef]
84. Craik, D.J.; Daly, N.L.; Bond, T.; Waine, C. Plant cyclotides: A unique family of cyclic and knotted proteins that defines the cyclic cystine knot structural motif. *J. Mol. Biol.* **1999**, *294*, 1327–1336. [CrossRef]
85. Rees, D.C.; Lipscomb, W.N. Refined crystal structure of the potato inhibitor complex of carboxypeptidase A at 2.5 Å resolution. *J. Mol. Biol.* **1982**, *160*, 475–498. [CrossRef]
86. Colgrave, M.L.; Craik, D.J. Thermal, chemical, and enzymatic stability of the cyclotide kalata B1: The importance of the cyclic cystine knot. *Biochemistry* **2004**, *43*, 5965–5975. [CrossRef]

87. Zhang, J.; Liao, B.; Craik, D.J.; Li, J.-T.; Hu, M.; Shu, W.-S. Identification of two suites of cyclotide precursor genes from metallophyte Viola baoshanensis: cDNA sequence variation, alternative RNA splicing and potential cyclotide diversity. *Gene* **2009**, *431*, 23–32. [CrossRef] [PubMed]
88. Gruber, C.W.; Čemažar, M.; Clark, R.J.; Horibe, T.; Renda, R.F.; Anderson, M.A.; Craik, D.J. A novel plant protein-disulfide isomerase involved in the oxidative folding of cystine knot defense proteins. *J. Biol. Chem.* **2007**, *282*, 20435–20446. [CrossRef] [PubMed]
89. Wang, C.K.L.; Kaas, Q.; Chiche, L.; Craik, D.J. CyBase: A database of cyclic protein sequences and structures, with applications in protein discovery and engineering. *Nucleic Acids Res.* **2007**, *36*, D206–D210. [CrossRef]
90. Qu, H.; Jackson, M.A.; Yap, K.; Harvey, P.J.; Gilding, E.K.; Craik, D.J. Production of a structurally validated cyclotide in rice suspension cells is enabled by a supporting biosynthetic enzyme. *Planta* **2020**, *252*, 97. [CrossRef]
91. James, A.M.; Haywood, J.; Leroux, J.; Ignasiak, K.; Elliott, A.G.; Schmidberger, J.W.; Fisher, M.F.; Nonis, S.G.; Fenske, R.; Bond, C.S.; et al. The macrocyclizing protease butelase 1 remains autocatalytic and reveals the structural basis for ligase activity. *Plant J.* **2019**, *98*, 988–999. [CrossRef]
92. Huang, Y.-H.; Kan, M.-W.; Craik, D.J. Protocols for measuring the stability and cytotoxicity of cyclotides. In *Methods in Enzymology*; Hicks, L.M., Ed.; Academic Press: Cambridge, MA, USA, 2022; Volume 663, pp. 619–640.
93. Lee, M.-H.; Jackson, M.A.; Rehm, F.B.H.; Barkauskas, D.S.; Ho, W.L.; Yap, K.; Craik, D.J.; Gilding, E.K. Proximity labelling confirms the Involvement of papain-like cysteine proteases and chaperones in cyclotide biosynthesis. *Plant Mol. Biol. Rep.* **2024**, *42*, 611–623. [CrossRef]
94. Fisher, M.F.; Payne, C.D.; Rosengren, K.J.; Mylne, J.S. An orbitide from *Ratibida columnifera* seed containing 16 amino acid residues. *J. Nat. Prod.* **2019**, *82*, 2152–2158. [CrossRef] [PubMed]
95. Barber, C.J.S.; Pujara, P.T.; Reed, D.W.; Chiwocha, S.; Zhang, H.; Covello, P.S. The two-step biosynthesis of cyclic peptides from *Linear Precursors* in a member of the plant family *Caryophyllaceae* Involves cyclization by a serine protease-like enzyme. *J. Biol. Chem.* **2013**, *288*, 12500–12510. [CrossRef]
96. Jackson, M.A.; Nguyen, L.T.T.; Gilding, E.K.; Durek, T.; Craik, D.J. Make it or break it: Plant AEPs on stage in biotechnology. *Biotechnol. Adv.* **2020**, *45*, 107651. [CrossRef] [PubMed]
97. Ortega, M.A.; Van Der Donk, W.A. New insights into the biosynthetic logic of ribosomally synthesized and post-translationally modified peptide natural products. *Cell Chem. Biol.* **2016**, *23*, 31–44. [CrossRef]
98. Seidel, V. Plant-derived chemicals: A source of inspiration for new drugs. *Plants* **2020**, *9*, 1562. [CrossRef]
99. Imtiaz, I.; Schloss, J.; Bugarcic, A. Traditional and contemporary herbal medicines in management of cancer: A scoping review. *J. Ayurveda Integr. Med.* **2024**, *15*, 100904. [CrossRef]
100. Bajpai, P.; Usmani, S.; Kumar, R.; Prakash, O. Recent advances in anticancer approach of traditional medicinal plants: A novel strategy for cancer chemotherapy. *Intell. Pharm.* **2024**, *2*, 291–304. [CrossRef]
101. Ravichandran, S.; Bhargavi, K.M.; Rai, A.; Pandey, T.; Rajput, J.; Sri, R.M.M. Medicinal plants for curing human diseases. *Insight Chin. Med.* **2023**, *6*, 570. [CrossRef]
102. Sheng-Ji, P. Ethnobotanical approaches of traditional medicine studies: Some experiences from Asia. *Pharm. Biol.* **2001**, *39* (Suppl. 1), 74–79. [PubMed]
103. Fisher, M.F.; Payne, C.D.; Chetty, T.; Crayn, D.; Berkowitz, O.; Whelan, J.; Rosengren, K.J.; Mylne, J.S. The genetic origin of evolidine, the first cyclopeptide discovered in plants, and related orbitides. *J. Biol. Chem.* **2020**, *295*, 14510–14521. [CrossRef] [PubMed]
104. Ficker, C.E.; Arnason, J.T.; Vindas, P.S.; Alvarez, L.P.; Akpagana, K.; Gbeassor, M.; De Souza, C.; Smith, M.L. Inhibition of human pathogenic fungi by ethnobotanically selected plant extracts. *Mycoses* **2003**, *46*, 29–37. [CrossRef]
105. Mayr, L.M.; Bojanic, D. Novel trends in high-throughput screening. *Curr. Opin. Pharmacol.* **2009**, *9*, 580–588. [CrossRef]
106. Mayr, L.M.; Fuerst, P. The future of high-throughput screening. *J. Biomol. Screen.* **2008**, *13*, 443–448. [CrossRef]
107. Fang, X.; Zheng, Y.; Duan, Y.; Liu, Y.; Zhong, W. Recent advances in design of fluorescence-based assays for high-throughput screening. *Anal. Chem.* **2019**, *91*, 482–504. [CrossRef]
108. Henrich, C.J.; Beutler, J.A. Matching the power of high throughput screening to the chemical diversity of natural products. *Nat. Prod. Rep.* **2013**, *30*, 1284–1298. [CrossRef] [PubMed]
109. Kriger, D.; Pasquale, M.A.; Ampolini, B.G.; Chekan, J.R. Mining raw plant transcriptomic data for new cyclopeptide alkaloids. *Beilstein J. Org. Chem.* **2024**, *20*, 1548–1559. [CrossRef]
110. Smit, S.J.; Lichman, B.R. Plant biosynthetic gene clusters in the context of metabolic evolution. *Nat. Prod. Rep.* **2022**, *39*, 1465–1482. [CrossRef]
111. Alami, M.M.; Ouyang, Z.; Zhang, Y.; Shu, S.; Yang, G.; Mei, Z.; Wang, X. The current developments in medicinal plant genomics enabled the diversification of secondary metabolites' biosynthesis. *Int. J. Mol. Sci.* **2022**, *23*, 15932. [CrossRef] [PubMed]
112. Mehta, A.; Hasija, Y. Bioinformatics approaches for genomics and post genomics applications of anticancer plants. In *Anticancer Plants: Mechanisms and Molecular Interactions*; Akhtar, M.S., Swamy, M.K., Eds.; Springer: Singapore, 2018; Volume 4, pp. 283–317.

113. Kautsar, S.A.; Suarez Duran, H.G.; Medema, M.H. Genomic Identification and Analysis of Specialized Metabolite Biosynthetic Gene Clusters in Plants Using PlantiSMASH. In *Plant Chemical Genomics: Methods and Protocols*; Fauser, F., Jonikas, M., Eds.; Springer: New York, NY, USA, 2018; pp. 173–188.
114. Chavali, A.K.; Rhee, S.Y. Bioinformatics tools for the identification of gene clusters that biosynthesize specialized metabolites. *Brief. Bioinform.* **2018**, *19*, 1022–1034. [CrossRef] [PubMed]
115. Lorenzo de los Santos, E.; Challis, G. ClusterTools: Functional element identification for the in silico prioritization of biosynthetic gene clusters. *Access Microbiol.* **2019**, *1*, 301. [CrossRef]
116. Horner, D.S.; Pavesi, G.; Castrignano, T.; De Meo, P.D.; Liuni, S.; Sammeth, M.; Picardi, E.; Pesole, G. Bioinformatics approaches for genomics and post genomics applications of next-generation sequencing. *Brief. Bioinform.* **2010**, *11*, 181–197. [CrossRef]
117. Zhang, Y.; Chen, M.; Bruner, S.D.; Ding, Y. Heterologous production of microbial ribosomally synthesized and post-translationally modified peptides. *Front. Microbiol.* **2018**, *9*, 1801. [CrossRef]
118. Voutquenne-Nazabadioko, L.; Gevrenova, R.; Borie, N.; Harakat, D.; Sayagh, C.; Weng, A.; Thakur, M.; Zaharieva, M.; Henry, M. Triterpenoid saponins from the roots of *Gypsophila trichotoma* Wender. *Phytochemistry* **2013**, *90*, 114–127. [CrossRef] [PubMed]
119. Gevrenova, R.; Joubert, O.; Mandova, T.; Zaiou, M.; Chapleur, Y.; Henry, M. Cytotoxic effects of four Caryophyllaceae species extracts on macrophage cell lines. *Pharm. Biol.* **2014**, *52*, 919–925. [CrossRef]
120. Timité, G.; Mitaine-Offer, A.C.; Miyamoto, T.; Ramezani, M.; Rustaiyan, A.; Mirjolet, J.F.; Duchamp, O.; Lacaille-Dubois, M.A. Structure elucidation of new oleanane-type glycosides from three species of *Acanthophyllum*. *Magn. Reson. Chem.* **2010**, *48*, 370–374. [CrossRef] [PubMed]
121. Luo, J.-G.; Chen, X.; Kong, L.-Y. Three new triterpenoid saponins from *Dianthus superbus*. *Chem. Pharm. Bull.* **2011**, *59*, 518–521. [CrossRef]
122. Yu, J.-O.; Liao, Z.-X.; Lei, J.-C.; Hu, X.-M. Antioxidant and cytotoxic activities of various fractions of ethanol extract of *Dianthus superbus*. *Food Chem.* **2007**, *104*, 1215–1219. [CrossRef]
123. Hsieh, P.-W.; Chang, F.-R.; Wu, C.-C.; Wu, K.-Y.; Li, C.-M.; Chen, S.-L.; Wu, Y.-C. New cytotoxic cyclic peptides and dianthramide from *Dianthus superbus*. *J. Nat. Prod.* **2004**, *67*, 1522–1527. [CrossRef]
124. Morita, H.; Shishido, A.; Kayashita, T.; Shimomura, M.; Takeya, K.; Itokawa, H. Cyclic peptide from higher plants. part 14. two novel cyclic peptides, Yunnanins A and B from *Stellaria yunnanensis*. *Chem. Lett.* **1994**, *26*, 2415–2418. [CrossRef]
125. Houshdar Tehrani, M.H.; Gholibeikian, M.; Bamoniri, A.; Mirjalili, B.B.F. Cancer treatment by Caryophyllaceae-type cyclopeptides. *Front. Endocrinol.* **2020**, *11*, 600856. [CrossRef] [PubMed]
126. Morita, H.; Kayashita, T.; Shimomura, M.; Takeya, K.; Itokawa, H. Cyclic peptides from higher plants. 24. yunnanin C, a novel cyclic heptapeptide from *Stellaria yunnanensis*. *J. Nat. Prod.* **1996**, *59*, 280–282. [CrossRef] [PubMed]
127. Lee, J.; Seo, Y.; Lee, J.; Ju, J. Antioxidant activities of *Dianthus chinensis* L. extract and its inhibitory activities against nitric oxide production and cancer cell growth and adhesion. *J. Korean Soc. Food Sci. Nutr.* **2016**, *45*, 44–51. [CrossRef]
128. Li, H.-y.; Koike, K.; Ohmoto, T.; Ikeda, K. Dianchinenosides A and B, two new saponins from *Dianthus chinensis*. *J. Nat. Prod.* **1993**, *56*, 1065–1070. [CrossRef]
129. Lee, J.W.; Kim, J.G.; Han, J.S.; Cho, Y.B.; Lee, Y.J.; Lee, D.; Shin, D.H.; Hong, J.T.; Lee, M.K.; Hwang, B.Y. Dianthiamides A-E, proline-containing orbitides from *Dianthus chinensis*. *Molecules* **2021**, *26*, 7275. [CrossRef]
130. Son, J.K.; Jung, J.H.; Lee, C.S.; Moon, D.C.; Choi, S.W.; Min, B.S.; Woo, M.H. DNA Topoisomerases I and II inhibition and cytotoxicity of constituents from the roots of *Rubia cordifolia*. *Bull. Korean Chem. Soc.* **2006**, *27*, 1231–1234. [CrossRef]
131. Itokawa, H.; Mihara, K.; Takeya, K. Studies on a novel anthraquinone and its glycosides isolated from *Rubia cordifolia* and *R. akane*. *Chem. Pharm. Bull.* **1983**, *31*, 2353–2358. [CrossRef]
132. Son, J.K.; Jung, S.J.; Jung, J.H.; Fang, Z.; Lee, C.S.; Seo, C.S.; Moon, D.C.; Min, B.S.; Kim, M.R.; Woo, M.H. Anticancer constituents from the roots of *Rubia cordifolia* L. *Chem. Pharm. Bull.* **2008**, *56*, 213–216. [CrossRef]
133. Tessier, A.; Delaveau, P.; Champion, B. Nouvelles anthraquinones des racines de *Rubia cordifolia*. *Planta Med.* **1981**, *41*, 337–343. [CrossRef]
134. Zengin, G.; Degirmenci, N.S.; Alpsoy, L.; Aktumsek, A. Evaluation of antioxidant, enzyme inhibition, and cytotoxic activity of three anthraquinones (alizarin, purpurin, and quinizarin). *Hum. Exp. Toxicol.* **2016**, *35*, 544–553. [CrossRef]
135. Lee, J.-E.; Hitotsuyanagi, Y.; Fukaya, H.; Kondo, K.; Takeya, K. New cytotoxic bicyclic hexapeptides, RA-XXIII and RA-XXIV, from *Rubia cordifolia* L. *Chem. Pharm. Bull.* **2008**, *56*, 730–733. [CrossRef]
136. Balachandran, P.; Ibrahim, M.A.; Zhang, J.; Wang, M.; Pasco, D.S.; Muhammad, I. Crosstalk of cancer signaling pathways by cyclic hexapeptides and anthraquinones from *Rubia cordifolia*. *Molecules* **2021**, *26*, 735. [CrossRef] [PubMed]
137. Wang, Z.; Zhao, S.-M.; Hu, Y.-Y.; Feng, L.; Zhao, L.-M.; Di, Y.-T.; Tan, N.-H. Rubipodanones AD, naphthohydroquinone dimers from the roots and rhizomes of *Rubia podantha*. *Phytochemistry* **2018**, *145*, 153–160. [CrossRef]
138. Wang, Z.; Zhao, S.-M.; Zhao, L.-M.; Chen, X.-Q.; Zeng, G.-Z.; Tan, N.-H. Rubipodanin A, the first natural N-desmonomethyl Rubiaceae-type cyclopeptide from *Rubia podantha*, indicating an important role of the N 9-methyl group in the conformation and bioactivity. *PLoS ONE* **2015**, *10*, e0144950. [CrossRef] [PubMed]

139. Hu, Y.Y.; Feng, L.; Wang, J.; Zhang, X.J.; Wang, Z.; Tan, N.H. Rubipodanin B, a new cytotoxic cyclopeptide from *Rubia podantha*. *Chem. Biodivers.* **2019**, *16*, e1800438. [CrossRef] [PubMed]
140. Fan, J.-T.; Chen, Y.-S.; Xu, W.-Y.; Du, L.; Zeng, G.-Z.; Zhang, Y.-M.; Su, J.; Li, Y.; Tan, N.-H. Rubiyunnanins A and B, two novel cyclic hexapeptides from *Rubia yunnanensis*. *Tetrahedron Lett.* **2010**, *51*, 6810–6813. [CrossRef]
141. Tao, J.; Morikawa, T.; Ando, S.; Matsuda, H.; Yoshikawa, M. Bioactive constituents from chinese natural nedicines. XI. inhibitors on NO production and degranulation in RBL-2H3 from *Rubia yunnanensis*: Structures of rubianosides II, III, and IV, rubianol-g, and rubianthraquinone. *Chem. Pharm. Bull.* **2003**, *51*, 654–662. [CrossRef] [PubMed]
142. Fan, J.-T.; Kuang, B.; Zeng, G.-Z.; Zhao, S.-M.; Ji, C.-J.; Zhang, Y.-M.; Tan, N.-H. Biologically active arborinane-type triterpenoids and anthraquinones from *Rubia yunnanensis*. *J. Nat. Prod.* **2011**, *74*, 2069–2080. [CrossRef] [PubMed]
143. Liou, M.-J.; Wu, T.-S. Triterpenoids from *Rubia yunnanensis*. *J. Nat. Prod.* **2002**, *65*, 1283–1287. [CrossRef]
144. Fan, J.-T.; Su, J.; Peng, Y.-M.; Li, Y.; Li, J.; Zhou, Y.-B.; Zeng, G.-Z.; Yan, H.; Tan, N.-H. Rubiyunnanins C–H, cytotoxic cyclic hexapeptides from *Rubia yunnanensis* inhibiting nitric oxide production and NF-κB activation. *Bioorg. Med. Chem.* **2010**, *18*, 8226–8234. [CrossRef]
145. Intahphuak, S.; Panthong, A.; Kanjanapothi, D.; Taesotikul, T.; Krachangchaeng, C.; Reutrakul, V. Anti-inflammatory and analgesic activities of *Mallotus spodocarpus* Airy Shaw. *J. Ethnopharmacol.* **2004**, *90*, 69–72. [CrossRef]
146. Sawektreeratana, N.; Krachangchaeng, C.; Pittayanurak, P.; Betterley, N.M.; Chairoungdua, A.; Wongpan, A.; Panvongsa, W.; Janthakit, P.; Nalaoh, P.; Promarak, V. Mallotumides A–C: Potent cytotoxic cycloheptapeptides from the roots of *Mallotus spodocarpus*. *Org. Lett.* **2023**, *25*, 8183–8187. [CrossRef]
147. Cordeiro, K.W.; Felipe, J.L.; Malange, K.F.; do Prado, P.R.; de Oliveira Figueiredo, P.; Garcez, F.R.; de Cássia Freitas, K.; Garcez, W.S.; Toffoli-Kadri, M.C. Anti-inflammatory and antinociceptive activities of *Croton urucurana* Baillon bark. *J. Ethnopharmacol.* **2016**, *183*, 128–135. [CrossRef] [PubMed]
148. Lara, L.L.; Nascimento, V.A.; Fernandes, C.C.; Forim, M.R.; Cazal, C.M. Chemical composition and antifungal activity of *Zanthoxylum riedelianum* stem bark essential oil. *Nat. Prod. Res.* **2022**, *36*, 1653–1658. [CrossRef] [PubMed]
149. Peres, M.T.L.P.; Pizzolatti, M.G.; Yunes, R.A.; Delle Monache, F. Clerodane diterpenes of *Croton ururucana*. *Phytochemistry* **1998**, *49*, 171–174. [CrossRef]
150. Candido-Bacani, P.d.M.; Figueiredo, P.d.O.; Matos, M.d.F.; Garcez, F.R.; Garcez, W.S. Cytotoxic orbitide from the latex of *Croton urucurana*. *J. Nat. Prod.* **2015**, *78*, 2754–2760. [CrossRef] [PubMed]
151. Islam, S.; Shajib, M.S.; Ahmed, T. Antinociceptive effect of methanol extract of *Celosia cristata* Linn. in mice. *BMC Complement. Altern Med.* **2016**, *16*, 400. [CrossRef] [PubMed]
152. Gholizadeh, A.; Kumar, M.; Balasubrahmanyam, A.; Sharma, S.; Narwal, S.; Lodha, M.; Kapoor, H. Antioxidant activity of antiviral proteins from *Celosia cristata*. *J. Plant Biochem. Biotechnol.* **2004**, *13*, 13–18. [CrossRef]
153. Wang, Y.; Lou, Z.; Wu, Q.-B.; Guo, M.-L. A novel hepatoprotective saponin from *Celosia cristata* L. *Fitoterapia* **2010**, *81*, 1246–1252. [CrossRef]
154. Liu, X.; Zhang, J.; Guo, K.; Jia, A.; Zhang, M.; Shi, Y.; Liu, C.; Xiao, L.; Sun, Z. Three new oleanane-type triterpenoid saponins from the seeds of *Celosia cristata* L. *Nat. Prod. Res.* **2018**, *32*, 167–174. [CrossRef] [PubMed]
155. Xu, X.; Jiang, N.; Liu, S.; Jin, Y.; Cheng, Y.; Xu, T.; Wang, X.; Liu, Y.; Zhang, M.; Du, S. Moroidin, a cyclopeptide from the seeds of *Celosia cristata* that induces apoptosis in A549 human lung cancer cells. *J. Nat. Prod.* **2022**, *85*, 1918–1927. [CrossRef]
156. Chen, C.-Y.; Chang, F.-R.; Pan, W.-B.; Wu, Y.-C. Four alkaloids from *Annona cherimola*. *Phytochemistry* **2001**, *56*, 753–757. [CrossRef] [PubMed]
157. Quílez, A.; Fernández-Arche, M.; García-Giménez, M.; De la Puerta, R. Potential therapeutic applications of the genus Annona: Local and traditional uses and pharmacology. *J. Ethnopharmacol.* **2018**, *225*, 244–270. [CrossRef] [PubMed]
158. Wélé, A.; Zhang, Y.; Ndoye, I.; Brouard, J.-P.; Pousset, J.-L.; Bodo, B. A cytotoxic cyclic heptapeptide from the seeds of *Annona cherimola*. *J. Nat. Prod.* **2004**, *67*, 1577–1579. [CrossRef]
159. Bitchi, M.B.; Magid, A.A.; Kabran, F.A.; Yao-Kouassi, P.A.; Harakat, D.; Morjani, H.; Tonzibo, F.Z.; Voutquenne-Nazabadioko, L. Isolation and structure elucidation of cyclopeptide alkaloids from the leaves of *Heisteria parvifolia*. *Phytochemistry* **2019**, *167*, 112081. [CrossRef]
160. Mseddi, K.; Alimi, F.; Noumi, E.; Veettil, V.N.; Deshpande, S.; Adnan, M.; Hamdi, A.; Elkahoui, S.; Alghamdi, A.; Kadri, A. *Thymus musilii* Velen. as a promising source of potent bioactive compounds with its pharmacological properties: In vitro and in silico analysis. *Arabian J. Chem.* **2020**, *13*, 6782–6801. [CrossRef]
161. Noumi, E.; Ahmad, I.; Bouali, N.; Patel, H.; Ghannay, S.; ALrashidi, A.A.; Abdulhakeem, M.A.; Patel, M.; Ceylan, O.; Badraoui, R. *Thymus musilii* velen. methanolic extract: In vitro and in silico screening of its antimicrobial, antioxidant, anti-quorum sensing, antibiofilm, and anticancer activities. *Life* **2022**, *13*, 62. [CrossRef]
162. Salehi, B.; Abu-Darwish, M.S.; Tarawneh, A.H.; Cabral, C.; Gadetskaya, A.V.; Salgueiro, L.; Hosseinabadi, T.; Rajabi, S.; Chanda, W.; Sharifi-Rad, M. *Thymus* spp. plants-food applications and phytopharmacy properties. *Trends Food Sci. Technol.* **2019**, *85*, 287–306. [CrossRef]

163. Fernandes, C.C.; Vieira, P.C.; Silva, V.C.d.; Dall'Oglio, E.L.; Silva, L.E.d.; Sousa Jr, P.T.d. 6-Acetonyl-N-methyl-dihydrodecarine, a new alkaloid from *Zanthoxylum riedelianum*. *J. Braz. Chem. Soc.* **2009**, *20*, 379–382. [CrossRef]
164. Ombito, J.O. Phytochemistry and pharmacology of the genus Zanthoxylum (Rutaceae): A review. *J. Nat. Prod.* **2021**, *11*, 21–43. [CrossRef]
165. Lee, S.-S.; Chen, W.-C.; Chen, C.-H. New jujubogenin glycosides from *Colubrina asiatica*. *J. Nat. Prod.* **2000**, *63*, 1580–1583. [CrossRef] [PubMed]
166. Sangsopha, W.; Lekphrom, R.; Schevenels, F.T.; Kanokmedhakul, K.; Kanokmedhakul, S. Two new bioactive triterpenoids from the roots of *Colubrina asiatica*. *Nat. Prod. Res.* **2020**, *34*, 482–488. [CrossRef] [PubMed]
167. Nadzir, M.M.; Ibrahim, N.E.; Idris, F.N.; Hisham, S.F. Biosynthesis of silver nanoparticles mediated by *Colubrina Asiatica* aqueous extract. *Mater. Today Proc.* **2019**, *16*, 2403–2407. [CrossRef]
168. Sangsopha, W.; Kanokmedhakul, K.; Lekphrom, R.; Kanokmedhakul, S. Chemical constituents and biological activities from branches of *Colubrina asiatica*. *Nat. Prod. Res.* **2018**, *32*, 1176–1179. [CrossRef] [PubMed]
169. Chaudhry, G.-e.-S.; Md Akim, A.; Sung, Y.Y.; Sifzizul, T.M.T. Cancer and apoptosis: The apoptotic activity of plant and marine natural products and their potential as targeted cancer therapeutics. *Front. Pharmacol.* **2022**, *13*, 842376. [CrossRef] [PubMed]
170. Vucic, D.; Fairbrother, W.J. The inhibitor of apoptosis proteins as therapeutic targets in cancer. *Clin. Cancer Res.* **2007**, *13*, 5995–6000. [CrossRef] [PubMed]
171. Gali-Muhtasib, H.; Hmadi, R.; Kareh, M.; Tohme, R.; Darwiche, N. Cell death mechanisms of plant-derived anticancer drugs: Beyond apoptosis. *Apoptosis* **2015**, *20*, 1531–1562. [CrossRef] [PubMed]
172. Nagini, S.; Kaur, S. Caspases: Moonlighting proteins with theranostic potential. In *Proteases in Human Diseases*; Chakraborti, S., Chakraborti, T., Dhalla, N.S., Eds.; Springer: Singapore, 2017; pp. 375–393.
173. Esmaeili, M.A.; Abagheri-Mahabadi, N.; Hashempour, H.; Farhadpour, M.; Gruber, C.W.; Ghassempour, A. Viola plant cyclotide vigno 5 induces mitochondria-mediated apoptosis via cytochrome C release and caspases activation in cervical cancer cells. *Fitoterapia* **2016**, *109*, 162–168. [CrossRef]
174. Zou, X.-G.; Li, J.; Sun, P.-L.; Fan, Y.-W.; Yang, J.-Y.; Deng, Z.-Y. Orbitides isolated from flaxseed induce apoptosis against SGC-7901 adenocarcinoma cells. *Int. J. Food Sci. Nutr.* **2020**, *71*, 929–939. [CrossRef] [PubMed]
175. de Matos Cândido-Bacani, P.; Ezan, F.; de Oliveira Figueiredo, P.; Matos, M.d.F.C.; Garcez, F.R.; Garcez, W.S.; Baffet, G. [1–9-NαC]-crourorb A1 isolated from *Croton urucurana* latex induces G2/M cell cycle arrest and apoptosis in human hepatocarcinoma cells. *Toxicol. Lett.* **2017**, *273*, 44–54. [CrossRef] [PubMed]
176. Peng, C.; Li, J.; Zhao, A.; Yu, S.; Zheng, L.; Deng, Z.Y. Non-oxidized and oxidized flaxseed orbitides differently induce HepG2 cell apoptosis: Involvement of cellular uptake and membrane death receptor DR4. *J. Sci. Food Agric.* **2024**, *104*, 4296–4308. [CrossRef]
177. Zou, X.-G.; Hu, J.-N.; Li, J.; Yang, J.-Y.; Du, Y.-X.; Yu, Y.-F.; Deng, Z.-Y. iCellular uptake of [1–9-NαC]-linusorb B2 and [1–9-NαC]-linusorb B3 isolated from flaxseed, and their antitumor activities in human gastric SGC-7901 cells. *J. Funct. Foods* **2018**, *48*, 692–703. [CrossRef]
178. Sung, N.Y.; Jeong, D.; Shim, Y.Y.; Ratan, Z.A.; Jang, Y.-J.; Reaney, M.J.; Lee, S.; Lee, B.-H.; Kim, J.-H.; Yi, Y.-S. The anti-cancer effect of linusorb B3 from flaxseed oil through the promotion of apoptosis, inhibition of actin polymerization, and suppression of Src activity in glioblastoma cells. *Molecules* **2020**, *25*, 5881. [CrossRef]
179. Sun, H.; Yang, J.; Fan, B.; Ren, M.; Wang, Y.; Chen, G.; Cheng, G. Genome-wide analysis of BURP domain-containing gene family in *Solanum lycopersicum* and functional analysis of *SlRD1* under drought and salt stresses. *Int. J. Mol. Sci.* **2024**, *25*, 12539. [CrossRef] [PubMed]
180. Yang, J.; Yang, T.; Yan, W.; Li, D.; Wang, F.; Wang, Z.; Guo, Y.; Bai, P.; Tan, N.; Chen, L. TAK1 inhibition by natural cyclopeptide RA-V promotes apoptosis and inhibits protective autophagy in Kras-dependent non-small-cell lung carcinoma cells. *RSC Adv.* **2018**, *8*, 23451–23458. [CrossRef] [PubMed]
181. Fang, X.-Y.; Chen, W.; Fan, J.-T.; Song, R.; Wang, L.; Gu, Y.-H.; Zeng, G.-Z.; Shen, Y.; Wu, X.-F.; Tan, N.-H. Plant cyclopeptide RA-V kills human breast cancer cells by inducing mitochondria-mediated apoptosis through blocking PDK1–AKT interaction. *Toxicol. Appl. Pharmacol.* **2013**, *267*, 95–103. [CrossRef] [PubMed]
182. Song, L.; Wang, Z.; Wang, Y.; Guo, D.; Yang, J.; Chen, L.; Tan, N. Natural cyclopeptide RA-XII, a new autophagy inhibitor, suppresses protective autophagy for enhancing apoptosis through AMPK/mTOR/P70S6K pathways in HepG2 cells. *Molecules* **2017**, *22*, 1934. [CrossRef] [PubMed]
183. Dutta, H.; Jain, N. Post-translational modifications and their implications in cancer. *Front. Oncol.* **2023**, *13*, 1240115. [CrossRef]
184. Walsh, G.; Jefferis, R. Post-translational modifications in the context of therapeutic proteins. *Nat. Biotechnol.* **2006**, *24*, 1241–1252. [CrossRef]
185. Gu, W.; Schmidt, E.W. Three principles of diversity-generating biosynthesis. *Acc. Chem. Res.* **2017**, *50*, 2569–2576. [CrossRef]
186. Montalban-Lopez, M.; Scott, T.A.; Ramesh, S.; Rahman, I.R.; van Heel, A.J.; Viel, J.H.; Bandarian, V.; Dittmann, E.; Genilloud, O.; Goto, Y.; et al. New developments in RiPP discovery, enzymology and engineering. *Nat. Prod. Rep.* **2021**, *38*, 130–239. [CrossRef] [PubMed]

187. Fujita, M.; Tanabata, T.; Urano, K.; Kikuchi, S.; Shinozaki, K. RIPPS: A plant phenotyping system for quantitative evaluation of growth under controlled environmental stress conditions. *Plant Cell Physiol.* **2018**, *59*, 2030–2038. [CrossRef]
188. Song, Z.-M.; Cai, C.; Gao, Y.; Lin, X.; Wu, G.; Liang, H.; Zhuo, Q.; Zhang, J.; Cai, P.; Liu, W.; et al. Deciphering the chemical landscape and potential ecological function of RiPPs from the untapped Archaea domain. *bioRxiv* **2024**. [CrossRef]
189. Alfi, A.; Popov, A.; Kumar, A.; Zhang, K.Y.; Dubiley, S.; Severinov, K.; Tagami, S. Cell-free mutant analysis combined with structure prediction of a lasso peptide biosynthetic protease B2. *ACS Synth. Biol.* **2022**, *11*, 2022–2028. [CrossRef]
190. Li, Y.; Han, Y.; Zeng, Z.; Li, W.; Feng, S.; Cao, W. Discovery and bioactivity of the novel lasso peptide microcin Y. *J. Agric. Food Chem.* **2021**, *69*, 8758–8767. [CrossRef]
191. Li, C.; Jin, K. Chemical strategies towards the development of effective anticancer peptides. *Curr. Med. Chem.* **2024**, *31*, 1839–1873. [CrossRef]
192. Jia, Z.; Zhu, X.; Zhou, Y.; Wu, J.; Cao, M.; Hu, C.; Yu, L.; Xu, R.; Chen, Z. Polypeptides from traditional Chinese medicine: Comprehensive review of perspective towards cancer management. *Int. J. Biol. Macromol.* **2024**, *260*, 129423. [CrossRef]
193. Colalto, C. Aspects of complexity in quality and safety assessment of peptide therapeutics and peptide-related impurities. a regulatory perspective. *Regul. Toxicol. Pharmacol.* **2024**, *153*, 105699. [CrossRef]
194. Comert Onder, F.; Ay, M. Recent developments in natural bioactive peptides: Anticancer potential and structure–activity relationships. In *Studies in Natural Products Chemistry*; Atta ur, R., Ed.; Elsevier: Amsterdam, The Netherlands, 2022; Volume 75, pp. 329–365.
195. Fujii, I. Heterologous expression systems for polyketide synthases. *Nat. Prod. Rep.* **2009**, *26*, 155–169. [CrossRef] [PubMed]
196. Watts, A.; Sankaranarayanan, S.; Watts, A.; Raipuria, R.K. Optimizing protein expression in heterologous system: Strategies and tools. *Meta Gene* **2021**, *29*, 100899. [CrossRef]

current issues in molecular biology

Review

Modulation of Multidrug Resistance Transporters by Food Components and Dietary Supplements: Implications for Cancer Therapy Efficacy and Safety

Agnieszka Brodzicka [1], Agnieszka Galanty [2] and Paweł Paśko [1,*]

[1] Department of Food Chemistry and Nutrition, Faculty of Pharmacy, Jagiellonian University Medical College, Medyczna 9, 30-688 Cracow, Poland

[2] Department of Pharmacognosy, Faculty of Pharmacy, Jagiellonian University Medical College, Medyczna 9, 30-688 Cracow, Poland; agnieszka.galanty@uj.edu.pl

* Correspondence: p.pasko@uj.edu.pl

Abstract: The aim of this review is to explore how diet and dietary supplements influence the activity of key multidrug resistance (MDR) transporters—MRP2, BCRP, and P-gp. These transporters play a crucial role in drug efflux from cancer cells and significantly affect chemotherapy outcomes. This review focuses on how dietary phytochemicals, such as catechins and quercetin, impact the expression and function of these transporters. Both in vitro and in vivo experiments were examined to assess changes in drug bioavailability and intracellular drug accumulation. The findings show that certain dietary components—such as catechins, flavonoids, resveratrol, curcumin, terpenoids, sterols, and alkaloids—can either inhibit or induce MDR transporter activity, thus influencing the effectiveness of chemotherapy. These results highlight the importance of understanding diet–drug interactions in cancer therapy to improve treatment outcomes and reduce side effects. In conclusion, dietary modifications and supplements should be carefully considered in cancer treatment plans to optimize therapeutic efficacy.

Keywords: MRP2; BCRP; P-gp; natural products; dietary supplements; anticancer drugs; drugs carriers

1. Introduction

The effectiveness and safety of anticancer therapy can be significantly influenced by different active compounds not only included in the daily diet but also in dietary supplements, which play crucial roles in modulating the activity of multidrug resistance (MDR) transporters. These transporters, such as multidrug resistance protein 2 (MRP2), breast cancer resistance protein (BCRP), and P-glycoprotein (P-gp), are pivotal in mediating drug efflux from cancer cells, thus contributing to the development of chemotherapy resistance [1]. Dietary components and supplements can either inhibit or induce these transporters, impacting drug bioavailability and therapeutic outcomes. The inhibition can lead to increased intracellular concentrations of chemotherapeutic agents, enhancing their cytotoxic effects on cancer cells [2,3]. Conversely, some dietary supplements may induce the expression of MDR transporters, potentially reducing the effectiveness of chemotherapy. Understanding the intricate interactions between diet, dietary supplements, and MDR transporters is crucial for optimizing cancer therapy. This knowledge can help in the development of dietary guidelines and supplement recommendations for patients undergoing chemotherapy, ensuring enhanced efficacy and reduced adverse effects [4,5].

The primary aim of this study is to investigate the impact of diet and dietary supplements on the function and expression of key MDR transporters, namely, MRP2, BCRP, and P-gp. Specifically, this study seeks to achieve the following: (i) elucidate the mechanisms: understand how various dietary components and supplements modulate the activity and expression of MRP2, BCRP, and P-gp in vitro and in vivo; (ii) evaluate the effects: assess the impact of these dietary factors on drug bioavailability, intracellular drug accumulation, and overall therapeutic outcomes in cancer treatment; and (iii) identify potential interactions: investigate potential beneficial or adverse interactions between dietary supplements and chemotherapeutic agents, with a focus on enhancing drug efficacy while minimizing toxicity.

2. Methods

A review of publications was conducted based on the PubMed and Google Scholar databases, together with reference lists of all chosen articles. The keywords used to search for publications were combinations of the following words: "food–drug interactions", "inhibition", "induction", "natural compounds", "drug transporters", "P-gp", "MRP2", "BCRP", "multidrug resistance", "cancer". The selection was limited to in vitro and in vivo studies using anticancer drugs and natural substances found in the daily diet, which could reverse multidrug resistance in cancer. Particular attention was given to studies describing the structure–activity relationship. A time limit covering the period 2017–2024 was introduced. No language constraints were introduced. All figures were made using ChemDraw 22.2.0 software.

3. Function of Selected Carriers Involved in Transport of Anticancer Drugs

3.1. *Multidrug Resistance-Associated Protein 2—MRP2*

Multidrug resistance-associated protein 2 (MRP2) is a member of the C subfamily of the superfamily of ATP-binding cassette (ABC), encoded by the *ABCC2* gene. It consists of 1545 amino acids forming three transmembrane domains and two ATP-binding domains. MRP2 is mostly expressed in the apical membrane of the tubular epithelial cells of the liver, kidney, and small intestine (Figure 1A). It is one of the efflux transporters and its main role is to pump out endogenous and exogenous substances from the cells. Its expression in the intestine limits the absorption of xenobiotics from the gastrointestinal tract, while in the liver, it facilitates the elimination of positively charged drugs and bilirubin glucuronate into the bile. It reduces the bioavailability of the drugs that are its substrates, including methotrexate, cisplatin, irinotecan, doxorubicin, ceftriaxone, ampicillin, and saquinavir. Its expression is increased in tumor tissues (including lung cancer, liver cancer, gastric cancer, squamous cell carcinoma of head and neck, and ovarian cancer), where it contributes to multidrug resistance by reducing intracellular drug accumulation [6,7].

In recent years, in vitro and in vivo studies have been conducted to find dietary-derived compounds that can affect the activity of the MRP2 transporter and help overcome multidrug resistance in cancer, what is discussed below.

3.2. *Breast Cancer Resistance Protein—BCRP*

Breast cancer resistance protein (BCRP) belongs to the ABC superfamily of transporters. It is encoded by the *ABCG2* gene and consists of 655 amino acids forming six α-helices. In the human body, it is localized on the apical side of enterocytes, hepatocytes, renal proximal tubule cells, and blood–brain barrier endothelial cells (Figure 1B). As an efflux transporter, it plays an important role in protecting cells from toxic compounds. In cancer cells, it is responsible for pumping drugs outside the cell, thereby contributing to multidrug resistance. Substrates of this transporter are endogenous compounds including urea, estrone-3-sulfate, and dehydroepiandrosterone sulfate and drugs including rosuvastatin, topotecan, sunitinib, grepafloxacin, acyclovir, cimetidine, methotrexate, and sulfasalazine [8,9].

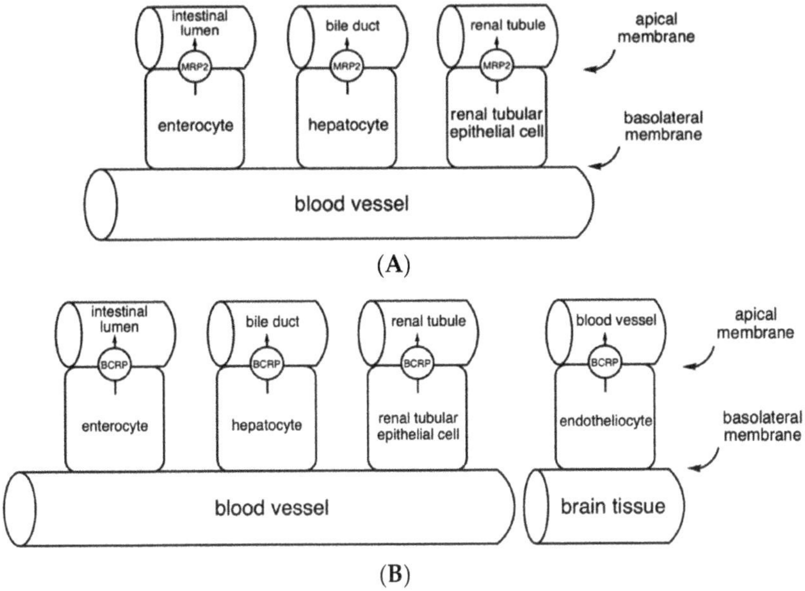

Figure 1. Localization of the MRP2 (**A**) and BCRP (**B**) transporters and the transport direction of their substrates in cells of the intestine, liver, kidney (**A**,**B**), and blood–brain barrier cells (**B**) according to [7,9].

3.3. *P-Glycoprotein—P-gp*

One of the best-studied and described xenobiotic transporters is P-glycoprotein (P-gp, ABCB1, MDR1), a member of the ABC family. P-gp is a glycosylated and phosphorylated protein composed of 1280 amino acids of 170 kDa occurring in several isoforms. It consists of two units, each containing an intracellular hydrophilic nucleotide-binding domain (NBD1 and NBD2) and a transmembrane domain (TMD1 and TMD2) composed of six hydrophobic α-helices (TM1-12). Within the NBD domain, ATP is hydrolyzed to ADP and Pi, used to translocate molecules across the cell membrane, while the TMD domains are responsible for substrate recognition and transport pathway determination [10–12]. P-gp is thought to have at least three substrate-binding sites and one allosteric regulatory site [10]. It is a transporter for many substrates that differ in molecular weight, structure, and function. It transports both low-mass molecules, such as amino acids, carbohydrates, and organic cations, and macromolecules, including proteins and polysaccharides [10,12]. Most substrates are lipid-soluble and have slightly amphipathic and hydrophobic properties. Often, substrates contain a positively charged nitrogen atom and aromatic rings [12]. P-gp substrates include digoxin, fexofenadine, loperamide, quinidine, or vinblastine [13], and they are localized in many tissues; of particular importance are the barrier tissues. Its presence has been found in the endothelium of cerebral vessels, kidneys, liver, lungs, ovaries, stomach, enterocytes of intestinal villi, and intestinal mucosa, as well as in the vascular endothelium of cancerous tumors [11]. P-gp is an efflux transporter and thus has a primarily protective function of shedding endogenous and exogenous toxic compounds outside the cell, thereby reducing the availability of xenobiotics. It also influences the development of multidrug resistance in antineoplastic, anticancer, and antiepileptic drug therapies. Its overexpression is associated with drug-resistant epilepsy and cancers of the hematopoietic system, brain, intestine, and kidney [11,12].

4. Influence of Polyphenolic Compounds on MDR Transporters

4.1. Catechins

Catechins are flavan derivatives, predominantly found in green tea (*Camellia sinensis* L. (Kuntze)). The most abundant green tea catechin is epigallocatechin gallate (EGCG), known for its antioxidant properties. Green tea is widely consumed both as a beverage and in dietary supplement form, where it is marketed for its potential benefits in supporting cardiovascular health, weight management, and antioxidant protection. The high concentration of catechins in green tea makes it a popular choice for people seeking natural antioxidant supplements [14]. Additionally, cocoa and dark chocolate are rich sources of catechins, particularly epicatechin (EC). These compounds contribute to the antioxidant capacity of cocoa products and are linked to various health benefits, including improved cardiovascular function and reduced risk of chronic diseases [15].

Some studies have highlighted the role of stereochemistry of green tea catechins in regulating the efflux transport rather than the absorption transport in the Caco-2 monolayers. Better transcellular permeability in the efflux transport was shown by trans catechins when compared to the corresponding cis (epi) catechins. In addition, after incubation with catechins, a significant increase in the expression of MRP2 and BCRP and decrease in the expression of P-gp in Caco-2 cells was observed [16]. Another study showed the combined effect of catechins and other phytochemicals present in green tea, namely, caffeine and theanine but also serine and glycine, on Caco-2 monolayers. The cells were incubated with EGCG, epicatechin gallate (ECG), or EC, which are substrates for MRP2, combined with caffeine, theanine, serine, or glycine. The MRP2 expression in the cells treated with EGCG and EC was increased 1.58- and 2.98-fold, respectively, while no significant changes were seen for ECG. The addition of caffeine, theanine, serine, and glycine caused a decrease in MRP2 expression, increased by EGCG. Only glycine caused a decrease in EC-enhanced MRP2 expression. The results of the study suggest that caffeine, theanine, glycine, and serine in tea may increase catechin transport by decreasing the expression of the catechin-enhanced efflux transporter MRP2 [17].

A study on Caco-2 cells was performed with BCRP substrate H33342 and BCRP inhibitor Ko143 with sodium fluoride. The cells pretreated with a green tea infusion, ECG, and EGCG, showed a significant increase in intracellular accumulation of the substrate, while the increase for EC and epigallocatechin (EGC) was not statistically significant. An analogous study was also conducted using aflatoxin B1 as a substrate of BCRP. The ejection rate of the aflatoxin B1 after preincubation with a green tea infusion and ECG, EGC, and EGCG was significantly reduced. The results suggest an inhibitory effect of the catechins present in green tea on the activity of the BCRP transporter [18].

The effect of EGCG on pharmacokinetics of tacrolimus and cyclosporine A was investigated in an in vivo study. The compounds were administered to rats (n = 42), with or without EGCG. Coadministration of EGCG caused a reduction in the C_{max} and AUC of tacrolimus, and distribution/elimination profiles were enhanced. The C_{max} and AUC of cyclosporine A were increased by ECGC at a dose of 3–30 mg/kg but decreased at a dose of 100 mg/kg. To investigate the underlying mechanism, the rats were administered EGCG (3, 10, 30, and 100 mg/kg for 7 days) or CYP3A (ketoconazole, 75 mg/kg) or P-gp (verapamil, 24 mg/kg) inhibitors. The mRNA levels of the drug-metabolizing enzymes, drug transporters (including MRP2), and nuclear receptors were then examined. Compared to the control, untreated group, a reduction in the amount of mRNA of MRP2 was observed in liver cells by 21.13, 47, 60, 40.41, and 25.22%, respectively. In the intestinal cells, a reduction in the amount of mRNA of MRP2 was also noted by 13.89, 47.77, 36.11, and 13.50%, respectively. This suggests an inhibitory effect of EGCG on MRP2 expression [19].

4.2. Quercetin and Its Derivatives

Quercetin is one of the most widespread plant flavonoids. It is found in vegetables such as onions and tomatoes, in fruits such as berries, apples, and grapes, and medicinal plants such as ginkgo biloba and St. John's wort. Quercetin and its derivatives are available in numerous dietary supplements designed to enhance immune function and reduce oxidative stress. These supplements often combine quercetin with vitamin C or bromelain to improve absorption and efficacy [20,21]. Quercetin exhibits many health-promoting properties, such as cardioprotective, anti-inflammatory, antioxidant, and antianaphylactic, and these make it a popular and widely available dietary supplement. These products typically contain 200–1500 mg of quercetin aglycone per tablet or capsule, and the manufacturers' recommended daily dose is 150–4000 mg. Compared to supplementation, the average daily intake of quercetin from food is 5–40 mg, which is up to 100 times lower than the value recommended by manufacturers [22–24].

Mohos V. et al. [22] investigated the effects of quercetin and its metabolites, quercetin 3′-sulfate, quercetin 3-glucuronide, isorhamnetin, and isorhamnetin 3-glucuronide, on the activity of the MRP2 transporter in an inverted insect cell membrane vesicles model, and CDCF was used as the substrate for MRP2. A statistically significant decrease in the transport of CDCF by MRP2 was observed when each flavonoid was administered at a concentration of 20 μM. Isorhamnetin 3-glucuronide, quercetin 3′-sulfate, and quercetin 3-glucuronide showed stronger impacts on the MRP2 activity (IC_{50} = 14.9, 19.6, and 24.2 μM, respectively) than hydrophobic compounds—quercetin and isorhamnetin (IC_{50} > 30 μM). In the same study, the effect of these flavonoids on the activity of BCRP was also examined. A statistically significant decrease in the transport of a specific fluorescent substrate (lucifer yellow) was induced by 0.05 μM of quercetin, 0.2 μM of quercetin-3′-sulfate, 1.0 μM of quercetin-3-glucuronide, 0.05 μM of isorhamnetin, and 20 μM of isorhamnetin-3-glucuronide. Quercetin and isorhamnetin were potent inhibitors of BCRP (IC_{50} = 0.13 and 0.06 μM, respectively); quercetin-3′-sulfate also showed strong inhibition (IC_{50} = 3.20 μM), whereas the glucuronides quercetin-3-glucuronide and isorhamnetin-3-glucuronide were weak inhibitors (IC_{50} = 13.5 μM, IC_{50} > 30 μM, respectively).

MDCKII-MRP2 is a specialized cell line derived from Madin-Darby canine kidney (MDCK) cells, which is a widely used model for studying epithelial cell functions. This specific cell line has been genetically engineered to overexpress the human MRP2. The cells were treated with phenolsulfonphtalein (MRP2 substrate), probenecid (MRP2 inhibitor), or 5 or 10 μM quercetin. Quercetin showed a statistically significant inhibitory effect on the MRP2 transporter at the higher concentration tested. The human colon adenocarcinoma cells (LS174T) were treated with vincristine (an MRP2 inducer) or quercetin. Quercetin at a concentration of 50 μM increased MRP2 mRNA expression three-fold compared to the control group and showed a stronger activating effect than vincristine [23].

In the in vivo study, the rats (n = 18) received the following: phosphate buffer (control group) or ketoconazole (CYP3A4 inhibitor) or verapamil (P-gp inhibitor) or a low (2.5 mg/kg), medium (5 mg/kg), or high (10 mg/kg) dose of quercetin 3-O-β-D-glucoside for 7 days. The amount of MRP2 transporter mRNA was significantly reduced by quercetin 3-O-β-D-glucoside at low, medium, and high doses by 66.03, 34.53, and 28.66% in the small intestine, respectively, and in the liver by 68.86, 32.70, and 20.44%, respectively, compared to the control group. In the groups with low, middle, and high doses of quercetin 3-O-β-D-glucoside, the amount of BCRP mRNA was reduced by 63.83, 27.52, and 43.68%, respectively, in the small intestine. However, in the liver, the middle- and high-dose quercetin 3-O-β-D-glucoside groups decreased the BCRP mRNA expression levels by 29.23 and 29.23%, respectively, and only the low-dose quercetin 3-O-β-D-glucoside group showed a significant reduction (56.15%). The effect was not dose-dependent. A low dose of quercetin 3-O-β-D-glucoside showed the strongest inhibitory effect on the MRP2 and BCRP transporter. Similar results were obtained when MRP2 and BCRP protein expression was examined. Quercetin 3-O-β-D-glucoside at low, medium, and high doses reduced MRP2 protein expression by 75.95, 42.60, and 50.84%, respectively, in the intestine compared to the control group, while in the liver, only the low dose of the substance showed a statistically significant 70.70% reduction in expression. In the low-, middle-, and high-dose quercetin 3-O-β-D-glucoside groups, BCRP protein expression was decreased by 70.61, 32.93, and

36.44%, respectively, in the small intestine and by 69.78, 27.73, and 30.86%, respectively, in the liver. The effect was also not dose-dependent [24].

Oral administration of quercetin (50, 100, and 250 mg/kg) to rats for 7 days had no effect on mRNA expression in the liver and kidney, while in the intestine, after administration of 100 mg/kg quercetin, mRNA expression was 15.4 times higher compared to the control group. The difference in MRP2 mRNA expression in different organs may have been due to higher concentrations of quercetin in the intestine than in the liver and kidney as a result of the first-pass effect. A further study using phenolsulfonphthalein and orally administered quercetin once or for 7 days at doses of 50, 100, and 250 mg/kg showed no significant changes in the pharmacokinetics of phenolsulfonphthalein [23]. In a recent in vivo experiment, the control group was orally administered docetaxel, and the study group was orally administered quercetin (100 mg/kg) and docetaxel. A significant increase in AUCinf was observed in the study group from 141.35 ± 35 to 251 ± 65, suggesting an inhibitory effect of quercetin on MRP2 transporter activity. The concentration of quercetin in the intestine was 18.1 mM, which may be a concentration higher than the IC_{50} of P-gp and CYP3A4 for quercetin. This suggests that the increased AUCinf may also have been due to the inhibition of P-gp and CYP3A4 activity. The total plasma concentration of quercetin was 78.1 μM, but its free plasma concentration was predicted to be much lower than the IC_{50} value against MRP2 (higher than 50 μM). It is caused by quercetin binding to plasma protein extensively. This might be the reason for incoherent results between in vitro and in vivo studies. The authors suggest that quercetin modulates the function and expression of MRP2 in vitro, while under in vivo conditions, there is little likelihood of the interaction [23].

4.3. Apigenin

Apigenin is a flavonoid predominantly found in parsley, celery, and chamomile tea. It is also present in significant amounts in fruits like oranges and certain herbs such as thyme and oregano. Apigenin is widely studied for its potential health benefits, including anti-inflammatory, antioxidant, and anticancer effects. Dietary supplements containing apigenin are marketed for their potential to support immune function, reduce inflammation, and promote relaxation and sleep [25].

The inhibitory potential of apigenin was investigated in a sole study. Oral administration of dasatinib after seven days' pretreatment of apigenin (40 mg/kg) significantly increased the plasma concentration of dasatinib compared to dasatinib alone. The significant inhibition of the BCRP protein (66.77% inhibition in hepatic cells and 41.06% inhibition in intestinal cells) was noted in the apigenin-pretreated rats compared to dasatinib alone. The bioavailability of dasatinib was enhanced by the significant inhibition of CYP3A2, P-gp, and BCRP1 expression and the suppression of its hepatic and intestinal metabolism [26].

4.4. Licochalcone A

Licochalcone A is a chalconoid predominantly found in the root of different licorice species. This compound is noted for its anti-inflammatory, antioxidant, and antimicrobial properties. It is used in various traditional medicines and is also being studied for its potential therapeutic applications in modern medicine. Licochalcone A is present in dietary supplements aimed at promoting skin health and reducing inflammation. These supplements often source licochalcone A from licorice root extracts, taking advantage of its potential benefits in managing skin conditions and enhancing overall wellness [27,28].

The effect of licochalcone A on the efflux transporters in the multidrug resistance cancer cells was examined using R482-HEK293 cells—a genetically engineered cell line derived from the human embryonic kidney 293 (HEK293) cells, overexpressing the R482 variant of the human BCRP. The cells were treated with different doses of mitoxantrone or topotecan and with nontoxic concentrations of licochalcone A (0.5, 1, 2, and 3 μM). Licochalcone A significantly restored the chemosensitivity of the cells to mitoxantrone and topotecan in a concentration-dependent manner (mitoxantrone: IC_{50} = 18.75, 7.09, 7.83, and 6.22 nM, respectively; topotecan: IC_{50} = 90.05, 51.47, 44.11, and 42.41 nM, respectively). It also significantly reversed BCRP-mediated mitoxantrone and topotecan resistance in a concentration-dependent manner in S1-M1-80 (mitoxantrone: IC_{50} = 39.47, 6.80, 2.63, and 1.53 μM, respectively; topotecan: IC_{50} = 1.03, 0.61, 0.41, and 0.31 μM) and H460-MX20 cell lines (mitoxantrone: IC_{50} = 441.96, 86.46, 74.77, and 69.86 nM, respectively; topotecan: IC_{50} = 366.91, 143.89, 147.56, and 130.38 nM, respectively) [29].

4.5. Miscellaneous Flavonoids

Some studies have also focused on flavonoids, which are commonly found in plants used for their beneficial effect on human health. These included ginkgo and St. John's wort (e.g., amentoflavone, apigenin, sciadopitysin), red clover (biochanin A), Chinese skullcap (e.g., oroxylin A), citrus fruits (e.g., diosmin, naringenin, isosinensetin, tangeretin, and sinensetin), kale, spinach, and broccoli (e.g., kaempferol, kaempferide) or propolis (e.g., chrysin, genkwanin). These compounds are incorporated into dietary supplements for their antioxidant, anti-inflammatory, and potential therapeutic properties and for metabolic health [30–33].

The effect of almost 100 flavonoids on BCRP transporter activity was investigated using mitoxantrone as a substrate. The flavonoids at 50 μM or the highest nontoxic concentration applied to MDCKII-BCRP cells showed significant, over 50%, inhibition of BCRP transporter activity. Next, the concentration–inhibitory effect relationship of the flavonoids was studied. The strongest inhibitor was amentoflavone (IC_{50} = 4 ± 1 μM), followed by kaempferide (IC_{50} = 5 ± 1 μM), kaempferol (IC_{50} = 15 ± 2 μM), diosmin (IC_{50} = 17 ± 3 μM), naringenin (IC_{50} = 19 ± 2 μM), chrysin (IC_{50} = 20 ± 3 μM), apigenin (IC_{50} = 24 ± 3 μM), biochanin A (IC_{50} = 24 ± 4 μM), licochalcone A (IC_{50} = 33 ± 8 μM), and genkwanin (IC_{50} = 37 ± 5 μM). The study was further conducted on rats (n = 39), which received a single dose of amentoflavone, licochalcone A, diosmin, chrysin, or naringenin at 30 mg/kg; genkwanin at 10 mg/kg; apigenin, biochanin A, kaempferol, or kaempferide at 25 mg/kg; or Ko143 at 25 mg/kg (positive control group), followed by the administration of mitoxantrone after 30 min. A 25.62% increase in the AUC0-t value of mitoxantrone was observed in the positive control group. After the administration of apigenin, naringenin, licochalcone A, kaempferol, and chrysin, an increase in AUC0-t values was observed by 30.10–81.97%, which was higher than that of the positive control group. The results indicate a significant inhibitory effect on the BCRP transporter activity of 11 of the 99 flavonoids tested [34]. A similar in vivo study on naringenin was also performed in rats (n = 12), which were provided with a single oral dose of dasatinib, with or without naringenin pretreatment (150 mg/kg daily for 7 days). The plasma mean concentration of dasatinib was significantly enhanced in the pretreated group compared with the non-pretreated animals [35].

A total of 75 flavonoids were examined towards their inhibitory effect on P-gp using MDR1–MDCKII cells. The concentration range of flavonoids screened was 0–100 μM except for tangeretin, isosinensetin, sciadopitysin, and oroxylin A, which were screened at 0–150 μM for further IC_{50} assay. Isosinensetin, tangeretin, sinensetin, sciadopitysin, and oroxylin A showed significant inhibition with the following IC_{50} values: 4.2, 12.66, 18.9, 53.42, and 78.33 μM, respectively. The wild cancer cells MX-1 and taxol-resistant MX-1/T cells were used to investigate the effect of P-gp inhibition by flavonoids (isosinensetin 8.4 μM, tangeretin 25.3 μM, sinensetin 37.8 μM, sciadopitysin 106.8 μM, oroxylin A 155.6 μM) on taxol (75μM) cytotoxicity. All flavonoids mentioned before and verapamil increased taxol toxicity in both cell lines, and tangeretin, oroxylin A, and sciadopitysin showed a much stronger reduction in cell viability than verapamil. Tangeretin and sciadopitysin significantly augmented taxol cytotoxicity in MX-1/T cells compared with MX-1 cells, and these might be used to reverse multidrug resistance in cancer [36].

An interesting study compared the activity of a number of polyphenols present in sour cherry (*Prunus cerasus*) fruits. The compounds were tested for their impact on the P-gp activity on the NIH 3T3 mouse fibroblast cell line and its human P-gp-overexpressing analogue, NIH 3T3 MDR1. The results showed that quercetin, quercetin-3-glucoside, narcissoside, and ellagic acid lowered the ATPase activity of P-gp and increased the accumulation of calcein and daunorubicin by P-gp-positive cells. Cyanidin-3O-sophoroside, catechin, naringenin, kuromanin, and caffeic acid also augmented the ATPase activity of P-gp, but they had a weaker impact on the intracellular accumulation of calcein and daunorubicin. Polyphenols such as epicatechin, trans-ferulic acid, oenin, malvin, and chlorogenic acid presented no effect. What is interesting is that two stereoisomers, catechin and epicatechin, showed different effects. The application of quercetin, naringenin, or ellagic acid with verapamil, a P-gp inhibitor, led to an additive or synergistic inhibitory effect that might be used in further studies to reverse multidrug resistance [37].

4.6. Sinapic Acid

Sinapic acid is a phenolic compound found in various fruits, vegetables, and grains. It is particularly abundant in canola (rapeseed) oil, mustard seeds, and certain berries like blueberries and cranberries. Sinapic acid is known for its antioxidant and anti-inflammatory properties, and it is increasingly incorporated into dietary supplements aimed at promoting cardiovascular health and reducing oxidative stress [38].

A sole study examined the impact of sinapic acid on BCRP protein. A single dose of dasatinib was given to rats (n = 6), with or without sinapic acid pretreatment (20 mg/kg per day for 7 days). A significant inhibition of the BCRP protein (51.44% inhibition in hepatic cells and 50.48% inhibition in intestinal cells) was observed in the pretreated rats compared with the animals given dasatinib alone. An increase in the bioavailability of dasatinib was found via modulation of CYP3A2, P-gp, and BCPR protein expression [39].

4.7. Resveratrol

Resveratrol is a stilbenoid found in a variety of foods, most notably in the peels of red grapes, translating to its presence in red wine and contributing to its potential health benefits. Additionally, resveratrol can be sourced from peanuts, dark chocolate, and certain types of Japanese knotweed (*Polygonum cuspidatum*), which is often used in supplements [40,41].

The effect of resveratrol on the expression of genes associated with multidrug resistance and the proteins encoded by these genes, including the *ABCB1* gene encoding P-gp, was investigated. Human gastric cancer cell lines were used for the study: two daunorubicin-resistant (EPG85-257RDB; RDB) and mitoxantrone-resistant (EPG85-257RNOV; RNOV) and one cytostatic-sensitive (EPG85-257P, a control cell line). Cells were treated with 30 or 50 μM resveratrol for 72 h. Resveratrol at both concentrations showed a statistically significant reduction in the expression of the *ABCB1* gene, among others. In the RDB cell line, a reduction in the expression of all the genes tested and selected proteins, including P-gp, was observed. Based on the results, it can be concluded that resveratrol, after long exposure, can reduce multidrug resistance in cancer cells by decreasing gene and protein expression [42]. Another study was conducted to evaluate the effects of resveratrol on the expression and function of P-gp on Caco-2 in CEM/ADR5000 cell lines. Resveratrol at concentrations of 10–100 μM inhibited P-gp efflux function by causing the accumulation of rhodamine 123 with calcein in a dose-dependent manner. In the rhodamine 123 assay, the potency of P-gp inhibition by resveratrol was 2.11–3.90 times higher than that caused by verapamil, which served as a positive control. In a calcein assay, the inhibitory potency was 1.64–4.6 times stronger than that caused by verapamil. Administration of 20 μM resveratrol also resulted in a significant increase in the cytotoxicity of doxorubicin, allowing the dose of the drug to be reduced while maintaining the effect. The cytotoxicity of doxorubicin combined with resveratrol was IC_{50} = 1.23 μM, compared to IC_{50} = 4.15 μM for doxorubicin alone. A 48 h observation of the Caco-2 cell line also noted significantly lower P-gp mRNA levels due to the presence of 20 μM resveratrol. The results of the study confirmed the inhibitory effect of resveratrol on the efflux activity of ABC transporters, including P-gp, as well as their expression [43].

4.8. Curcumin

Curcumin is a bioactive compound predominantly found in turmeric, a spice derived from the root of the *Curcuma longa* plant. It is widely used in traditional Indian and Southeast Asian cuisines and is the primary ingredient in curry powder, contributing to its distinctive yellow color and potential health benefits, such as anti-inflammatory and antioxidant effects [44,45].

An in vitro study was performed to examine how natural compounds can control BCRP expression in mixed conditions. Human oral squamous carcinoma OECM1 and head/neck cancer SASL90d cell lines were used in the experiment. Curcumin at the doses of 5, 10, and 15 µM and EGCG at the doses of 20, 30, and 50 µM significantly decreased BCRP levels and BCRP protein expression compared with the control group. The therapeutic effect of the tested compounds was also examined. Protoporphyrin IX accumulation was enhanced in EGCG- and curcumin-treated cells in a dose-dependent manner and was inversely correlated with the cell viability [46].

The study conducted on Caco-2, CEM/ADR5000, and CCRF-CEM cell lines was to test whether the combination of polyphenols, including curcumin, with doxorubicin showed synergistic effects in anticancer treatment. The results showed a beneficial effect of combining polyphenols with doxorubicin on the sensitization of cancer cells. The ability of the polyphenols used to inhibit P-gp activity was also investigated. The evaluation was based on the concentration of doxorubicin inside the cell. All polyphenols showed an increase in doxorubicin concentration. The results of the study presented evidence of curcumin's inhibitory effect on P-gp in the Caco-2 and CEM/ADR5000 cell lines. A study on the CCRF-CEM cell line showing low expression of ABC transporters confirmed the absence of P-gp transporter activity [47]. The ability of curcumin to reverse multidrug resistance was also investigated on doxorubicin-resistant colon cancer cells of the SW620/Ad300 line. Curcumin administration showed an increase in doxorubicin-induced cytotoxicity and cell apoptosis, which was due to the reversal of resistance mediated by P-gp action. Further studies indicated an increase in doxorubicin accumulation in resistant cells after curcumin administration due to its inhibitory effect on P-gp activity. No changes were observed in the doxorubicin-sensitive SW620 cell line. The above data suggest the ability of curcumin to reverse multidrug resistance during anticancer treatment [48].

5. Effect of Terpenoids and Sterols on MDR Transporters

Menthol, geraniol, caryophyllene, and carnosol are naturally occurring terpenoid compounds with notable health benefits. Menthol is a monoterpene primarily found in the essential oils of different mint plants, such as peppermint (*Mentha × piperita*), and is widely used in foods, beverages, and topical products for its cooling and soothing effects. Geraniol, a monoterpene alcohol, is abundant in essential oils of roses, geraniums, and citronella and contributes to their fragrance. Caryophyllene, a sesquiterpene, is present in black pepper, cloves, and cinnamon, known for its spicy aroma and potential anti-inflammatory properties. Carnosol is a diterpenoid, found in rosemary (*Rosmarinus officinalis*) and sage (*Salvia officinalis*) and is noted for its antioxidant and cytotoxic activities [49,50].

5.1. Menthol

An in vitro study on HepG2 cells was conducted to evaluate the effect of menthol on the expression of MRP2 and its impact on the cytotoxicity of epirubicin and cisplatin. Exposure of the cells to menthol at concentrations of 50 and 100 µM increased the expression of MRP2 mRNA and led to a decrease in the intracellular accumulation of epirubicin and in the intracellular concentration of the epirubicin remaining. Menthol at a concentration of 10 µM had no significant effect on the expression of MRP2. Treatment with MK-571 (MRP2 inhibitor), but not verapamil (P-gp inhibitor), significantly attenuated the reduced intracellular accumulation of epirubicin. Both epirubicin and cisplatin had cytotoxic effects on HepG2 cells, but the decline in cell viability was significantly suppressed by 24 h exposure to menthol. These findings show that menthol leads hepatocellular carcinoma to develop resistance to anticancer treatments, such as epirubicin and cisplatin, through the induction of MRP2 [51].

5.2. Geraniol

The potential effect of geraniol supplementation on restoring MRP2 activity inhibited by fructose as an inductor of metabolic syndrome was examined. Wistar rats were used to investigate the effects of geraniol on metabolic syndrome (MetS)-like conditions [52]. The animals were fed a standard commercial diet and received plain tap water (control group) or tap water with 10% fructose (FRU group) for 21 days to induce MetS-like conditions. In the geraniol treatment protocol, both control and MetS rats were administered either Tween 80 (control) or geraniol in Tween 80 (250 mg/kg/day). Supplementation with this natural compound restored MRP2 activity in fructose-fed rats [14].

5.3. β-Caryophyllene Oxide

Interesting in vitro studies were performed to investigate the ability of β-caryophyllene oxide (CRYO) at nontoxic doses to suppress efflux transporters and augment the response of hepatocellular carcinoma cells to sorafenib. Flow cytometry of fluorescent substrates' export revealed that CRYO inhibited the efflux of rhodamine 123 (MDR1) and calcein (MRP1 and MRP2) but did not inhibit fluorescein (MRP3, MRP4, MRP5). Treatment of human liver Alexander cell sublines, both WT (wild-type) and R (with enhanced multidrug resistance), with sorafenib caused cell death, which was more marked in WT cells than in R cells. The IC_{50} value was lower in WT cells (1.2 ± 0.4 μM) than in R cells (3.3 ± 0.3 μM). An in vivo study in mice showed that CRYO inhibited sorafenib efflux, favored its intracellular accumulation, and enhanced its cytotoxic response [53]. In the in vivo study, Hepa1-6 wild-type (WT) and Hepa1-6/R (resistant) liver cancer cells were implanted in mice to evaluate the efficacy of sorafenib and its combination with CRYO. After 28 days, tumors developed with a final volume (FTV) of 7.9 ± 0.4 cm^3 in the WT group and 6.6 ± 0.3 cm^3 in the resistant group. Treatment with sorafenib alone reduced the tumor volume in WT cells by 38% (to 4.9 ± 0.5 cm^3) and was less effective in resistant cells, showing a 20% reduction (to 5.3 ± 0.6 cm^3), which was not statistically significant. However, the combination of sorafenib with CRYO significantly enhanced the treatment's efficacy, reducing tumor volumes by approximately 65% and 58% in WT and in the resistant cells, respectively. Tumor weights at the study's conclusion corresponded with these volume measurements. Additionally, high-performance liquid chromatography–mass spectrometry (HPLC-MS/MS) analysis revealed that coadministration of CRYO increased the intratumoral concentration of sorafenib. In WT tumors, sorafenib levels increased from 67 ± 6 nmol/g tissue to 87 ± 5 nmol/g with CRYO. In resistant tumors, sorafenib accumulation was initially lower (31 ± 3 nmol/g) but increased significantly (to 94 ± 5 nmol/g) with the addition of CRYO, suggesting CRYO enhances sorafenib's accumulation and efficacy in tumor tissue.

In a study on human cholangiocarcinoma EGI-1 and TFK-1 cell lines, the loading value of 25 μM mitoxantrone was higher when it was administered with the BCRP inhibitor fumitremorgin C compared to mitoxantrone alone. A similar effect was observed with mitoxantrone and CRYO. The compound significantly increased the cytotoxicity caused by cisplatin, mitoxantrone, sorafenib, and 7-ethyl-10-hydroxy-camptothecin in EGI-1 and TFK-1 cell lines. It showed little or no effect with gemcitabine, 5-fluorouracil, and oxaliplatin. A further in vivo study was performed in mice (n = 15) treated with 50 mg/kg CRYO, cisplatin, or a combination of both substances. A significant inhibitory effect on the BCRP transporter was observed only in the third group [54].

5.4. Carnosic Acid and Carnosol

Carnosic acid, carnosol, and rosemary extract (containing 23.2% carnosic acid and 12.4% carnosol) at concentrations up to 100 μg/mL were applied to a HepG2 cell line model for 24 h. Carnosic acid significantly increased the expression of the MRP2 transporter in contrast to rosemary extract and carnosol, which increased the expression only slightly. Increasing the expression of the MRP2 transporter may be one of the methods used in chemoprevention [55].

5.5. Beta-Sitosterol

Beta-sitosterol, a plant sterol with cholesterol-lowering properties, is naturally present in a variety of foods including nuts, seeds, and plant-based oils. Significant sources include peanuts, almonds, and avocados. It is also found in high amounts in wheat germ and soy products. These dietary sources contribute to its potential benefits in managing cholesterol levels and supporting heart health. In dietary supplements, beta-sitosterol is often derived from plant sources such as soybeans, corn, and pine trees. These supplements are commonly marketed for their benefits in reducing cholesterol levels and alleviating symptoms of benign prostatic hyperplasia (BPH). They provide a concentrated source of beta-sitosterol compared to typical dietary intake [56].

An in vitro study was conducted on HCT116/OXA cells, human colon cancer cells resistant to oxaliplatin. A significant decrease in the IC_{50} values of oxaliplatin was observed after administration of β-sitosterol at concentrations of 12.5, 25, and 50 μM, suggesting the sensitization of cells to its effects, with IC_{50} values of 222.74 ± 9.53, 98.29 ± 5.65, and 72.06 ± 4.52 μM, respectively, compared to 279.81 ± 11.69 μM in the control group. In further studies to determine which transporter associated with multidrug resistance is affected by β-sitosterol, the intracellular accumulations of mitoxantrone (BCRP substrate), rhodamine 123 (P-gp substrate), and CDCF (MRP2 substrate) were evaluated. β-sitosterol did not affect the intracellular accumulation of rhodamine 123 and CDCF but significantly dose-dependently increased the accumulation of mitoxantrone, indicating an inhibitory effect of β-sitosterol on BCRP transporter activity. BCRP expression in cells with oxaliplatin applied was not significantly reduced. The combination of oxaliplatin with 50 μM β-sitosterol showed significant inhibition of the expression of this transporter. The researchers also conducted an in vivo study on mice (n = 24) inoculated with HCT116/OXA cells to induce tumors and administered with β-sitosterol at 10 mg/kg, oxaliplatin, or the two substances combined. In the oxaliplatin group, a slight inhibition of tumor growth was observed. No changes were observed in the β-sitosterol-only group compared to the control group. Significant inhibition from day 12 of therapy was noted in mice given oxaliplatin combined with β-sitosterol, with a tumor volume 87% smaller compared to the control group. The results suggest that the combined use of oxaliplatin with β-sitosterol may have a beneficial effect on the treatment of colorectal cancer [57].

6. Effect of Alkaloids on MDR Transporters

6.1. Berberine

Berberine is an alkaloid predominantly found in several traditional medicinal plants, including Berberis species (such as *Berberis vulgaris*), *Coptis chinensis* (golden thread), and *Phellodendron amurense* (Amur cork tree). These plants are commonly used in traditional Chinese medicine for their antimicrobial, anti-inflammatory, and blood-sugar-lowering effects. Berberine is commonly present in dietary supplements recommended for hyperglycemia and atherosclerosis [58].

An in vitro study on the MCF-7/DOXFluc breast cancer cell line showed that berberine administered with doxorubicin in a 2:1 ratio optimally enhanced the antiproliferative effects of doxorubicin by increasing its concentration and retention time in tumor cells as a result of facilitating its uptake by inhibiting P-gp activity. The group treated with a combination of berberine (Ber) and doxorubicin (DOX) showed a smaller tumor volume compared to the other groups. While the group that received only Ber (10 mg/kg) or only DOX displayed a slight decrease in tumor growth compared to the control group, the combination treatment resulted in a significantly greater inhibition of tumor growth. Notably, the body weight of the nude mice in the DOX-only group significantly decreased, likely due to the toxicities and side effects associated with DOX. An in vivo study in mice using D-luciferin sodium indicated that berberine could significantly reduce P-gp activity.

Berberine use caused the down-regulation of P-gp, as determined by Western blot and immunohistochemical tests. Based on the results of high-performance liquid chromatography, an increase in the distribution of doxorubicin into tumor tissues was observed after the administration of berberine. The above data suggest that berberine is an inhibitor of P-gp and causes a down-regulation of its expression [59]. Different results were observed by Yu et al. [60], who performed a study with berberine-rich *Coptidis rhizoma*. The rats were administered cyclosporine, a known substrate for P-gp, and were pretreated with a decoction of *Coptidis rhizoma* (1 g/2 mL/kg) 0.5 h before cyclosporine administration or the decoction twice a day, and the seventh dose was given 0.5 h before cyclosporine. The dose of *Coptidis rhizoma* corresponded to the average daily dose of 10 g used in clinical practice in humans. The results indicated that the administration of one and seven doses of *Coptidis rhizoma* decoction significantly reduced the C_{max} of cyclosporine by 56.9% and 70.4%, respectively, and the AUC0-t by 56.4% and 68.7%, respectively. A study on LS 180 human colon cancer cells showed a significant reduction in the intracellular accumulation of rhodamine 123 after administration of 2.5, 5.0, and 10 μM berberine. The results described indicate that P-gp is activated after oral ingestion of *Coptidis rhizoma* decoction.

6.2. Capsaicin

Capsaicin is the active compound responsible for the spicy heat in chili peppers (*Capsicum* species). It is most abundantly found in varieties such as cayenne, jalapeño, and habanero peppers. Capsaicin contributes to the characteristic pungency of these peppers and is recognized for its potential health benefits, including analgesic, anti-inflammatory, and metabolic effects. In dietary supplements, capsaicin is commonly included in formulations designed to support weight loss, enhance metabolism, and relieve pain [61].

A sole study described the effect of capsaicin on MRP2 transporter. The rats (n = 36) were orally administered capsaicin (3.0 mg/kg), MRP2 transporter inhibitor—cyclosporine A, or olive oil as the control group. On the last day of treatment, all individuals were given vinblastine. The AUC0-t value of vinblastine in rats after capsaicin treatment was 1.3 times higher and 1.7 times higher after cyclosporine A treatment compared to the control group. A significant decrease in MRP2 expression (mRNA analysis) was also observed. The study suggests an inhibitory effect of capsaicin on the MRP2 transporter in rats [62].

6.3. Piperine

Piperine is an alkaloid found primarily in black (*Piper nigrum*) and long (*Piper longum*) peppers. It is well-known for its role in enhancing the bioavailability of various nutrients and drugs by inhibiting certain drug-metabolizing enzymes. Black pepper is the most common dietary source of piperine, and it is often included in dietary supplements aimed at improving nutrient absorption. Studies show that piperine can significantly increase the absorption of curcumin, a compound found in turmeric, which highlights its role in enhancing the effectiveness of dietary supplements [63].

The inhibitory effect of piperine on MRP2 transporter and/or BCRP transporter was evaluated in vivo. The rats (n = 16) received a single oral dose of silybin (50 mg/kg) or piperine (10 mg/kg) combined with silybin. The measured C_{max} values of silybin were 1.49 times higher for silybin A and 1.39 times higher for silybin B in the piperine-treated group. AUC0-t values were also higher by 146% and 181% for silybin A and silybin B, respectively. To investigate the mechanism by which the bioavailability of silybin was increased after piperine treatment, an in vitro study was conducted on models of the Caco-2, MDCKII-BCRP, and MDCKII-MRP2 cell lines. Caco-2 cells were incubated with silybin (10 μM) and piperine (up to 40 μM). The rate of silybin transport was higher in the direction from the basolateral side to the apical side than in the opposite direction and was 5.04 ± 0.48, respectively, for silybin A and 4.61 ± 0.39 for silybin B. A significant increase in transport from the apical to the basolateral side and a decrease in the silybin efflux ratio after piperine administration was observed. This suggests the inhibition of MRP2 and/or BCRP transporter activity by piperine in Caco-2 cells. In a study on the

MDCKII-MRP2 cell line, a concentration-dependent, significant reduction in the efflux ratio of the CDCFDA compound (substrate for MRP2) was observed from 3.58 ± 0.52 to 1.40 ± 0.02 after piperine administration. This suggests that piperine is an inhibitor of the MRP2 transporter, which may have been the mechanism responsible for the increased bioavailability of silybin in the Caco-2 cells. Piperine concentration-dependently decreased the efflux ratio of silybin A from 2.34 ± 0.17 to 1.55 ± 0.38 and silybin B from 2.05 ± 0.22 to 1.32 ± 1.32 in the MDCKII-BCRP cell line. This suggests the inhibition of BCRP transporter activity by piperine, which may have been a mechanism for the increased bioavailability of silybin [64].

In the study by Kim et al. [65], the mice received piperine (10 mg/kg), capsaicin (5 mg/kg), and [6]-gingerol (5 mg/kg), a compound found in ginger. The substances were administered in two subsequent doses every 60 min (piperine) or every 30 min (capsaicin and [6]-gingerol), and then the animals received doxorubicin. None of the substances significantly affected the plasma concentration of doxorubicin. Based on the calculated tissue-to-plasma partition coefficients, it can be concluded that piperine significantly increased the level of distribution of doxorubicin to the kidney and liver, and capsaicin to the kidney, liver, and brain. [6]-gingerol did not affect the distribution of doxorubicin. The inhibition of P-gp may have caused a decrease in the secretion of doxorubicin into the urine and bile, which may have affected its accumulation in the previously mentioned organs.

7. Effect of Plant Juices on MDR Transporters

7.1. Rocket Juice

Diet–drug interactions with rocket (*Eruca vesicaria*) were explored. The rats (n = 64) were given the juice of fresh rocket leaves at doses of 1.0, 1.4, and 2.0 g/kg for 14 days. On the fifteenth day, half of each group was treated with cyclophosphamide or control saline solution. No changes in MRP2 protein expression were observed 24 h after cyclophosphamide administration. However, a significant increase was observed in MRP2 expression in liver cells after the administration of the highest dose of rocket leaf juice in both male and female rats. It should be considered that the consumption of rocket might negatively affect treatments with drugs whose pharmacokinetics depend on the action of ABC transporters and drugs that induce DNA damage [66].

7.2. Cranberry Juice

An in vitro study examined the impact of cranberry juice on BCRP transporter, using the MDCKII-BCRP cell line model, mitoxantrone as a substrate, and Ko143 (a BCRP inhibitor) as a positive control group. Administration of cranberry juice at concentrations of 5.0, 2.5, and 1.3 mg/mL resulted in a decrease in the intracellular accumulation of mitoxantrone by 22, 17, and 15%, respectively. Quercetin, isorhamnetin, myricetin, cyanidin, protocatechuic acid, and scopoletin were detected in this juice, and cyanidin was the major constituent. Metabolites of these compounds, such as glucuronides and sulfates, showed an increase in intracellular accumulation of mitoxantrone by 19%. The results suggest that cranberry juice activates the BCRP transporter. The researchers also conducted an in vivo study examining the interaction between warfarin and cranberry juice. They found that consuming cranberry juice 0.5 h before taking racemic warfarin significantly lowered the maximum concentration (C_{max}) and area under the curve ($AUC_{0\text{-}t}$) for S-warfarin by 48% and 34%, respectively. Similarly, the C_{max} and AUC0-t for R-warfarin were reduced by 51% and 52%. Moreover, the area under the curve from time 0 to 10 h ($AUC_{0–10}$) for both S- and R-warfarin decreased by 52% and 54%, respectively. In a different part of the study, administering cranberry juice 10 h after warfarin did not alter the C_{max} and $AUC_{0–t}$ of either enantiomer. However, the half-life (t1/2) and the AUC from 48 to 96 h ($AUC_{48–96}$) for S-warfarin increased significantly, by 267% and 126%, respectively. The results suggest that cranberry juice activated BCRP during absorption and inhibited the activity of this transporter during the elimination process [67].

Another study examined cranberry juice in rats. The animals (n = 12) were given gefitinib alone, or combined with cranberry juice (5 g/kg of cranberry as juice). Coadministration of gefitinib and cranberry juice caused a significant increase in C_{max} and AUC0-t values (28 and 55%, respectively). LS 180 cell line (intestinal human cancer adenocarcinoma) was used to evaluate the effect of cranberry juice on the activity of P-gp. Cranberry juice significantly reduced the intracellular accumulation of the P-gp substrate rhodamine 123 by 27%. The protein level of P-gp in rat enterocytes was decreased by 28%, and in hepatocytes it was increased by 39%. The protein levels of BCRP, CYP3A4, and CYP2D6 were decreased in both enterocytes (by 22, 24, and 38%, respectively) and hepatocytes (by 40, 25, and 30%, respectively). The authors suggest that the influence of cranberry juice on the absorption of gefitinib by modulating P-gp is negligible because of the opposite effects of cranberry juice on P-gp activity and its protein levels. Changes in the activities and protein levels of BCRP, CYP3A4, and CYP2D6 might explain the effect of cranberry juice on the pharmacokinetics of gefitinib [68].

8. Structure–Activity Relationship

Despite the importance of the interaction between the natural compounds and different MDR transporters, only a few studies described the impact of the structural elements of the studied compounds on their activity towards the transporters. As far as BCRP transporter is concerned, a sole study was performed for flavonoids, based on the computational docking model. The results indicated that the presence of an aromatic ring, hydrophobic groups, and hydrogen bond acceptors was necessary for the inhibition of the BCRP transporter. Compounds containing in their structure an aromatic ring B (marked in orange in Figure 2A), a methoxyl group at the 4′ position (marked in blue in Figure 2A), hydroxyl and/or hydrophobic substituents at positions 5 and 7 (marked in green in Figure 2A) showed greater inhibitory activity. It was observed that the substitution at these positions with large substituents such as glucose could reduce the inhibitory effect or cause it to disappear [69]. Some more data exist on the effect observed towards P-gp activity, including the compounds representing different chemical classes discussed within this review.

It is believed that flavonoids can interact with different sites on P-gp (substrate-binding site, other drug-binding sites, ATP-binding site, allosteric site, steroid-interacting region). In cellular studies, most flavonoids affected P-gp activity at concentrations of at least 10 μM but usually at higher values. Such levels are only achievable in the gut, probably after oral supplementation with these compounds. Flavonoid metabolites present in human plasma, due to their hydrophilic properties, cannot interact with P-gp. Therefore, there is little likelihood of the interaction between P-gp and flavonoids in other tissues. Thanks to numerous studies on cells, it was possible to identify the elements of the flavonoid structure responsible for inhibiting P-gp (Figure 2B). These include hydroxyl groups at the C3 and C5 positions, a double bond between the carbons at C2 and C3, a phenyl substituent at C2, a carbonyl group at C4, and hydrophobic groupings on the A or B ring. Hydrophobicity is essential for P-gp inhibition [69], and the optimal number of hydroxyl groups is three. However, flavonoids with four hydroxyl groups did not show as strong a P-gp inhibitory activity as did the flavonoids with more groups [70].

The curcumin molecule is composed of two parts: a seven-atom linker with a β-diketone in the middle and aromatic rings that are located at the ends of the chain. The same main structures are found among two other P-gp inhibitors: tetrahydrocurcumin and verapamil (Figure 2C). It is suggested that the diketone structure is not necessary to provide multidrug resistance reversal activity in cancer treatment, and in addition, compounds with stronger activity have shorter linkers [71,72].

In the case of alkaloids, in silico studies have shown that piperine can interact with P-gp at both the drug-binding site and NBD, causing its inhibition [73]. Hydrophobic interactions with P-gp, specifically with Leu339, Met69, Met986, Phe72, Phe336, Phe728, Phe983, Tyr953, Val982, and hydrogen bonds with Tyr307 are responsible for its inhibition [73,74]. A structural similarity has been noted between piperine's 1,3-benzodioxol ring system and 4-chloro-7-nitrobenzofurazan, which is an inhibitor of P-gp that forms bonds with magnesium ions at the ATP-binding site (Figure 2D).

It has been shown that both structures having two electron acceptor groups can interact with divalent cations. The alkenyl side chain of piperine may have some effect on reducing the affinity compared to 4-chloro-7-nitrobenzofurazan, which has additional C=N and NO_2 groups [75]. Some phytochemicals having a 1,3-benzodioxol ring, including piperine, showed inhibitory effects on both P-gp and CYP3A4 [76].

Studies also have shown a high correlation between the amount of hydrogen bonds formed by the structural elements of berberine and its metabolites (berberrubine, thalifendine, demethyleneberberine, jatrorrhizine, columbamine) with P-gp and the affinity for binding to the extracellular part of P-gp. During the early binding stage, hydrophobic and electrostatic interactions are the main determinant, while during the late release stage, electrostatic interactions are of primary importance. Potent substrates for P-gp that are its competitive inhibitors should have high hydrophobicity to dissolve in the hydrophobic medium of the membrane [77]. The structure of berberine, along with the labeled structures responsible for forming each type of bond, is shown in Figure 2E [78].

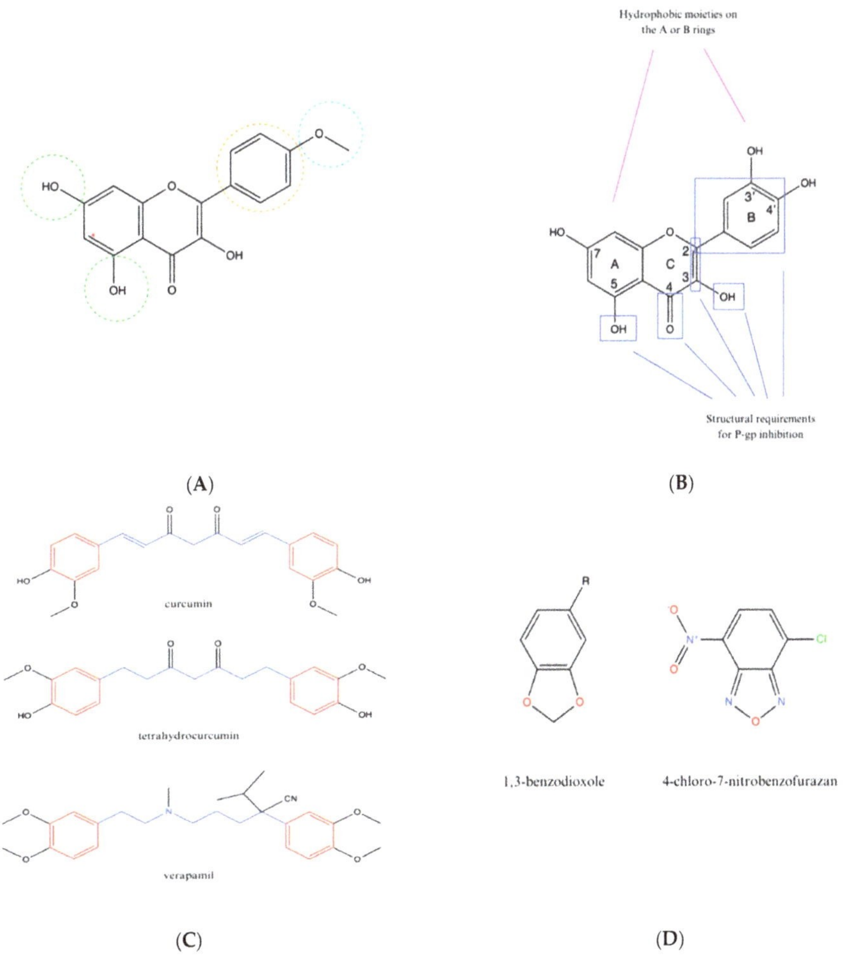

Figure 2. *Cont.*

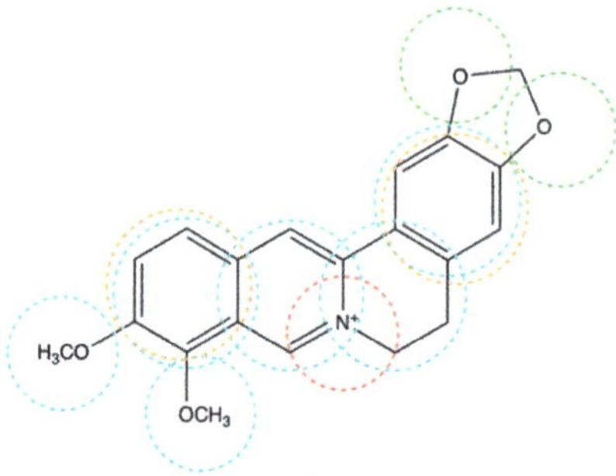

(E)

Figure 2. The structural requirements of natural compounds for inhibition of selected transporters. (**A**) The chemical structure of kaempferide (BCRP inhibitor), with the hydroxyl groups at positions 5 and 7, being hydrogen bond acceptors, in green, the aromatic ring B in orange, and the methoxyl hydrophobic group at the 4′ position in blue—prepared according to [34]. (**B**) Structural requirements in flavonoids for P-gp inhibition—prepared according to [69]. (**C**) Similarity of chemical structures of curcumin, tetrahydrocurcumin, and verapamil; the red color indicates the aromatic rings at the ends of the chains, and the blue color indicates the linker—prepared according to [72]. (**D**) Similarity of chemical structures of 1,3-benzodioxole and 4-chloro-7-nitrobenzofurazan—prepared according to [75]. (**E**) Structure of berberine with labeled structures responsible for bond formation. Aromatic rings are marked in orange, hydrophobic elements in blue, cations in red, hydrogen bond acceptors in green—prepared according to [78].

9. The Study Limitations

Despite the comprehensive analysis provided, this study has several limitations that must be acknowledged. Firstly, the in vitro and in vivo studies conducted on animal models may not fully replicate the complexity of human physiology and cancer biology. While these models provide valuable insights, the extrapolation of results to human subjects should be approached with caution. Another limitation is the variability in the bioavailability and metabolism of dietary compounds. Factors such as individual genetic differences, gut microbiota composition, and overall health status can influence the absorption and efficacy of these compounds. This variability can lead to inconsistent results and may affect the generalizability of the findings. Furthermore, this study primarily focuses on a limited range of dietary compounds and supplements. The vast diversity of phytochemicals and their potential interactions with MDR transporters warrant further investigation. Comprehensive studies encompassing a broader spectrum of dietary components are needed to fully elucidate their roles in modulating drug resistance. Lastly, the potential side effects and toxicity of combining dietary supplements with chemotherapeutic agents were not extensively addressed. While certain supplements may enhance drug efficacy, they may also pose the risks of adverse interactions and toxicity. Future research should aim to establish safe and effective dosages and combinations for clinical use.

In summary, while this study provides significant insights into the influence of diet and dietary supplements on MDR transporters and anticancer therapy, further research is needed to validate these findings in clinical settings and expand the scope of dietary compounds investigated and the wide range of used anticancer drugs.

10. Conclusions

The findings of this study underscore the critical role of dietary modifications in enhancing the efficacy of chemotherapy (Figure 3). Our results indicate that specific dietary interventions can significantly impact the outcomes of chemotherapy treatments, suggesting that diet should be considered an integral component of cancer care.

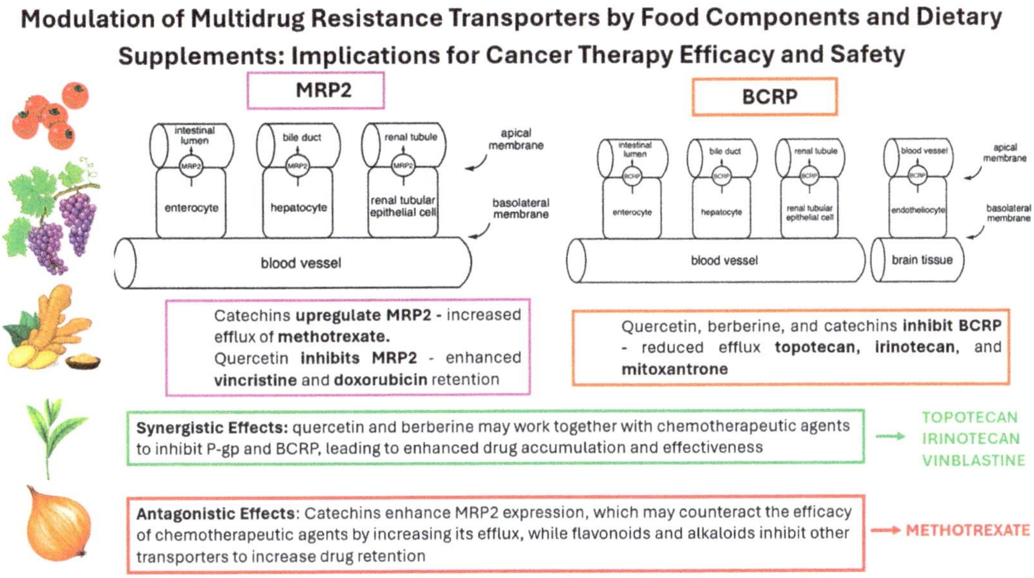

Figure 3. The summary of potential effects of interactions between MDR transporters and selected natural compounds on chemotherapy efficacy.

Key implications of our research include the following:

- Enhanced efficacy through targeted nutrients: Incorporating a diet rich in specific nutrients, e.g., antioxidants, has been shown to improve specific aspects of chemotherapy efficacy, e.g., tumor response in in vitro or animal studies. However, patients undergoing chemotherapy should be careful in increasing the intake of these nutrients, especially when taken as dietary supplements, and consult healthcare professionals.
- Potential dietary modifications: Based on our findings, we recommend that patients should discuss the possibility of dietary modifications with their oncologists with the help of a clinical pharmacist and clinical dietician. These changes could potentially optimize the effectiveness of chemotherapy and improve overall patient well-being.
- Personalized dietary plans: It is essential for dietary recommendations to be tailored to the individual patient, considering factors such as specific type of cancer, treatment regimen, and personal health conditions. Personalized dietary plans should be developed in collaboration with nutritionists and healthcare providers to ensure the best possible outcomes.

In conclusion, integrating targeted dietary modifications into chemotherapy regimens holds promise for enhancing treatment efficacy and supporting patient health. Future research should continue to explore these dietary interactions to further refine recommendations and improve cancer treatment protocols.

Author Contributions: Conceptualization, P.P.; methodology, P.P., A.B. and A.G.; software, A.B. and P.P.; formal analysis, A.B.; investigation, A.B., P.P. and A.G.; resources, A.B. and P.P.; data curation, A.B.; writing—original draft preparation, A.B., P.P. and A.G.; writing—review and editing, P.P. and A.G.; visualization, A.B.; supervision, P.P. and A.G.; project administration, P.P.; funding acquisition, P.P. All authors have read and agreed to the published version of the manuscript.

Funding: This research received no external funding.

Institutional Review Board Statement: Not applicable.

Informed Consent Statement: Not applicable.

Data Availability Statement: Data availability on the request.

Conflicts of Interest: The authors declare no conflicts of interest.

References

1. Escribano-Ferrer, E.; Reglero, G.; Santoyo, S. Polyphenols as Modulators of Multidrug Resistance Proteins: Potential Clinical Applications. *Nutrients* **2020**, *12*, 559.
2. Noguchi, K.; Katayama, K.; Mitsuhashi, J.; Sugimoto, Y. Dietary Flavonoids and Multidrug Resistance in Cancer Chemotherapy: A Comprehensive Review. *Front. Pharmacol.* **2021**, *12*, 741116.
3. Li, W.; Lu, Y.; Chen, M.; Zeng, G. Natural Products Modulating P-gp and BCRP in Cancer Therapy: Potential Applications in Chemotherapy. *Curr. Med. Chem.* **2021**, *28*, 3170–3185.
4. Tan, H.-Y.; Wang, N.; Tsao, S.-W.; Che, C.-M.; Yuen, M.-F.; Feng, Y. Dietary Supplements and Chemotherapy: Potential Roles and Mechanisms in Modulating Drug Resistance. *J. Clin. Med.* **2021**, *10*, 1936.
5. Goh, D.-L.; Li, J.; Zhu, Y.; Feng, Y. The Influence of Diet on Drug Transporter Expression and Function in Cancer Therapy. *Pharmacol. Rev.* **2020**, *72*, 759–796.
6. Fang, Y.; Cao, W.; Liang, F.; Xia, M.; Pan, S.; Xu, X. Structure Affinity Relationship and Docking Studies of Flavonoids as Substrates of Multidrug-Resistant Associated Protein 2 (MRP2) in MDCK/MRP2 Cells. *Food Chem.* **2019**, *291*, 101–109. [CrossRef]
7. Zhang, L.; Liang, C.; Xu, P.; Liu, M.; Xu, F.; Wang, X. Characterization of In Vitro Mrp2 Transporter Model Based on Intestinal Organoids. *Regul. Toxicol. Pharmacol.* **2019**, *108*, 104449. [CrossRef]
8. Banik, A.; Ghosh, K.; Patil, U.K.; Gayen, S. Identification of Molecular Fingerprints of Natural Products for the Inhibition of Breast Cancer Resistance Protein (BCRP). *Phytomedicine* **2021**, *85*, 102375. [CrossRef]
9. Safar, Z.; Kis, E.; Erdo, F.; Zolnerciks, J.K.; Krajcsi, P. ABCG2/BCRP: Variants, Transporter Interaction Profile of Substrates and Inhibitors. *Expert Opin. Drug Metab. Toxicol.* **2019**, *15*, 313–328. [CrossRef]
10. Yakusheva, E.N.; Titov, D.S. Structure and Function of Multidrug Resistance Protein 1. *Biochemistry* **2018**, *83*, 907–929. [CrossRef]
11. Smolik, M.; Suraj, J.; Kurpinska, A.; Walczak, M. ABC Membrane Transporters and Their Multifunctional Nature. *Postepy Hig. Med. Dosw.* **2018**, *72*, 606–622. [CrossRef]
12. Silva, V.; Gil-Martins, E.; Silva, B.; Rocha-Pereira, C.; Sousa, M.E.; Remião, F.; Silva, R. Xanthones as P-glycoprotein Modulators and Their Impact on Drug Bioavailability. *Expert Opin. Drug Metab. Toxicol.* **2021**, *17*, 441–482. [CrossRef]
13. Drug Development and Drug Interactions | Table of Substrates, Inhibitors and Inducers | FDA [Internet]. Available online: https://www.fda.gov/drugs/drug-interactions-labeling/drug-development-and-drug-interactions-table-substrates-inhibitors-and-inducers (accessed on 18 May 2024).
14. Cabrera, C.; Artacho, R.; Giménez, R. Beneficial Effects of Green Tea—A Review. *J. Am. Coll. Nutr.* **2006**, *25*, 79–99. [CrossRef] [PubMed]
15. Keen, C.L.; Holt, R.R.; Oteiza, P.I.; Fraga, C.G.; Schmitz, H.H. Cocoa Antioxidants and Cardiovascular Health. *Am. J. Clin. Nutr.* **2005**, *81*, 298S–303S. [CrossRef] [PubMed]
16. Ai, Z.; Liu, S.; Qu, F.; Zhang, H.; Chen, Y.; Ni, D. Effect of Stereochemical Configuration on the Transport and Metabolism of Catechins from Green Tea Across Caco-2 Monolayers. *Molecules* **2019**, *24*, 1185. [CrossRef] [PubMed]
17. Wang, Y.; Zuo, Y.; Deng, S.; Zhu, F.; Liu, Q.; Wang, R.; Li, T.; Cai, H.; Wan, X.; Xie, Z.; et al. Using Caffeine and Free Amino Acids to Enhance the Transepithelial Transport of Catechins in Caco-2 Cells. *J. Agric. Food Chem.* **2019**, *67*, 5477–5485. [CrossRef]
18. Tuntiteerawit, P.; Jarukamjorn, K.; Porasuphatana, S. The Effect of Green Tea Catechins on Breast Cancer Resistance Protein Activity and Intestinal Efflux of Aflatoxin B1 via Breast Cancer Resistance Protein in Caco-2 Cells. *Toxicol. Res.* **2020**, *36*, 293–300. [CrossRef]
19. Huang, X.; Zhang, R.; Yang, T.; Wei, Y.; Yang, C.; Zhou, J.; Liu, Y.; Shi, S. Inhibition Effect of Epigallocatechin-3-gallate on the Pharmacokinetics of Calcineurin Inhibitors, Tacrolimus, and Cyclosporine A, in Rats. *Expert Opin. Drug Metab. Toxicol.* **2021**, *17*, 121–134. [CrossRef]
20. Boots, A.W.; Haenen, G.R.; Bast, A. Health Effects of Quercetin: From Antioxidant to Nutraceutical. *Eur. J. Pharmacol.* **2008**, *585*, 325–337. [CrossRef]
21. Li, Y.; Yao, J.; Han, C.; Yang, J.; Chaudhry, M.T.; Wang, S.; Liu, H.; Yin, Y. Quercetin, Inflammation and Immunity. *Nutrients* **2016**, *8*, 167. [CrossRef]
22. Mohos, V.; Fliszár-Nyúl, E.; Ungvári, O.; Kuffa, K.; Needs, P.W.; Kroon, P.A.; Telbisz, Á.; Özvegy-Laczka, C.; Poór, M. Inhibitory Effects of Quercetin and Its Main Methyl, Sulfate, and Glucuronic Acid Conjugates on Cytochrome P450 Enzymes, and on OATP, BCRP and MRP2 Transporters. *Nutrients* **2020**, *12*, 2306. [CrossRef] [PubMed]
23. Oh, J.H.; Lee, J.H.; Lee, Y.J. Evaluation of the Mrp2-mediated Flavonoid-Drug Interaction Potential of Quercetin in Rats and In Vitro Models. *Asian J. Pharm. Sci.* **2019**, *14*, 621–630. [CrossRef] [PubMed]
24. Yang, T.; Liu, Y.; Huang, X.; Zhang, R.; Yang, C.; Zhou, J.; Zhang, Y.; Wan, J.; Shi, S. Quercetin-3-O-β-D-glucoside Decreases the Bioavailability of Cyclosporin A Through Regulation of Drug Metabolizing Enzymes, Transporters and Nuclear Receptors in Rats. *Mol. Med. Rep.* **2018**, *18*, 2599–2612. [CrossRef]
25. Shukla, S.; Gupta, S. Apigenin: A Promising Molecule for Cancer Prevention. *Pharm. Res.* **2010**, *27*, 962–978. [CrossRef] [PubMed]

26. Raish, M.; Ahmad, A.; Shahid, M.; Jardan, Y.A.B.; Ahad, A.; Kalam, M.A.; Ansari, M.A.; Iqbal, M.; Ali, N.; Alkharfy, K.M.; et al. Effects of Apigenin on Pharmacokinetics of Dasatinib and Probable Interaction Mechanism. *Molecules* **2023**, *28*, 1602. [CrossRef]
27. Fu, Y.; Chen, J.; Li, Y.J.; Zheng, Y.F.; Li, P. Antioxidant and Anti-inflammatory Activities of Six Flavonoids Separated from Licorice. *Food Chem.* **2005**, *96*, 669–674. [CrossRef]
28. Haraguchi, H.; Ishikawa, H.; Mizutani, K.; Tamura, Y.; Kinoshita, T. Antioxidative and Superoxide Scavenging Activities of Retrochalcones in Glycyrrhiza inflata. *Bioorg. Med. Chem.* **1998**, *6*, 339–347. [CrossRef]
29. Wu, C.P.; Lusvarghi, S.; Hsiao, S.H.; Liu, T.C.; Li, Y.Q.; Huang, Y.H.; Ambudkar, S.V. Licochalcone A Selectively Resensitizes ABCG2-Overexpressing Multidrug-Resistant Cancer Cells to Chemotherapeutic Drugs. *J. Nat. Prod.* **2020**, *83*, 1461–1472. [CrossRef]
30. Wang, T.Y.; Li, Q.; Bi, K.S. Bioactive Flavonoids in Medicinal Plants: Structure, Activity and Biological Fate. *Asian J. Pharm. Sci.* **2018**, *13*, 12–23. [CrossRef]
31. Panche, A.N.; Diwan, A.D.; Chandra, S.R. Flavonoids: An Overview. *J. Nutr. Sci.* **2016**, *5*, e47. [CrossRef]
32. Li, S.; Lo, C.Y.; Ho, C.T. Hydroxylated Polymethoxyflavones and Methylated Flavonoids in Sweet Orange (Citrus sinensis) Peel. *J. Agric. Food Chem.* **2006**, *54*, 4176–4185. [CrossRef] [PubMed]
33. Zhao, Q.; Chen, X.Y.; Martin, C. Scutellaria baicalensis, the golden herb from the garden of Chinese medicinal plants. *Sci. Bull.* **2016**, *61*, 1391–1398. [CrossRef] [PubMed]
34. Fan, X.; Bai, J.; Zhao, S.; Hu, M.; Sun, Y.; Wang, B.; Ji, M.; Jin, J.; Wang, X.; Hu, J.; et al. Evaluation of inhibitory effects of flavonoids on breast cancer resistance protein (BCRP): From library screening to biological evaluation to structure-activity relationship. *Toxicol. In Vitro* **2019**, *61*, 104642. [CrossRef]
35. Raish, M.; Ahmad, A.; Karim, B.A.; Jardan, Y.A.B.; Ahad, A.; Iqbal, M.; Alkharfy, K.M.; Al-Jenoobi, F.I.; Mohammed, O.M. Pharmacokinetics of Dasatinib in Rats: A Potential Food–Drug Interaction with Naringenin. *Eur. J. Drug Metab. Pharmacokinet.* **2024**, *49*, 239–247. [CrossRef] [PubMed]
36. Bai, J.; Zhao, S.; Fan, X.; Chen, Y.; Zou, X.; Hu, M.; Wang, B.; Jin, J.; Wang, X.; Hu, J.; et al. Inhibitory effects of flavonoids on P-glycoprotein in vitro and in vivo: Food/herb-drug interactions and structure–activity relationships. *Toxicol. Appl. Pharmacol.* **2019**, *369*, 49–59. [CrossRef] [PubMed]
37. Singh, K.; Tarapcsák, S.; Gyöngy, Z.; Ritter, Z.; Batta, G.; Bosire, R.; Remenyik, J.; Goda, K. Effects of polyphenols on p-glycoprotein (Abcb1) activity. *Pharmaceutics* **2021**, *13*, 2062. [CrossRef]
38. Nićiforović, N.; Abramovič, H. Sinapic acid and its derivatives: Natural sources and bioactivity. *Compr. Rev. Food Sci. Food Saf.* **2014**, *13*, 34–51. [CrossRef]
39. Shahid, M.; Ahmad, A.; Raish, M.; Bin Jardan, Y.A.; Alkharfy, K.M.; Ahad, A.; Kalam, M.A.; Ansari, M.A.; Iqbal, M.; Ali, N.; et al. Herb-drug interaction: Effect of sinapic acid on the pharmacokinetics of dasatinib in rats. *Saudi Pharm. J.* **2023**, *31*, 101819. [CrossRef]
40. Aggarwal, B.B.; Shishodia, S. Molecular targets of dietary agents for prevention and therapy of cancer. *Biochem. Pharmacol.* **2006**, *71*, 1397–1421. [CrossRef]
41. Baur, J.A.; Sinclair, D.A. Therapeutic potential of resveratrol: The in vivo evidence. *Nat. Rev. Drug Discov.* **2006**, *5*, 493–506. [CrossRef]
42. Mieszala, K.; Rudewicz, M.; Gomulkiewicz, A.; Ratajczak-Wielgomas, K.; Grzegrzolka, J.; Dziegiel, P.; Borska, S. Expression of genes and proteins of multidrug resistance in gastric cancer cells treated with resveratrol. *Oncol. Lett.* **2018**, *15*, 5825–5832. [CrossRef]
43. El-Readi, M.Z.; Eid, S.Y.; Abdelghany, A.A.; Al-Amoudi, H.S.; Efferth, T.; Wink, M. Resveratrol mediated cancer cell apoptosis, and modulation of multidrug resistance proteins and metabolic enzymes. *Phytomedicine* **2019**, *55*, 269–281. [CrossRef] [PubMed]
44. Prasad, S.; Gupta, S.C.; Tyagi, A.K.; Aggarwal, B.B. Curcumin, a component of golden spice: From bedside to bench and back. *Biotechnol. Adv.* **2014**, *32*, 1053–1064. [CrossRef] [PubMed]
45. Hewlings, S.J.; Kalman, D.S. Curcumin: A review of its' effects on human health. *Foods* **2017**, *6*, 92. [CrossRef]
46. Yang, H.; Wei, Y.C.; Li, W.C.; Chen, H.Y.; Lin, H.Y.; Chiang, C.P.; Chen, H.M. Natural compounds modulate drug transporter mediated oral cancer treatment. *Biomolecules* **2020**, *10*, 1335. [CrossRef] [PubMed]
47. Li, H.; Krstin, S.; Wink, M. Modulation of multidrug resistant in cancer cells by EGCG, tannic acid and curcumin. *Phytomedicine* **2018**, *50*, 213–222. [CrossRef]
48. Zhang, N.; Gao, M.; Wang, Z.; Zhang, J.; Cui, W.; Li, J.; Zhu, X.; Zhang, H.; Yang, D.H.; Xu, X. Curcumin reverses doxorubicin resistance in colon cancer cells at the metabolic level. *J. Pharm. Biomed. Anal.* **2021**, *201*, 114129. [CrossRef]
49. Burt, S. Essential oils: Their antibacterial properties and potential applications in foods—A review. *Int. J. Food Microbiol.* **2004**, *94*, 223–253. [CrossRef]
50. Kamran, S.; Sinniah, A.; Abdulghani, M.A.; Alshawsh, M.A. Therapeutic potential of certain terpenoids as anticancer agents: A scoping review. *Cancers* **2022**, *14*, 1100. [CrossRef]
51. Nagai, K.; Tamura, M.; Murayama, R.; Fukuno, S.; Ito, T.; Konishi, H. Development of multi-drug resistance to anticancer drugs in HepG2 cells due to MRP2 upregulation on exposure to menthol. *PLoS ONE* **2023**, *18*, e0291822. [CrossRef]
52. Zecchinati, F.; Barranco, M.M.; Arana, M.R.; Tocchetti, G.N.; Domínguez, C.J.; Perdomo, V.G.; Ruiz, M.L.; Mottino, A.D.; García, F.; Villanueva, S.S.M. Reversion of down-regulation of intestinal multidrug resistance-associated protein 2 in fructose-fed rats by geraniol and vitamin C: Potential role of inflammatory response and oxidative stress. *J. Nutr. Biochem.* **2019**, *68*, 7–15. [CrossRef] [PubMed]

53. Di Giacomo, S.; Briz, O.; Monte, M.J.; Sanchez-Vicente, L.; Abete, L.; Lozano, E.; Mazzanti, G.; Di Sotto, A.; Marin, J.J. Chemosensitization of hepatocellular carcinoma cells to sorafenib by β-caryophyllene oxide-induced inhibition of ABC export pumps. *Arch. Toxicol.* **2019**, *93*, 623–634. [CrossRef]
54. Ortiz-Rivero, S.; Peleteiro-Vigil, A.; Abete, L.; Lozano, E.; Hammer, H.S.; Di Giacomo, S.; Abad, M.; Boix, L.; Forner, A.; Reig, M.; et al. Sensitization of cholangiocarcinoma cells to chemotherapy through BCRP inhibition with β-caryophyllene oxide. *Biomed. Pharmacother.* **2024**, *170*, 116038. [CrossRef] [PubMed]
55. Tong, X.P.; Ma, Y.X.; Quan, D.N.; Zhang, L.; Yan, M.; Fan, X.R. Rosemary Extracts Upregulate Nrf2, Sestrin2, and MRP2 Protein Level in Human Hepatoma HepG2 Cells. *Evid.-Based Complement. Alternat. Med.* **2017**, *207*, 7359806. [CrossRef]
56. Bin Sayeed, M.S.; Ameen, S.S. Beta-sitosterol: A promising but orphan nutraceutical to fight against cancer. *Nutr. Cancer* **2015**, *67*, 1216–1222. [CrossRef]
57. Wang, Z.; Zhan, Y.; Xu, J.; Wang, Y.; Sun, M.; Chen, J.; Liang, T.; Wu, L.; Xu, K. β-Sitosterol Reverses Multidrug Resistance via BCRP Suppression by Inhibiting the p53-MDM2 Interaction in Colorectal Cancer. *J. Agric. Food Chem.* **2020**, *68*, 3850–3858. [CrossRef]
58. Gómez-Garduño, J.; León-Rodríguez, R.; Alemón-Medina, R.; Pérez-Guillé, B.E.; Soriano-Rosales, R.E.; González-Ortiz, A.; Chávez-Pacheco, J.L.; Solorio-López, E.; Fernandez-Pérez, P.; Rivera-Espinosa, L. Phytochemicals that interfere with drug metabolism and transport, modifying plasma concentration in humans and animals. *Dose-Response* **2022**, *20*, 15593258221120485. [CrossRef] [PubMed]
59. Qian, K.; Tang, C.Y.; Chen, L.Y.; Zheng, S.; Zhao, Y.; Ma, L.S.; Xu, L.; Fan, L.H.; Yu, J.D.; Tan, H.S.; et al. Berberine Reverses Breast Cancer Multidrug Resistance Based on Fluorescence Pharmacokinetics in Vitro and in Vivo. *ACS Omega* **2021**, *6*, 10645–10654. [CrossRef]
60. Yu, C.P.; Huang, C.Y.; Lin, S.P.; Hou, Y.C. Activation of P-glycoprotein and CYP 3A by Coptidis Rhizoma in vivo: Using cyclosporine as a probe substrate in rats. *J. Food Drug Anal.* **2018**, *26*, S125–S132. [CrossRef]
61. Whiting, S.; Derbyshire, E.; Tiwari, B.K. Capsaicinoids and capsinoids. A potential role for weight management? A systematic review of the evidence. *Appetite* **2012**, *59*, 341–348. [CrossRef]
62. Zhai, X.; Feng, Y.; Liu, J.; Li, J.; Zong, Y.; Tuo, Z.; Gao, S.; Lv, Y. Pharmacokinetic effects of capsaicin on vinblastine in rats mediated by CYP3A and Mrp2. *Fundam. Clin. Pharmacol.* **2019**, *33*, 376–384. [CrossRef] [PubMed]
63. Shoba, G.; Joy, D.; Joseph, T.; Majeed, M.; Rajendran, R.; Srinivas, P.S. Influence of piperine on the pharmacokinetics of curcumin in animals and human volunteers. *Planta Med.* **1998**, *64*, 353–356. [CrossRef]
64. Bi, X.; Yuan, Z.; Qu, B.; Zhou, H.; Liu, Z.; Xie, Y. Piperine enhances the bioavailability of silybin via inhibition of efflux transporters BCRP and MRP2. *Phytomedicine* **2019**, *54*, 98–108. [CrossRef]
65. Kim, T.H.; Shin, S.; Yoo, S.D.; Shin, B.S. Effects of phytochemical P-glycoprotein modulators on the pharmacokinetics and tissue distribution of doxorubicin in mice. *Molecules* **2018**, *23*, 349. [CrossRef] [PubMed]
66. Roma, M.I.; Schiariti Lampropulos, V.E.; Ayllón-Cabrera, I.; Salazar Sanabria, A.N.; López Nigro, M.M.; Peroni, R.N.; Carballo, M.A. Modulation of hepatic ABC transporters by Eruca vesicaria intake: Potential diet-drug interactions. *Food Chem. Toxicol.* **2019**, *133*, 110797. [CrossRef] [PubMed]
67. Yu, C.P.; Yang, M.S.; Hsu, P.W.; Lin, S.P.; Hou, Y.C. Bidirectional influences of cranberry on the pharmacokinetics and pharmacodynamics of warfarin with mechanism elucidation. *Nutrients* **2021**, *13*, 3219. [CrossRef] [PubMed]
68. Yu, C.P.; Tsai, P.L.; Li, P.Y.; Hsu, P.W.; Lin, S.P.; Lee, C.P.D.; Hou, Y.C. Cranberry Ingestion Modulated Drug Transporters and Metabolizing Enzymes: Gefitinib Used as a Probe Substrate in Rats. *Molecules* **2022**, *27*, 5772. [CrossRef]
69. Miron, A.; Aprotosoaie, A.C.; Trifan, A.; Xiao, J. Flavonoids as modulators of metabolic enzymes and drug transporters. *Ann. N. Y. Acad. Sci.* **2017**, *1398*, 152–167. [CrossRef]
70. Ferreira, A.; Pousinho, S.; Fortuna, A.; Falcão, A.; Alves, G. Flavonoid compounds as reversal agents of the P-glycoprotein-mediated multidrug resistance: Biology, chemistry, and pharmacology. *Phytochem. Rev.* **2015**, *14*, 233–272. [CrossRef]
71. Sagnou, M.; Novikov, F.N.; Ivanova, E.S.; Alexiou, P.; Stroylov, V.S.; Titov, I.Y.; Tatarskiy, V.V.; Vagida, M.S.; Pelecanou, M.; Shtil, A.A.; et al. Novel curcumin derivatives as P-glycoprotein inhibitors: Molecular modeling, synthesis, and sensitization of multidrug-resistant cells to doxorubicin. *Eur. J. Med. Chem.* **2020**, *198*, 112331. [CrossRef]
72. El-Araby, M.E.; Omar, A.M.; Khayat, M.T.; Assiri, H.A.; Al-Abd, A.M. Molecular mimics of classic P-glycoprotein inhibitors as multidrug resistance suppressors and their synergistic effect on paclitaxel. *PLoS ONE* **2017**, *12*, e0170186. [CrossRef]
73. Syed, S.B.; Arya, H.; Fu, I.H.; Yeh, T.K.; Periyasamy, L.; Hsieh, H.P.; Coumar, M.S. Targeting P-glycoprotein: Investigation of piperine analogs for overcoming drug resistance in cancer. *Sci. Rep.* **2017**, *7*, 7972. [CrossRef] [PubMed]
74. Tinoush, B.; Shirdel, I.; Wink, M. Phytochemicals: Potential Lead Molecules for MDR Reversal. *Front. Pharmacol.* **2020**, *11*, 832. [CrossRef] [PubMed]
75. Morsy, M.A.; El-Sheikh, A.A.K.; Ibrahim, A.R.N.; Khedr, M.A.; Al-Taher, A.Y. In silico comparisons between natural inhibitors of ABCB1/P-glycoprotein to overcome doxorubicin-resistance in the NCI/ADR-RES cell line. *Eur. J. Pharm. Sci.* **2018**, *112*, 87–94. [CrossRef] [PubMed]
76. Syed, S.B.; Lin, S.Y.; Arya, H.; Fu, I.H.; Yeh, T.K.; Charles, M.R.C.; Periyasamy, L.; Hsieh, H.P.; Coumar, M.S. Overcoming vincristine resistance in cancer: Computational design and discovery of piperine-inspired P-glycoprotein inhibitors. *Chem. Biol. Drug Des.* **2021**, *97*, 51–66. [CrossRef]

77. Zhang, Y.T.; Yu, Y.Q.; Yan, X.X.; Wang, W.J.; Tian, X.T.; Wang, L.; Zhu, W.L.; Gong, L.K.; Pan, G.Y. Different structures of berberine and five other protoberberine alkaloids that affect P-glycoprotein-mediated efflux capacity. *Acta Pharmacol. Sin.* **2019**, *40*, 133–142. [CrossRef]
78. Chu, M.; Chen, X.; Wang, J.; Guo, L.; Wang, Q.; Gao, Z.; Kang, J.; Zhang, M.; Feng, J.; Guo, Q.; et al. Polypharmacology of berberine based on multi-target binding motifs. *Front. Pharmacol.* **2018**, *9*, 801. [CrossRef]

current issues in molecular biology

Review

Ashwagandha-Induced Programmed Cell Death in the Treatment of Breast Cancer

Renata Kołodziejska [1,*], Agnieszka Tafelska-Kaczmarek [2], Mateusz Pawluk [1], Krzysztof Sergot [3], Lucyna Pisarska [1], Alina Woźniak [1,*] and Hanna Pawluk [1]

1 Department of Medical Biology and Biochemistry, Faculty of Medicine, Collegium Medicum in Bydgoszcz, Nicolaus Copernicus University in Toruń, Karłowicza 24, 85-092 Bydgoszcz, Poland; pawluk.mateusz23@gmail.com (M.P.); lucyna.pisarska@cm.umk.pl (L.P.); hannapawluk1@wp.pl (H.P.)
2 Department of Organic Chemistry, Faculty of Chemistry, Nicolaus Copernicus University, Gagarina 7, 87-100 Toruń, Poland; tafel@umk.pl
3 Laboratory of Laser Molecular Spectroscopy, Institute of Applied Radiation Chemistry, Faculty of Chemistry, Lodz University of Technology, Wroblewskiego 15, 93-590 Lodz, Poland; krzysztofsergot@gmail.com
* Correspondence: renatakol@poczta.fm (R.K.); alina-wozniak@wp.pl (A.W.)

Abstract: The aim of this review is to provide experimental evidence for the programmed-death activity of Ashwagandha (*Withania somnifera*) in the anti-cancer therapy of breast cancer. The literature search was conducted using online electronic databases (Google Scholar, PubMed, Scopus). Collection schedule data for the review article covered the years 2004–2024. Ashwagandha active substances, especially Withaferin A (WA), are the most promising anti-cancer compounds. WS exerts its effect on breast cancer cells by inducing programmed cell death, especially apoptosis, at the molecular level. Ashwagandha has been found to possess a potential for treating breast cancer, especially estrogen receptor/progesterone receptor (ER/PR)-positive and triple-negative breast cancer.

Keywords: *Withania somnifera*; Withaferin A; breast cancer; apoptosis; cell death

1. Introduction

Cancer affects both women and men and constitutes a serious clinical problem, as cancer incidence and mortality rates are increasing every year. According to the International Agency for Research on Cancer (IARC), almost 20 million new cancer cases and 9.7 million cancer-related deaths were reported in 2022. Estimates show that approximately 1 in 9 men and 1 in 12 women die from cancer. In 2022, the most frequently diagnosed cancer was lung cancer, corresponding to 12.4% of all cancers in the world, followed by breast cancer in women (11.6%), colorectal cancer (9.6%), prostate cancer (7.3%), and stomach (4.9%) [1].

The 2024 Cancer Statistics Update from the American Cancer Society estimates that 2,001,140 new cases of cancer and 611,720 cancer deaths are projected to occur in the United States. Incidence rates from 2015 to 2019 increased by 0.6–1% per year for breast, pancreatic, and endometrial cancers and by 2–3% per year for papillomavirus-related prostate, liver, kidney, and oral cancers and melanoma [2,3].

The main causes of cancer, apart from genetics, may be increasing environmental pollution, improper diet, low physical activity, alcohol abuse or smoking. Exposure of ancestors to toxic substances, stress, or improper nutrition may influence the occurrence of epigenetic intergenerational inheritance of cancer and the emergence of a variable patient phenotype. Breast cancer (BC) is the most common malignant tumor and the main cause of death in women, and pathogenic variants in BC susceptibility genes constitute the strongest hereditary risk factor for the development of the disease, especially in the context of early-onset breast cancer (EOBC), which is inherited in approximately 10–20% [4,5]. BC is a heterogeneous group of tumors that differ in their morphological appearance, clinical course, and prognosis. The following molecular subtypes of breast cancer are distinguished:

luminal A (60–70%), luminal B (10–20%), human epidermal growth factor (HER2) positive (13–15%), and triple-negative breast cancer (TNBC; 10–15%). In routine practice, molecular forms of breast cancer are defined on the basis of immunohistochemical examination, assessing the expression of the following proteins: estrogen receptor (ER), progesterone receptor (PR), and HER2 receptor [6,7].

There is a great need to develop effective and easily accessible methods for early detection of this disease. The mammography examination (MMG) used so far is not sensitive enough to detect all cases of breast cancer, although it is still a standard examination and the most frequently used in diagnostics. In addition to MMG, other imaging methods are used to diagnose breast cancer, ultrasound (USG), magnetic resonance imaging (MRI), and positron emission tomography (PET) [8–10].

The treatment system is based on clinical and pathological assessment, taking into account the histological type and degree of cancer malignancy, biomarker expression, advancement of the primary tumor location, and the extent of metastases. Apart from invasive treatment and chemotherapy, pharmacological treatment is used. The development of personalized medicine and immunotherapy in recent years has resulted in significant progress in breast cancer treatment [11].

Apart from conventional medicine, natural medicine is becoming more and more popular due to its lower toxicity and selectivity compared to conventional therapies. One of the medicinal plants used in traditional medicine is *Withania somnifera* (WS) [12]. Ashwagandha is mostly considered safe, but side effects are possible [13].

Preclinical experimental evidence shows that WS leaf and root extracts inhibit cancer [14–19]. Methanol and ethanol extracts of WS stems have been shown to be highly cytotoxic and inhibit the growth of the human breast cancer cell line [20]. Experimental studies on animals have proven that the use of WS root extract and intermittent fasting are a promising solution in the treatment of breast cancer to overcome cisplatin resistance [21]. In turn, a standardized Ashwagandha extract (Oncowithanib) showed effective therapeutic activity in MCF7 cells and is associated with suppression of the expression of key cellular kinases, such as RSK1, AKT1, and mTOR [22].

It is known that WS has anticancer properties, but the mechanism of its action is not fully understood. The inhibition of cancer cells by WA may be the result of the following molecular mechanisms: induction of apoptosis; induction of oxidative stress; reduction of NF-κB, STAT3, and estrogen receptor expression; inhibition of the cell cycle in the G2-M phase, proteasomes, and processes important for the spread of cancer cell metastases [16,23–51]. WA inhibits cancer metastasis by partially reversing the epithelial-to-mesenchymal pathway, targeting the urokinase-type plasminogen activator (uPA) and activating the transcription factors Notch2 and Notch4 and reducing Notch1 [39,41,43].

This review assessed the anti-tumor role of WS in breast cancer based on the available scientific literature. We tried to determine the involvement of one of the most active components of Ahwagandha, withaferin A (WA), in the induction of programmed cell death, one of the mechanisms of inhibiting cancer cell proliferation and metastasis.

2. Data Collection Methodology

This review is narrative in nature and presents the collected literature on Ashwagandha-induced programmed tumor-cell death in breast cancer. A comprehensive search strategy was employed across international databases like Google Scholar, PubMed, and Scopus using keywords and phrases, namely *Withania somnifera* L. Dunal in breast cancer; Withaferin A, Ashwagandha, Ashwaganddha in breast cancer; apoptosis by Ashwagandha in breast cancer; and programmatic death of breast cancer. The collection schedule data for the review article covered the years 2004–2024, with a total of 242 articles. The publication inclusion criteria were as follows: (1) articles on Ashwagandha in the treatment of breast cancer, with particular emphasis on the mechanism of promoted cancer cell death; (2) only article and review document types (preclinical and clinical research) and; and (3) only English-language articles. The exclusion criteria were as follows: (1) articles that did not concern the use of Ashwagandha in the treatment of breast cancer; (2) articles that have not been peer-reviewed.

3. *Withania somnifera*

Ashwagandha (*Withania somnifera* L. *Dunal*) is a species of plant from the Solanaceae family. It naturally occurs in dry regions of tropical and subtropical climates, i.e., in Africa, Asia, and southern Europe. The name "Ashwagandha" was derived from the Sanskrit terms "ashva", which means "horse," and "gandha", which means "smell", and denotes the root's aroma, which is similar to that of a horse. Synonyms of the name Ashwagandha are Indian winter cherry, Indian ginseng, and poison gooseberry. The plant has derived its names due to its certain features. Because of its pronounced anti-stress effects, the plant was ascribed its species name "somnifera", meaning "sleep-inducer" in Latin [52]. The roots, leaves, flowers, and fruits of this plant are used in Indian folk medicine (Ayurveda) and as a dietary supplement [53,54].

WS and its roots have a wide range of pharmacological effects due to their medically useful chemical composition. It is active, among others, with the following properties: anti-inflammatory, anti-arthritic, anti-cancer, anti-epileptic, anti-depressant, anti-Alzheimer's disease, anti-Parkinson's disease, analgesic, cardioprotective, neuroprotective, anti-microbial, anti-fungal, anti-oxidant, anti-diabetic agent, etc. [44,55].

Various chemical components are found in the different parts of the plant. The roots of WS contain alkaloids (withananine, withanine, somniferine, somnine, somniferinine), amino acids (alanine, cysteine, glycine, tyrosine), steroidal lactones (withaferin A, withanolides A, B, D, E, F, G, H, I, J, K, L, M), steroids (sitoindosides VII, VIII, IX, X), volatile oil, starch, reducing sugars, glycosides, hentriacontane, dulcitol, flavonoids, withaniol, withanicil, iron, withasomnine, withanosides I-VII, and many others [52,56–59]. Typically, WS roots are used for medicinal purposes in the form of root extract as well as powder. Ashwagandha leaves contain withaferin A; 12 withanolides, including withanolide A, B, D, and E; withanone, flavonoids; free amino acids; and also condensed tannins, chlorogenic acid, *N*-heterocyclic compounds, and others [52,57,58]. Fruits, flowers, and seeds contain compounds like withanolides, withanolide glycosides, withanone, amino acids, flavonoids, condensed tannins, proteolytic eznyme, and psoralen [52,57,58,60].

The major chemical constituents of Ashwagandha are withanolides, C28-steroidal lactones, having an ergostane skeleton, in which C-22 and C-26 are appropriately oxidized to form five- or six-membered lactone rings [57]. Moreover, various compounds were found in WS, which are the modifications or structural variants of withanolides such as withaferin A, withanone, ashwagandhanolide, and sitoindosides. The main components of Withania somnifera are shown in Figure 1.

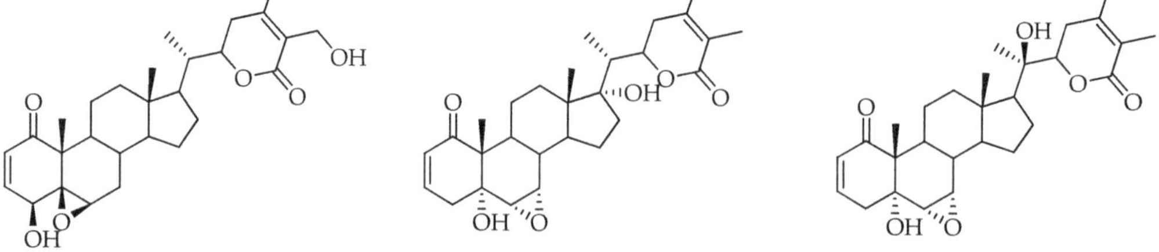

Withaferin A **Withanone** **Withanolide A**

Figure 1. Structures of key components present in *Withania somnifera*.

Withania somnifera extract has anti-oxidant and anti-microbial properties [61]. It has been found that WS shows activity against a variety of bacteria, viruses, and fungi, mainly due to the presence of withaferin A, withantolide A, and withanone [62–64]. Moreover, anti-inflammatory activity against protein denaturation in vitro results from Ashwagandha's alkaloids and withanolides [65]. Many studies have also confirmed that the main components of Ashwagandha are responsible for the neuroprotective and anti-neurodegenerative effects in diseases such as Alzheimer's, Parkinson's, Huntington's, and epilepsy [66–72]. Withaferin A from WS has been shown to help treat diabetes [73,74]. In turn, the alkaloids present in the WS plant have anti-stress activity [75,76]. Extensive research is also being conducted on the anti-cancer properties of Ashwagandha extract, especially its phytochemicals withanolides and withaferin A [17]. Activity has been found against cancer of prostate, kidney, bladder, gastric, colon, lung, breast, leukemia, and others [12,77,78].

4. Mechanism of Breast Cancer Cell Death by Ashwagandha

WS is involved in many biochemical processes, including apoptosis, which is a form of cell suicide that occurs not only as a result of cell damage or external stress but also during normal development and morphogenesis.

The mechanism of apoptosis mainly consists of two basic pathways involved in inducing apoptosis, intracellular (intrinsic apoptosis) or extracellular (extrinsic apoptosis) (Figure 2) [79].

In the intrinsic pathway, apoptosis occurs via mitochondrial mediation. Apoptotic signaling in the extrinsic pathway involves extracellular ligands such as tumor necrosis factor (TNF), Fas ligand (Fas-L), and TNF-related apoptosis-inducing ligand (TRAIL). These ligands are attached to the extracellular domain of transmembrane receptors (DRs), which include TNF type 1 receptor (TNFR1), Fas (also called CD95/Apo-1), and TRAIL receptors [80].

The intrinsic, mitochondrial pathway of apoptosis is triggered by various intracellular stressors. Proteins from the Bcl-2 family are responsible for regulating this pathway, including pro-apoptotic proteins (Bax, Bak, Bok, Bim, Bid, Bik, Bad, Bmf, Hrk, Noxa, Puma, Blk) and anti-apoptotic proteins (Bcl-2, Bcl-XL, Bcl-w, A1, Mcl-1). Internal cellular stress activates Bcl-2 proteins that have only one domain, the so-called BH3-only proteins (Bcl-2 homology 3), containing Bid, Bim, Bad, Bik, Noxa, Puma, and Hrk. These proteins neutralize the action of anti-apoptotic proteins or, acting directly, activate multi-domain apoptosis-inducing proteins, i.e., Bax or Bak [81–85].

Oligomerizing Bax or Bak create pores in the outer mitochondrial membrane, which results in its destabilization. Disruption of the integrity of mitochondrial potential results in the release of pro-apoptotic proteins into the cytosol. Proteins that are generally involved in intrinsic pathway include cytochrome C (called apoptotic protease-activating factor 1 (Apaf-2)), Smac/DIABLO, HtrA2/Omi and AIF, Endonuclease G and CAD. Cytochrome C (CytC) combines with Apaf-1 and procaspase-9 to form an apoptosome that releases caspase-9 (CASP9). In turn, the CASP9 initiator activates caspase-3 (CASP3) and caspase-7 (CASP7). Smac/DIABLO and HtrA2/Omi indirectly promote apoptosis by affecting caspase-3/7 activation through inhibition of inhibitor of apoptosis proteins (IAPs). Whereas, AIF, Endonuclease G, and CAD proteins travel directly to the cell nucleus, cutting DNA into short fragments [86].

In the intrinsic apoptosis pathway, the element of pro-apoptotic regulation is the p53 protein, the so-called guardian of the genome. Under stress conditions, the p53 protein moves to the mitochondria, where it forms a complex with Bcl-2 and Bcl-XL, causing their inactivation. As a result, the permeability of the mitochondrial membrane increases and CytC is released [87].

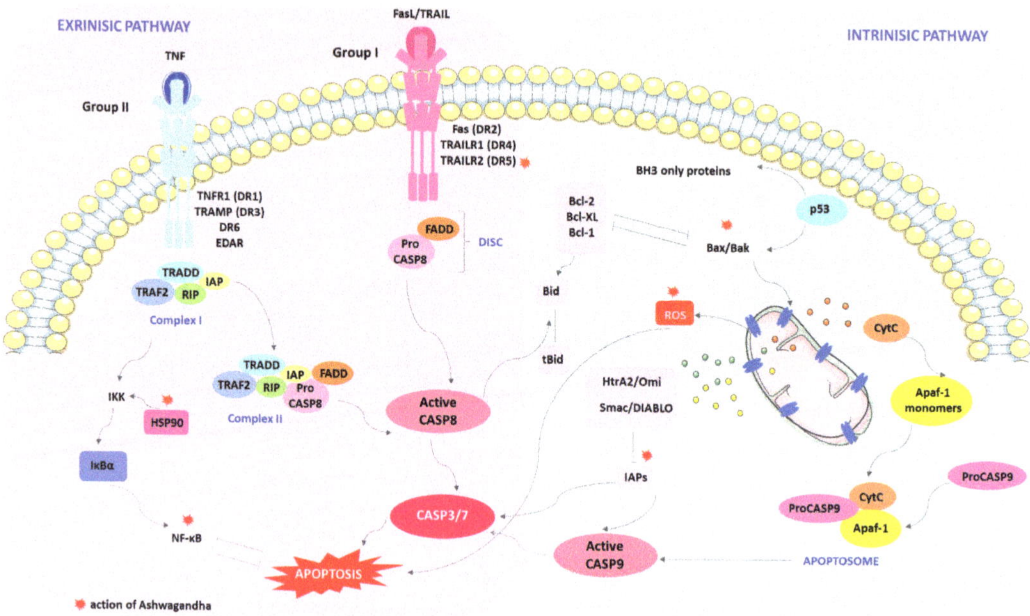

Figure 2. Internal and external pathways of apoptosis: the action of Ashwagandha. The effects of Ashwagandha on pathways of apoptosis are marked with a red asterisk. Active components of Ashwagandha induce apoptosis in both the internal and external pathways by mediating the production of reactive oxygen species and regulating the expression of Bcl-2 and IAP family proteins and the heat shock protein HSP90, as well as activating Death Receptor 5 (DR5) and inhibiting the IKK/NF-κB pathway. Abbreviations: Apaf-1—apoptotic protease activating factor 1; Bak, Bax, Bcl-1, Bcl-XL, Bid, tBid—Bcl-2 family proteins; BH3-only proteins—Bcl-2 homology 3; CASP3/7/8/9—caspase-3/7/8/9; CytC—cytochrome C; FADD—Fas-associated death domain; Fas-L—Fas ligand; IAPs—inhibitors of apoptosis proteins; HSP90—heat shock protein 90; HtrA2/Omi—apoptosis proteins; IκBα—nuclear factor of kappa light polypeptide gene enhancer in B-cells inhibitor alpha; IKK—kinase complex; NF-κB—nuclear factor-κB; ProCASP9—procaspase-9; Fas (DR2) TRAILR1 (DR4), TRAILR2 (DR5), TNFR1 (DR1), TRAMP (DR3), DR6 and EDAR—tumor necrosis factor receptor TNFR family; RIP—receptor-interacting protein kinase; ROS—reactive oxygen species; Smac/DIABLO—apoptosis proteins; TRAF2—TNF receptor associated factor-2; TRAIL—TNF-related apoptosis-inducing ligand; TNF—tumor necrosis factor; TRADD—TNF-related death domain. This figure was created using Servier Medical Art (available at https://smart.servier.com/, accessed on 12 April 2024).

In the extrinsic apoptosis pathway, the pro-apoptotic signal is transmitted via receptors from the tumor necrosis factor receptor TNFR family (Fas (DR2) TRAILR1 (DR4), TRAILR2 (DR5), TNFR1 (DR1), TRAMP (DR3), DR6 and EDAR). A feature of death receptors is the presence of an intracellular domain called the death domain (DD). After attaching the ligand to the receptor, it is activated through oligomerization and conformational changes, which then attaches an adapter protein such as Fas-associated death domain (FADD), tumor necrosis factor receptor-1-associated death domain (TRADD), or death domain-associated protein (Daxx)-containing death domains. The adapter protein further combines with procaspase-8 to form the death-inducing signaling complex (DISC). Attachment of an appropriate ligand to the receptor induces signal transmission through the death domain of the adapter protein to caspase-8 (CASP8). The consequence of this is the activation by autoproteolysis of procaspase-8, which is a direct activator of caspase 3/7 [80,81,84,88].

Fas (DR2), TRAILR1 (DR4), and TRAILR2 (DR5) receptors belong to the first group of death receptors activated by FasL and TRAIL. Once activated, these receptors recruit the DISC complex, which consists of FADD and CASP8. Due to the amount of activated CASP8, we can divide this phase into two types. In the type of stage when the amount of active CASP8 is higher, direct activation of CASP3 occurs. However, in the second type, when we are dealing with a low level of CASP3 activation via CASP8, caspase-8 activates the pro-apoptotic Bid protein into the active form tBid, which interacts with Bax/Bak proteins, and CytC is released [84,89,90].

The second group of death receptors includes the TNFR1 (DR1), TRAMP (DR3), DR6, and EDAR receptors. The apoptosis-inducing ligand is TNF. Once activated, the receptors recruit the TNF-related death domain (TRADD) as an adapter protein and bind to TNF receptor-related factors-2.5 (TRAF2.5), receptor-interacting protein kinase (RIP1 or RIPK1), and cellular inhibitors of apoptosis proteins (cIAP) [84].

Two distinct complexes may be formed for TNFR1. Complex I is the TNFR1 complex consisting of proteins containing DD TRADD, TNF-2 receptor-associated factor (TRAF2 (TNF)), cIAP1, and the receptor serine/threonine protein kinase 1 (RIP1). This complex activates nuclear factor-κB (NF-κB) and the c-Jun NH2-terminalkinase/Jun proto-oncogene/AP-1 transcription factor subunit (JNK/AP-1). NF-κB inhibits TNF-induced apoptosis. Complex II arises after the TRADD-based complex cleaves from the receptor and recruits FADD and the initiator CASP8. The balance between these complexes is dependent on the protein FLIP, a CASP8 inhibitor. Complex II mediates apoptosis when activation of the NF-κB pathway is inadequate [84].

In the classic way of NF-κB activation, after the action of an appropriate stimulating factor, e.g., pro-inflammatory cytokines (TNF), the IKK kinase complex is activated. The active IKK complex catalyzes the phosphorylation of IκBα, which leads to its degradation and the release of the NF-κB dimer. Then, the NF-κB dimer is translocated to the cell nucleus and activates the transcription of appropriate genes, the end products of which have the ability to inhibit apoptosis [91–93].

In addition to DR, apoptosis is influenced by growth factors through the phosphatidinositide-3-kinase (PI3K) and murine thymus virus oncogene homolog v-AKT (AKT) pathways. Growth factors bind to receptors and activate PI3K, which activates AKT. AKT is important in the regulation of Bad. Moreover, protein kinase-C (PKC) influences apoptosis by activating ribosomal S6 kinase (p90RSK) [94].

In healthy breast cells, a balance is maintained between cell proliferation and death. Once a balance is disrupted, an activated anti-apoptotic signaling pathway or a deficiency in the pro-apoptosis pathway can lead to uncontrolled cell proliferation [95,96].

Withaferin A and extracts from the Ayurvedic medicinal plant Withania somnifera can inhibit the proliferation of breast cancer cells by inducing apoptosis in both the intrinsic and extrinsic pathways. WA and/or WS root protein extract (WSPF) induces death in cultured MDA-MB-231 and MCF-7 cancer cells and MDA-MB-231 xenografts in vivo by mediating the production of reactive oxygen species (ROS) in the intrinsic apoptosis pathway (Figure 2) [28,97,98]. Selective killing of MCF-7 and MDA-MB-231 cancer cells by WA and/or WSPF is mediated by the induction of oxidative stress via ROS levels, DNA damage, mitochondrial structure, and membrane potential [97–99]. WA inhibits oxidative phosphorylation (OXPHOS) in Complex III, accompanied by apoptotic release of DNA fragments associated with histones in the cytosol [28,100,101]. However, the anti-cancer effect of WA was significantly attenuated in the presence of anti-oxidants, as it has been shown that ectopic expression of Cu and Zn-superoxide dismutase (SOD) significantly weakens its apoptotic properties [28]. Moreover, WA shows high selectivity, causing ROS production only in MDA-MB-231 and MCF-7 cells, but not in the normal human mammary epithelial cell line (HMEC) [28].

WA is involved in the regulation of the expression of Bcl-2 proteins, which are critical regulators of cell death, acting either as inhibitors or facilitators of apoptosis. Both Bax and Bak appear to contribute to the induction of apoptosis by WA (Figure 2). The active substance contained in Ashwagandha enhances the activation of these pro-apoptotic proteins in MDA-MB-231 and MCF-7 cells [28]. WA inhibits the survival of MCF-7 and MDA-MB-231 breast cancer cell lines in culture and delays the growth of MDA-MB-231 xenografts in vivo due to reduced cell proliferation and increased apoptosis. According to Stan et al., apoptosis by WA is probably mediated by forkhead box O3 (FOXO3a) and Bim proteins in both cancer cell lines. WA-induced apoptosis was accompanied by the induction of Bim-s and Bim-L in MCF-7 cells and the induction of Bim-s and Bim-EL isoforms in MDA-MB-231 cells [25].

WA also results in suppression of these IAP family proteins: XIAP, cIAP-2, and survivin in MDA-MB-231 and MCF-7 human breast cancer cells (Figure 2). IAP family proteins (IAP, cIAP1, cIAP2, NAIP, livin, and survivin) act as endogenous inhibitors of apoptosis and are involved in the cell's adaptive response to stress, differentiation, motility, and immune response. IAPs can inhibit both the intrinsic and extrinsic apoptosis pathways. The overexpression of IAP family proteins is observed in breast cancer, which results in improved survival of cancer cells, increased tumor growth and, consequently, metastases. Therefore, it seems that the reduction in the expression of these proteins by WA indicates its significant role in apoptosis [102].

In the extrinsic apoptosis pathway, the TRAIL pathway is considered the most attractive cancer therapy agent, which is non-toxic compared to the FasL and TNF-α pathways. Its safety in cancer patients has been confirmed in phase I and II clinical trials [103–106]. TRAIL is expressed mainly on the surface of immune cells and induces apoptosis in various cancer cell lines. In a group of patients with triple-negative breast cancer (TNBC), pre-clinical models have demonstrated the effectiveness of therapy targeting the TRAIL DR pathway [107]. WA inhibits breast tumor growth by upregulation of death receptor 5 (DR5, also known as TRAIL-R2/TRICK-2/KILLER/TNFRSF10B) (Figure 2) [107]. WA has been shown to activate phosphorylation of S6RSK in breast cancer cells via activation of cell signal-regulated kinase (ERK) [108]. Both RSK and ERK play a key role in breast cancer progression and metastasis [109]. WA induced a feed-forward loop of ERK and RSK, causing the simultaneous upregulation/activation of homology protein/C-EBP axis (CHOP) and ETS-like transcription factor 1 (Elk1). The recruitment of CHOP and Elk1 to the DR5 promoter leads to activation of the death receptor, DR5, which is responsible for the aggregation of proteins promoting apoptotic signal transduction [108].

The heat shock protein (HSP) transcription factor may also play an important role in apoptosis through WA by regulating survivin expression. In many types of cancer, heat shock factor 1 (HSF1) is a transcription factor activated under environmental stress, which leads to increased expression of HSP proteins. HSF1 is increased in expression and facilitates cancer transformation by modulating signaling pathways related to growth and proliferation, apoptosis, metabolism, and motility. WA induced HSF1 phosphorylation, which is probably due to a transient cellular defense response to WA-induced stress [110]. The level of HSP expression determines the fate of cells, because these biomolecules can direct them to the apoptosis or survival pathway. One of the HSP subfamily proteins, heat shock chaperone 90 (HSP90), has become an exciting target for cancer therapy due to its role in regulating cell proliferation, survival, and apoptosis. HSP90 can modulate the activity and stability of many transcription factors and kinases related to apoptosis, including NF-κB, p53, protein kinase B (PKB/AKT), Proto-Oncogene, Serine/Threonine Kinase (Raf-1), and stress-activated protein/kinase/Jun N-terminal kinase (SAPK/JAK). In the pathway involving NF-κB, cell survival is conditioned by the formation of an NF-κB complex with the kinase of the κB inhibitor kinase complex (IKK). KK is composed of IKKα and IKKβ and NF-κB essential modulator (NEMO) or IKKγ. IKKβ IKK kinase phosphorylates two specific serine residues in the N-terminal region of IκBα, causing proteasomal degradation of IκBα and nuclear translocation of canonical NF-κB members, mainly p50/RelA and p50/c-Rel dimers [111,112]. The active substances of Ashwagandha, 2,3-unsaturated double bond-containing withanolides, exhibit potent inhibitory effects on the activity of the Hsp90 chaperone by depleting several important signaling molecules involved in cell survival (Figure 2). Withanolides inhibited the IKK/NF-κB pathway in MDA-MB-23, an ER-negative human breast cancer cell line. They reduced the activity of anti-apoptotic proteins (Bcl-2, Bcl-xL, and c-FLIP) that are regulated by NF-κB [113].

Janus kinase (JAK)-signal transducer and activator of transcription (STAT) signaling also mediates apoptosis. STAT proteins (STAT 1A, 1B, 2, 3, 4, 5A, 5B, and 6) are a family of transcription factors, each of which performs a unique function in the transmission of extracellular and direct signals regulating the transcription of genes that are involved in cell survival, proliferation, chemoresistance, and angiogenesis. Signal transducers and activators of transcription proteins (STATs) are activated by binding to their receptors on the cell membrane. The phosphorylated receptor-kinase complex is the site of STAT attachment, which is then phosphorylated on tyrosine residues necessary for activation. Then, after dimerization, STAT translocated to the nucleus can influence cell apoptosis by regulating the transcription of target genes such as Bcl-xL, p21, and Myc [114–116].

In many human cancers, including breast cancer, STAT3 and STAT5 are persistently phosphorylated and overactivated [117]. STAT3 increases the expression of c-Myc and the metastasis regulator Twist genes and is, therefore, thought to induce breast cancer [118]. Aberrant STAT5 signaling promotes cyclin D, Bcl-2, and matrix metalloproteinase-2 (MMP-2) gene expression, resulting in increased cell proliferation, survival, and metastasis [119,120]. WA causes inactivation of STAT3 and STAT5 by inhibiting their recruitment to growth factor and cytokine receptors as well as tyrosine phosphorylation, nuclear translocation, and DNA binding. Furthermore, STAT3 inhibits Bcl-xL and Mcl-1. (Figure 3) [117].

Other studies have demonstrated the role of mitogen-activated protein kinases (MAPKs) in the regulation of apoptosis by WA (Figure 3). MCF-7 cell death resulted from the action of WA via pharmacological inhibition of ERK kinase and p38 MAPK [121]. The MAPK pathway, often called the RAS-RAF-MEK-ERK signaling cascade, serves to transmit upstream signals to downstream effectors to regulate physiological processes such as cell proliferation, differentiation, survival, and death [122]. It is the most frequently mutated signaling pathway in human cancers; therefore, this pathway may be a promising strategy in cancer therapy [123,124].

The mitogen-activated protein kinase (MAPK) cascade consists of serine/threonine kinases that convert extracellular molecules such as growth factors (EGF), insulin-like growth factor I (IGF-I), hormones, and differentiation factors into intracellular signals [123,124]. There are four core protein kinases in the Ras/Raf/MEK/ERK-signaling pathway: Ras, Raf, MEK, and ERK. Once the signaling molecules are attached, the receptors dimerize, which activates RAS proteins. Activated RAS protein recruits RAF protein from the cytosol to the cell membrane, leading to its activation. Active RAF kinase phosphorylates MEK1 and 2 proteins, which activate ERK1 and 2 proteins. After transmitting the signal to the cell nucleus, ERK kinases phosphorylate and activate many target molecules responsible for cell growth, migration, and survival [125,126].

WA also acts to reduce the level of estrogen receptor alpha (Erα), which consequently affects the induction of apoptosis and inhibition of the growth of ER-α-positive MCF-7 and T47D breast cancer cells [33].

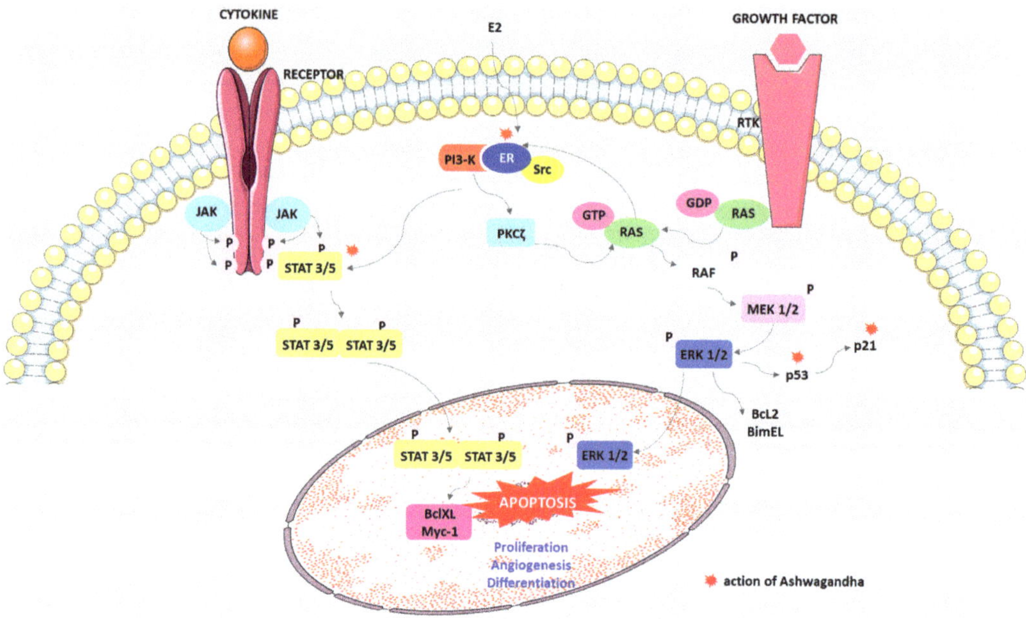

Figure 3. Mechanism of action of Ashwagandha. The effects of Ashwagandha on pathways of apoptosis is marked with a red asterisk. Active components of Ashwagandha induce apoptosis by inhibiting the recruitment of STAT3 and STAT5, regulating the MAPK pathway and the expression of p53 and p21 proteins and reducing the level of estrogen receptor alpha (Erα). Abbreviations: AKT—protein kinase B; Bcl-XL, BimEL, Myc-1—Bcl-2 family proteins; E2—17β-estradiol; ER—estrogen receptor; ERK—extracellular signal-regulated kinase; FOXO3a—forkhead transcription factor; GDP—guanosine diphosphate; GTP—guanosine-5′-triphosphate; JAK—janus kinase; MEK—mitogen-activated extracellular signal-regulated kinase; NF-κB—nuclear factor-κB; PI3-K—PI 3-kinase; p21 protein—Cyclin-dependent kinase inhibitor; p53 protein—transcription factor with tumor suppressor properties; RAF—rapidly accelerated fibrosarcoma kinase; RAS—cellular signal transduction protein; RTK—receptor tyrosine kinase; STAT—signal transducer and activator of transcription. This figure was created using Servier Medical Art (available at https://smart.servier.com/, accessed on 12 April 2024).

17β-estradiol (E2) exerts its effects on proliferation mainly through rapid non-genomic mechanisms derived from the binding of the hormone to Erα. Non-genomic signals are transmitted to the nucleus via various intracellular-signaling pathways such as MAPK/ERK and PI3K/AKT [127–129]. E2 induces the association of ERα with Src and the PI 3-kinase (PI3K) adapter subunit p85a. Estradiol-stimulated PI 3-kinase/PDK1 pathway activates PKCζ in MCF-7 cells, which controls Ras-dependent ERK activation. Furthermore, E2 phosphorylates STAT3 and STAT5 by an ER-dependent mechanism [130]. The ERβ isoform has also been shown to play an important role in the proliferative action of E2, which can act as a tumor suppressor by modulating the proliferative action of ERα [129]. The E2-ERβ complex activates p38/MAPK leading to apoptosis while E2-ERα activates transduction pathways involved in cell cycle progression. The E2-ERβ complex activates p38/MAPK leading to apoptosis while E2-ERα activates transduction pathways involved in cell cycle progression [129,131,132]. WA reduces ERα levels post-translationally, inducing ERα protein aggregation and degradation. The anti-cancer activity of WA is mediated by RET tyrosine kinase (RET) and p53, which inhibits growth and apoptosis [110,133]. While RET is overexpressed in ERα-positive breast cancer, its activation stimulates the proliferation, survival, and dispersal of MCF-7 breast cancer cells [134]. WA had anti-tumor effects through the downregulation of RET protein with parallel depletion of Erα coupled with increases in the expression of phosphorylated mitogen-activated protein kinase p38 (phospho-p38 MAPK), p53, and p21 (Figure 3) [14,110].

In addition to apoptosis, there are also other non-apoptotic modes of cell death including autophagy, necroptosis, paraptosis, and apoptosis-like programmed cell death.

Autophagy or autophagic cell death are referred to as type II cell death. This process plays an important role in the degradation of cellular components inside the dying cell in autophagic vacuoles. It helps maintain cellular energy supply and homeostasis in rapidly proliferating cancer cells. Cancer cells use this process to respond to various environmental stimuli and avoid anti-cancer therapy [135]. The anti-tumor effect of WA in many breast cancer subtypes, including luminal A, luminal B, basal, claudin-low, and HER2W subtypes, is related to impairment of lysosomal activity, causing blockage of autophagic flux, which results in energy depletion leading to growth inhibition and induction of apoptosis. WA is an activator of 5′AMP-activated protein kinase AMP (AMPK), which works synergistically with 2-deoxy-d-glucose (2-DG) to inhibit breast cancer growth and is also an inhibitor of lactate dehydrogenase (LDHA), a key enzyme catalyzing the conversion of pyruvate to lactate [136].

Inhibition of the WA-mediated proteasome degradation system and perturbation of autophagy causes the accumulation of ubiquitinated proteins, which in turn results in unfolded protein responses and ER stress-mediated proteotoxicity in the human breast cancer cell lines MCF-7 and MDA-MB-231 [137].

Another process involved in programmed cell death that is morphologically different from apoptosis and autophagy is paraptosis. WA acts on the mitochondrial membrane potential, causing its hyperpolarization and the formation of many cytoplasmic vesicles. In the human breast cancer cell lines MCF-7 and MDA-MB-231, mitochondrial swelling and fusion occur, and the endoplasmic reticulum (ER) expands. WA reduces the level of the native paraptosis inhibitor, actin-interacting protein-1 (Alix/AIP-1), indicating that WA promotes death in both MCF-7 and MDA-MB-231 cell lines through paraptosis through the action of ROS [138].

Summarizing pre-clinical studies, it can be concluded that Ashwagandha has anti-cancer activity in various experimental models. WS acts at many stages, leading to apoptosis, both in the extrinsic and intrinsic pathways. WA and/or its extracts induce death in cancer cell cultures in vivo by mediating ROS production [28,97–99]. WA regulates the expression of Bcl-2 proteins, reduces the expression of IAP proteins XIAP, cIAP-2, and survivin and apoptosis inhibitors [25,97,102]. It inhibits the growth of breast cancer cells by activating DR5 [108]. It affects the activity of the Hsp90 protein, the recruitment of STAT3 and STAT5, and the regulation of the MAPK pathway [107,117,121]. It influences the reduction of the level of estrogen receptor alpha [33,110]. WA inhibits autophagic flux and reduces the level of paraptosis inhibitor, inducing death in breast cancer cells via ROS [137,138].

Information regarding the mechanism of action of Ashwagandha on various cell lines, taking into account the concentrations of active components of the plant extract used, is presented in Table 1.

There is little information about clinical trials confirming the use of WS in the treatment of breast cancer, although they are crucial to confirm its effectiveness and safety. It has only been shown that WS reduces chemotherapy-induced fatigue and improves the quality of life after administering 2 g of WS root extract every 8 h, throughout the course of chemotherapy. Similarly, survival analysis showed that patients in the WS treatment group had a better 24-month survival rate of 76% compared to the control group, which had a survival rate of 56% [47,139,140].

Table 1. Effect of WA and Ashwagandha extract on various breast cancer cell lines.

Phytochemicals/ Concentration	Cell Lines	Mechanism of Action of Ashwagandha	Reference
WA/2.5 µM	MDA-MB-23 MCF-7 MDA-MB-231	ROS-mediated apoptotic induction due to inhibition of mitochondrial respiration.	[28]
WA/3.0 mg/mL	MCF-7 MDA-MB-231	ROS-mediated apoptotic induction. Dysregulation of Bax/Bcl-2, loss of mitochondrial membrane potential and caspase-3 activation.	[97]
Extract/6 µg/mL; WA/1 µM, witanonem/25 µg/mL	MCF-7	ROS-mediated apoptotic induction. DNA damage, mitochondrial structure, and membrane potential.	[98]
WA/2 µM	MCF-7 i SUM159	Changes the assembly of complex III. Inhibition of mitochondrial dynamics.	[99]
WA/IC50 < 2 µM	MCF-7 MDA-MB-231	Regulation of apoptosis involving FOXO3a and Bim. Induction of Bim-s and Bim-L in MCF-7 cells. Induction of Bim-s and Bim-EL isoforms in MDA-MB-231 cells.	[25]
WA/2.5 and 5 µM	MDA-MB-231 MCF-7	Decrease in the expression of XIAP, cIAP-2 and survivin proteins, apoptosis inhibitors.	[102]
WFA/5 µM	MCF7 MDA-MB-231	DR5 upregulation. Increased nuclear accumulation of Elk1 and CHOP.	[108]
WA/5 µM, 4β-Hydroxywithanolide (HW)/ 20 µM, Anomanolide A (AA)/20 µM, Peruvianolide H (PH)/20 µM)	MDA-MB-231 MCF-7	Inhibition of Hsp90.	[107]
WA/3 µM	MDA-MB-468	Inhibition of STAT3 and STAT5 recruitment.	[117]
WA/2.5 µM	MCF-7	Inhibition of ERK and p38 MAPK.	[121]
	MCF-7 T47D	Inhibition of estrogen receptor α expression.	[33]
WA/2.5, 5 µM	MCF-7		[110]
WA/5 µM	MCF7, MDA-MB-231, MDA-MB-468, T47D, SUM149, SUM159, SKBR3	Blocking the flow of autophagy and lysosomal proteolytic activity.	[136]
WA/4 µM	MCF-7 MDA-MB-231	Inhibition of the proteasome degradation system and disruption of autophagy.	[137]
	MCF-7 MDA-MB-231	ROS-mediated paraptosis induction.	[138]

Although Ashwagandha was considered safe in clinical trials, improper dosage or failure to take into account individual contraindications may lead to a number of health problems, ranging from nausea and vomiting to more serious complications, such as hypertension, liver dysfunction, and hyperbilirubinemia [141,142].

Additionally, people taking anti-diabetic, anti-hypertensive, or central nervous system medications should be careful, because WS may interact with these medications, enhancing or changing their effects. Ashwagandha may also affect thyroid hormone and testosterone levels [143–146].

There is also a lack of clear evidence on the safety of the long-term use of WS over many months or years. Ashwagandha was well tolerated at a dose of 300 mg per day in an eight-week study [147]. For insomnia, a dose of 600 milligrams per day has been found to be safe and effective [148]. This dosage has also been associated with improved memory [149].

The extensive exploratory studies demonstrate the potential of Ashwagandha in the treatment of breast cancer through its anti-cancer activity, safety profile, and combination therapy possibilities. However, due to inconsistent therapeutic results resulting from the widely varying composition of active components in the plant extract, the actual use of WS in the treatment of cancer is limited. Further research and standardization are needed to harness its full therapeutic potential.

5. Conclusions

Withaferin A (WA) and withanolides are the most promising anti-cancer compounds of Ashwagandha, which play a major role in the induction of the apoptosis of cancer cells. This review attempts to confirm its therapeutic properties, with a particular emphasis on its role in the treatment of breast cancer. The literature data indicate that compounds isolated from various parts of this plant, such as the root, stem, and leaves, have significant anti-cancer and immunomodulatory properties; therefore, they can be used alone or in combination with other chemotherapy drugs in the treatment of breast cancer. Reaching for natural medicine can complement the standard treatment of cancer patients without undesirable side effects and may also have a positive impact on reducing the feeling of fatigue and improving their quality of life [139].

Author Contributions: Conceptualization, R.K. and H.P.; writing—original draft preparation, R.K., H.P. and A.T.-K.; writing—review and editing, R.K., H.P., A.T.-K., M.P., K.S., L.P. and A.W.; visualization, R.K., K.S. and M.P.; supervision, R.K. and H.P.; project administration, R.K. and H.P.; funding acquisition, A.W. All authors have read and agreed to the published version of the manuscript.

Funding: This research received no external funding.

Conflicts of Interest: The authors declare no conflicts of interest.

References

1. Bray, F.; Laversanne, M.; Sung, H.; Jacques Ferlay, J.; Siegel, R.L.; Soerjomataram, I.; Jemal, A. Global cancer statistics 2022: GLOBOCAN estimates of incidence and mortality worldwide for 36 cancers in 185 countries. *CA Cancer J. Clin.* **2024**, *74*, 229–263. [CrossRef] [PubMed]
2. Siegel, R.L.; Giaquinto, A.N.; Jemal, A. Cancer statistics. *CA Cancer J. Clin.* **2024**, *74*, 12–49. [CrossRef] [PubMed]
3. Dizon, D.S.; Kamal, A.H. Cancer statistics 2024: All hands on deck. *CA Cancer J. Clin.* **2024**, *74*, 8–9. [CrossRef] [PubMed]
4. Siddig, A.; Tengku Din, T.A.D.A.; Mohd Nafi, S.N.; Yahya, M.M.; Sulong, S.; Wan Abdul Rahman, W.F. The unique biology behind the early onset of breast cancer. *Genes* **2021**, *12*, 372. [CrossRef] [PubMed]
5. Carmen Criscitiello, C.; Corti, C. Breast cancer genetics: Diagnostics and treatment. *Genes* **2022**, *13*, 1593. [CrossRef] [PubMed]
6. Harbeck, N.; Penault-Llorca, F.; Cortes, J.; Gnant, M.; Houssami, N.; Poortmans, P.; Ruddy, K.; Tsang, J.; Cardoso, F. Breast cancer. *Nat. Rev. Dis. Primers* **2019**, *5*, 1–31. [CrossRef] [PubMed]
7. Łukasiewicz, S.; Czeczelewski, M.; Forma, A.; Baj, J.; Sitarz, R.; Stanisławek, A. Breast cancer—Epidemiology, risk factors, classification, prognostic markers, and current treatment strategies—An updated review. *Cancers* **2021**, *13*, 4287. [CrossRef] [PubMed]
8. Mohi ud din, N.; Ahmad Dar, R.; Rasool, M.; Assad, A. Breast cancer detection using deep learning: Datasets, methods, and challenges ahead. *Comput. Biol. Med.* **2022**, *149*, 106073. [CrossRef]
9. Bhimani, C.; Matta, D.; Roth, R.G.; Liao, L.; Tinney, E.; Brill, K.; Germaine, P. Contrast-enhanced spectral mammography: Technique, indications, and clinical applications. *Acad. Radiol.* **2017**, *24*, 84–88. [CrossRef]
10. Krzakowski, M.; Rutkowski, P.; Jassem, J.; Zaucha, R.; Fijuth, J.; Słuszniak, J.; Jarząb, B.; Zegarski, W.; Małkowski, B.; Kawecki, A.; et al. Recommendations on the application of positron emission tomography in oncology. *Oncol. Clin. Pract.* **2015**, *11*, 155–171.
11. Debela, D.T.; Muzazu, S.G.Y.; Heraro, K.D.; Ndalama, M.N.; Mesele, B.W.; Haile, D.C.; Sophia Khalayi, S. New approaches and procedures for cancer treatment: Current perspectives. *SAGE Open Med.* **2021**, *9*, 20503121211034366. [CrossRef] [PubMed]
12. Mehta, V.; Chander, H.; Munshi, A. Mechanisms of anti-tumor activity of *Withania somnifera* (Ashwagandha). *Nutr. Cancer* **2021**, *73*, 914–926. [CrossRef] [PubMed]
13. National Center for Complementary and Integrative Health. Ashwagandha. Available online: https://www.nccih.nih.gov/health/ashwagandha#:~:text=What%20Have%20We%20Learned?,testosterone%20levels%20and%20sperm%20quality (accessed on 12 July 2024).
14. Widodo, N.; Kaur, K.; Shrestha, B.G.; Takagi, Y.; Ishii, T.; Wadhwa, R.; Kaul, S.C. Selective killing of cancer cells by leaf extract of ashwagandha: Identification of a tumor-inhibitory factor and the first molecular insights to its effect. *Clin. Cancer Res.* **2007**, *13*, 2298–2306. [CrossRef] [PubMed]

15. Padmavathi, B.; Rath, P.C.; Rao, A.R.; Singh, R.P. Roots of *Withania somnifera* inhibit forestomach and skin carcinogenesis in mice. *Evid. Based Complement. Alternat. Med.* **2005**, *2*, 99–105. [CrossRef] [PubMed]
16. Antony, M.L.; Lee, J.; Hahm, E.-R.; Kim, S.-H.; Marcus, A.I.; Kumari, V.; Ji, X.; Yang, Z.; Vowell, C.L.; Wipf, P.; et al. Growth arrest by the antitumor steroidal lactone withaferin A in human breast cancer cells is associated with down-regulation and covalent binding at cysteine 303 of β-tubulin. *J. Biol. Chem.* **2014**, *289*, 1852–1865. [CrossRef] [PubMed]
17. Dutta, R.; Khalil, R.; Green, R.; Mohapatra, S.S.; Mohapatra, S. *Withania somnifera* (Ashwagandha) and Withaferin A: Potential in integrative oncology. *Int. J. Mol. Sci.* **2019**, *20*, 5310. [CrossRef]
18. Singh, N.; Yadav, S.S.; Rao, A.S.; Nandal, A.; Kumar, S.; Ganaie, S.A.; Narasihman, B. Review on anticancerous therapeutic potential of *Withania somnifera* (L.) Dunal. *J. Ethnopharmacol.* **2021**, *270*, 113704. [CrossRef] [PubMed]
19. Govindaram, L.K.; Al Bratty, M.; Alhazmi, H.A.; Kandasamy, R.; Thangavel, N.; Ibrahim, A.M.; Mariya, G.A.; Kumar, P. Formulation, biopharmaceutical evaluation and in-vitro screening of polyherbal phytosomes for breast cancer therapy. *Drug Dev. Ind. Pharm.* **2022**, *48*, 552–565. [CrossRef]
20. Srivastava, A.N.; Ahmad, R.; Khan, M.A. Evaluation and comparison of the in vitro cytotoxic activity of *Withania somnifera* methanolic and ethanolic extracts against MDA-MB-231 and vero cell lines. *Sci. Pharm.* **2015**, *84*, 41–59. [CrossRef]
21. Jawarneh, S.; Talib, W.H. Combination of Ashwagandha water extract and intermittent fasting as a therapy to overcome cisplatin resistance in breast cancer: An in vitro and in vivo study. *Front. Nutr.* **2022**, *9*, 863619. [CrossRef]
22. Cavaleri, F.; Chattopadhyay, S.; Palsule, V.; Kar, P.K.; Chatterjee, R. Study of drug targets associated with oncogenesis and cancer cell survival and the therapeutic activity of engineered Ashwagandha extract having differential Withanolide constitutions. *Integr. Cancer Ther.* **2024**, *23*, 15347354231223499. [CrossRef]
23. Srinivasan, S.; Ranga, R.S.; Burikhanov, R.; Han, S.S.; Chendil, D. Par-4-dependent apoptosis by the dietary compound withaferin A in prostate cancer cells. *Cancer Res.* **2007**, *67*, 246–253. [CrossRef]
24. Ahmad, R.; Fatima, A.; Srivastava, A.N.; Ali Khan, M. Evaluation of apoptotic activity of Withania coagulans methanolic extract against human breast cancer and Vero cell lines. *J. Ayurveda Integr. Med.* **2017**, *8*, 177–183. [CrossRef]
25. Stan, S.D.; Hahm, E.R.; Warin, R.; Singh, S.V. Withaferin A causes FOXO3a- and Bim-dependent apoptosis and inhibits growth of human breast cancer cells in vivo. *Cancer Res.* **2008**, *68*, 7661–7669. [CrossRef] [PubMed]
26. Grover, A.; Singh, R.; Shandilya, A.; Priyandoko, D.; Agrawal, V.; Bisaria, V.S.; Wadhwa, R.; Kaul, S.C.; Sundar, D. Ashwagandha derived withanone targets TPX2-aurora A complex: Computational and experimental evidence to its anticancer activity. *PLoS ONE* **2012**, *7*, e30890. [CrossRef] [PubMed]
27. Samanta, S.K.; Lee, J.; Hahm, E.-R.; Singh, S.V. Peptidyl-prolyl cis/trans isomerase Pin1 regulates withaferin A-mediated cell cycle arrest in human breast cancer cells. *Mol. Carcinog.* **2018**, *57*, 936–946. [CrossRef]
28. Hahm, E.R.; Moura, M.B.; Kelley, E.E.; Van Houten, B.; Shiva, S.; Singh, S.V. Withaferin A-induced apoptosis in human breast cancer cells is mediated by reactive oxygen species. *PLoS ONE* **2011**, *6*, e23354. [CrossRef]
29. Gambhir, L.; Checker, R.; Sharma, D.; Thoh, M.; Patil, A.; Degani, M.; Vikram Gota, V.; Sandur, S.K. Thiol dependent NF-κB suppression and inhibition of T-cell mediated adaptive immune responses by a naturally occurring steroidal lactone Withaferin A. *Toxicol. Appl. Pharmacol.* **2015**, *289*, 297–312. [CrossRef]
30. Ichikawa, H.; Takada, Y.; Shishodia, S.; Jayaprakasam, B.; Nair, M.G.; Aggarwal, B.B. Withanolides potentiate apoptosis, inhibit invasion, and abolish osteoclastogenesis through suppression of nuclear factor-κB (NF-κB) activation and NF-κB-regulated gene expression. *Mol. Cancer Ther.* **2006**, *5*, 1434–1445. [CrossRef] [PubMed]
31. Kaileh, M.; Vanden Berghe, W.; Heyerick, A.; Horion, J.; Piette, J.; Libert, C.; De Keukeleire, D.; Essawi, T.; Haegeman, G. Withaferin a strongly elicits IκB kinase β hyperphosphorylation concomitant with potent inhibition of its kinase activity. *J. Biol. Chem.* **2007**, *282*, 4253–4264. [CrossRef]
32. Lee, J.; Hahm, E.R.; Singh, S.V. Withaferin A inhibits activation of signal transducer and activator of transcription 3 in human breast cancer cells. *Carcinogenesis* **2010**, *31*, 1991–1998. [CrossRef] [PubMed]
33. Hahm, E.R.; Lee, J.; Huang, Y.; Singh, S.V. Withaferin A suppresses estrogen receptor-α expression in human breast cancer cells. *Mol. Carcinog.* **2011**, *50*, 614–624. [CrossRef] [PubMed]
34. Stan, S.D.; Zeng, Y.; Singh, S.V. Ayurvedic medicine constituent withaferin A causes G2 and M phase cell cycle arrest in human breast cancer cells. *Nutr. Cancer* **2008**, *60*, 51–60. [CrossRef]
35. Meher, K.; Paithankar, H.; Hosur, R.V.; Lopus, M. Ashwagandha-polyphenols-functionalized gold nanoparticles facilitate apoptosis by perturbing microtubule assembly dynamics in breast cancer cells. *J. Drug Deliv. Sci. Technol.* **2022**, *70*, 103225. [CrossRef]
36. Yang, H.; Shi, G.; Dou, Q.P. The tumor proteasome is a primary target for the natural anticancer compound withaferin A isolated from "Indian winter cherry". *Mol. Pharmacol.* **2007**, *71*, 426–437. [CrossRef]
37. Mohan, R.; Hammers, H.J.; Bargagna-Mohan, P.; Zhan, X.H.; Herbstritt, C.J.; Ruiz, A.; Zhang, L.; Hanson, A.D.; Conner, B.P.; Rougas, J.; et al. Withaferin A is a potent inhibitor of angiogenesis. *Angiogenesis* **2004**, *7*, 115–122. [CrossRef]
38. Lee, J.; Hahm, E.-R.; Marcus, A.I.; Singh, S.V. Withaferin A inhibits experimental epithelial-mesenchymal transition in MCF-10a cells and suppresses vimentin protein level in vivo in breast tumors. *Mol. Carcinog.* **2015**, *54*, 417–429. [CrossRef]
39. Yang, Z.; Garcia, A.; Xu, S.; Powell, D.R.; Vertino, P.M.; Singh, S.; Marcus, A.I. *Withania somnifera* root extract inhibits mammary cancer metastasis and epithelial to mesenchymal transition. *PLoS ONE* **2013**, *8*, e75069. [CrossRef] [PubMed]

40. Thaiparambil, J.T.; Bender, L.; Ganesh, T.; Kline, E.; Patel, P.; Liu, Y.; Tighiouart, M.; Vertino, P.M.; Harvey, R.D.; Garcia, A.; et al. Withaferin A inhibits breast cancer invasion and metastasis at sub-cytotoxic doses by inducing vimentin disassembly and serine 56 phosphorylation. *Int. J. Cancer* **2011**, *129*, 2744–2755. [CrossRef]
41. Szarc vel Szic, K.; Op de Beeck, K.; Ratman, D.; Wouters, A.; Beck, I.M.; Declerck, K.; Heyninck, K.; Fransen, E.; Bracke, M.; De Bosscher, K.; et al. Pharmacological levels of withaferin A (*Withania somnifera*) trigger clinically relevant anticancer effects specific to triple negative breast cancer cells. *PLoS ONE* **2014**, *9*, e87850. [CrossRef]
42. Gao, R.; Shah, N.; Lee, J.-S.; Katiyar, S.P.; Li, L.; Oh, E.; Sundar, D.; Yun, C.-O.; Wadhwa, R.; Kaul, S.C. Withanone-rich combination of Ashwagandha withanolides restricts metastasis and angiogenesis through hnRNP-K. *Mol. Cancer Ther.* **2014**, *13*, 2930–2940. [CrossRef]
43. Lee, J.; Sehrawat, A.; Singh, S.V. Withaferin A causes activation of Notch2 and Notch4 in human breast cancer cells. *Breast Cancer Res. Treat.* **2012**, *136*, 45–56. [CrossRef] [PubMed]
44. Bashir, A.; Nabi, M.; Tabassum, N.; Afzal, S.; Ayoub, M. An updated review on phytochemistry and molecular targets of *Withania somnifera* (L.) Dunal (Ashwagandha). *Front. Pharmacol.* **2023**, *14*, 1049334. [CrossRef] [PubMed]
45. Ali, M.A.; Farah, M.A.; Al-Anazi, K.M.; Basha, S.H.; Bai, F.; Lee, J.; Al-Hemaid, F.M.A.; Mahmoud, A.H.; Hailan, W.A.Q. In silico elucidation of the plausible inhibitory potential of Withaferin A of *Withania somnifera* medicinal herb against Breast cancer targeting estrogen receptor. *Curr. Pharm. Biotechnol.* **2020**, *21*, 842–851. [CrossRef]
46. Hahm, E.-R.; Kim, S.-H.; Singh, K.B.; Singh, K.; Singh, S.V. A comprehensive review and perspective on anticancer mechanisms of withaferin A in breast cancer. *Cancer Prev. Res.* **2020**, *13*, 721–734. [CrossRef] [PubMed]
47. Vashi, R.; Patel, B.M.; Goyal, R.K. Keeping abreast about ashwagandha in breast cancer. *J. Ethnopharmacol.* **2021**, *269*, 113759. [CrossRef] [PubMed]
48. Mallipeddi, H.; Thyagarajan, A.; Sahu, R.P. Implications of Withaferin-A for triple-negative breast cancer chemoprevention. *Biomed. Pharmacother.* **2021**, *134*, 111124. [CrossRef] [PubMed]
49. Prasad, K.; Saggam, A.; Guruprasad, K.P.; Tillu, G.; Patwardhan, B.; Satyamoorthy, K. Molecular mechanisms of Asparagus racemosus willd. and *Withania somnifera* (L.) Dunal as chemotherapeutic adjuvants for breast cancer treatment. *J. Ethnopharmacol.* **2024**, *331*, 118261. [CrossRef] [PubMed]
50. Sivasankarapillai, V.S.; Nair, R.M.K.; Rahdar, A.; Bungau, S.; Zaha, D.C.; Aleya, L.; Tit, D.M. Overview of the anticancer activity of withaferin A, an active constituent of the Indian ginseng *Withania somnifera*. *Environ. Sci. Pollut. Res. Int.* **2020**, *27*, 26025–26035. [CrossRef]
51. Rahman, M.M.; Huixin Wu, H.; Tollefsbol, T.O. A novel combinatorial approach using sulforaphane- and withaferin A-rich extracts for prevention of estrogen receptor-negative breast cancer through epigenetic and gut microbial mechanisms. *Sci. Rep.* **2024**, *14*, 12091. [CrossRef]
52. Ahmad, M.; Dar, N.J. Withania somnifera: Ethnobotany, Pharmacology, and Therapeutic Functions. In *Sustained Energy for Enhanced Human Functions and Activity*; Academic Press: Cambridge, MA, USA, 2017; pp. 137–154. [CrossRef]
53. Kulkarni, S.K.; Dhir, A. *Withania somnifera*: An Indian ginseng. *Prog. Neuro-Psychopharmacol. Biol. Psychiatry* **2008**, *32*, 1093–1105. [CrossRef] [PubMed]
54. Winters, M. Ancient medicine, modern use: *Withania somnifera* and its potential role in integrative oncology. *Altern. Med. Rev.* **2006**, *11*, 269–277. [PubMed]
55. Bhat, J.A.; Akther, T.; Najar, R.A.; Rasool, F.; Hamid, A. *Withania somnifera* (L.) Dunal (Ashwagandha); current understanding and future prospect as a potential drug candidate. *Front. Pharmacol.* **2022**, *13*, 1029123. [CrossRef] [PubMed]
56. Sharifi-Rad, J.; Quispe, C.; Ayatollahi, S.A.; Kobarfard, F.; Staniak, M.; Stępień, A.; Czopek, K.; Sen, S.; Acharya, K.; Matthews, K.R.; et al. Chemical composition, biological activity, and health-promoting effects of *Withania somnifera* for pharma-food industry applications. *J. Food Qual.* **2021**, *2021*, 8985179. [CrossRef]
57. Gaurav, H.; Yadav, D.; Maurya, A.; Yadav, H.; Yadav, R.; Shukla, A.C.; Sharma, M.; Gupta, V.K.; Palazon, J. Biodiversity, biochemical profiling, and pharmaco-commercial applications of *Withania somnifera*: A Review. *Molecules* **2023**, *28*, 1208. [CrossRef] [PubMed]
58. Uddin, Q.; Samiulla, L.; Singh, V.K.; Jamil, S.S. Phytochemical and pharmacological profile of *Withania somnifera* Dunal: A Review. *J. Appl. Pharm. Sci.* **2012**, *2*, 170–175.
59. Visweswari, G.; Christopher, R.; Rajendra, W. Phytochemical screening of active secondary metabolites present in *Withania somnifera* root: Role in traditional medicine. *Int. J. Pharm. Sci. Res.* **2013**, *4*, 2770–2776. [CrossRef]
60. Bhatia, A.; Bharti, S.K.; Tewari, S.K.; Sidhu, O.P.; Roy, R. Metabolic profiling for studying chemotype variations in *Withania somnifera* (L.) Dunal fruits using GC–MS and NMR spectroscopy. *Phytochemistry* **2013**, *93*, 105–115. [CrossRef] [PubMed]
61. Alam, N.; Hossain, M.; Mottalib, M.A.; Sulaiman, S.A.; Gan, S.H.; Khalil, M.I. Methanolic extracts of *Withania somnifera* leaves, fruits and roots possess antioxidant properties and antibacterial activities. *BMC Complement. Altern. Med.* **2012**, *12*, 175. [CrossRef]
62. Ozeer, F.Z.; Nagandran, S.; Wu, Y.S.; Wong, L.S.; Stephen, A.; Lee, M.F.; Kijsomporn, J.; Guad, R.M.; Batumalaie, K.; Oyewusi, H.A.; et al. A comprehensive review of phytochemicals of *Withania somnifera* (L.) Dunal (Solanaceae) as antiviral therapeutics. *Discov. Appl. Sci.* **2024**, *6*, 187. [CrossRef]
63. Saleem, S.; Muhammad, G.; Hussain, M.A.; Altaf, M.; Bukhari, S.N.A. *Withania somnifera* L.: Insights into the phytochemical profile, therapeutic potential, clinical trials, and future prospective. *Iran J. Basic Med. Sci.* **2020**, *23*, 1501–1526. [CrossRef]

64. Bahira, S.; Moharana, T.; Sahu, R.R.; Raut, S.; Behera, S. In vitro study of the antibacterial activities of *Withania somnifera* leaf extract against human pathogenic bacteria. *Int. J. Pharm. Sci. Rev. Res.* **2019**, *56*, 139–145.
65. Chandra, S.; Chatterjee, P.; Dey, P.; Bhattacharya, S. Evaluation of anti-inflammatory effect of Ashwagandha: A preliminary study in vitro. *Pharmacogn. J.* **2012**, *4*, 47–49. [CrossRef]
66. Pandey, A.; Bani, S.; Dutt, P.; Satti, N.K.; Suri, K.A.; Qazi, G.N. Multifunctional neuroprotective effect of withanone, a compound from *Withania somnifera* roots in alleviating cognitive dysfunction. *Cytokine* **2018**, *102*, 211–221. [CrossRef] [PubMed]
67. Das, R.; Rauf, A.; Akhter, S.; Islam, M.N.; Emran, T.B.; Mitra, S.; Khan, I.N.; Mubarak, M.S. Role of withaferin A and its derivatives in the management of Alzheimer's disease: Recent trends and future perspectives. *Molecules* **2021**, *26*, 3696. [CrossRef]
68. Singh, M.; Ramassamy, C. In vitro screening of neuroprotective activity of Indian medicinal plant *Withania somnifera*. *J. Nutr. Sci.* **2017**, *6*, e54. [CrossRef]
69. Wongtrakul, J.; Thongtan, T.; Kumrapich, B.; Saisawang, C.; Ketterman, A.J. Neuroprotective effects of *Withania somnifera* in the SH-SY5Y Parkinson cell model. *Heliyon* **2021**, *7*, e08172. [CrossRef]
70. Kumar, P.; Kumar, A. Possible neuroprotective effect of *Withania somnifera* root extract against 3-nitropropionic acid-induced behavioral, biochemical, and mitochondrial dysfunction in an animal model of Huntington's disease. *J. Med. Food* **2009**, *12*, 591–600. [CrossRef] [PubMed]
71. Joshi, T.; Kumar, V.; Kaznacheyeva, E.V.; Jana, N.R. Withaferin A induces heat shock response and ameliorates disease progression in a mouse model of Huntington's disease. *Mol. Neurobiol.* **2021**, *58*, 3992–4006. [CrossRef] [PubMed]
72. Anju, T.R.; Smijin, S.; Jobin, M.; Paulose, C.S. Altered muscarinic receptor expression in the cerebral cortex of epileptic rats: Restorative role of *Withania somnifera*. *Biochem. Cell Biol.* **2018**, *96*, 433–440. [CrossRef]
73. SoRelle, J.A.; Itoh, T.; Peng, H.; Kanak, M.A.; Sugimoto, K.; Matsumoto, S.; Levy, M.S.; Lawrence, M.C.; Naziruddin, B. Withaferin A inhibits pro-inflammatory cytokine-induced damage to islets in culture and following transplantation. *Diabetologia* **2013**, *56*, 814–824. [CrossRef] [PubMed]
74. Gorelick, J.; Rosenberg, R.; Smotrich, A.; Hanuš, L.; Bernstein, N. Hypoglycemic activity of withanolides and elicitated *Withania somnifera*. *Phytochemistry* **2015**, *116*, 283–289. [CrossRef] [PubMed]
75. Auddy, B.; Hazra, J.; Mitra, A.; Abedon, B. A standardized *Withania somnifera* extract significantly reduces stress-related parameters in chronically stressed humans: A double-blind, randomized, placebo-controlled study. *J. Am. Neutraceut. Assoc.* **2008**, *11*, 50–56.
76. Majeed, M.; Nagabhushanam, K.; Mundkur, L. A standardized Ashwagandha root extract alleviates stress, anxiety, and improves quality of life in healthy adults by modulating stress hormones: Results from a randomized, double-blind, placebo-controlled study. *Medicine* **2023**, *102*, 41. [CrossRef] [PubMed]
77. Kashyap, V.K.; Peasah-Darkwah, G.; Dhasmana, A.; Jaggi, M.; Yallapu, M.M.; Chauhan, S.C. *Withania somnifera*: Progress towards a pharmaceutical agent for immunomodulation and cancer therapeutics. *Pharmaceutics* **2022**, *14*, 611. [CrossRef] [PubMed]
78. Palliyaguru, D.L.; Singh, S.V.; Kensler, T.W. *Withania somnifera*: From prevention to treatment of cancer. *Mol. Nutr. Food Res.* **2016**, *60*, 1342–1353. [CrossRef] [PubMed]
79. Suraweera, C.D.; Hinds, M.G.; Kvansakul, M. Poxviral strategies to overcome host cell ppoptosis. *Pathogens* **2020**, *10*, 6. [CrossRef] [PubMed]
80. Jan, R.; Chaudhry, G.-e.-S. Understanding apoptosis and apoptotic pathways targeted cancer herapeutics. *Adv. Pharm. Bull.* **2019**, *9*, 205–218. [CrossRef] [PubMed]
81. Elmore, S. Apoptosis: A review of programmed cell death. *Toxicol. Pathol.* **2007**, *35*, 495–516. [CrossRef]
82. Wang, C.; Youle, R.J. The Role of mitochondria in apoptosis. *Annu. Rev. Genet.* **2009**, *43*, 95–118. [CrossRef]
83. Galluzzi, L.; Kepp, O.; Trojel-Hansen, C.; Kroemer, G. Mitochondrial control of cellular life, stress, and death. *Circ. Res.* **2012**, *111*, 1198–1207. [CrossRef] [PubMed]
84. Cavalcante, G.C.; Schaan, A.P.; Cabral, G.F.; Santana-da-Silva, M.N.; Pinto, P.; Vidal, A.F.; Ribeiro-dos-Santos, Â.; Cell's Fate, A. An overview of the molecular biology and genetics of apoptosis. *Int. J. Mol. Sci.* **2019**, *20*, 4133. [CrossRef] [PubMed]
85. Lomonosova, E.; Chinnadurai, G. BH3-only proteins in apoptosis and beyond: An overview. *Oncogene* **2008**, *27*, 2–19. [CrossRef] [PubMed]
86. Yuan, S.; Akey, C.W. Apoptosome structure, assembly, and procaspase activation. *Structure* **2013**, *21*, 501–515. [CrossRef]
87. Schlereth, K.; Charles, J.P.; Bretz, A.C.; Stiewe, T. Life or death: p53-induced apoptosis requires DNA binding cooperativity. *Cell Cycle* **2010**, *15*, 4068–4076. [CrossRef]
88. Jin, Z.; El-Deiry, W.S. Overview of cell death signaling pathways. *Cancer Biol. Ther.* **2005**, *4*, 139–163. [CrossRef] [PubMed]
89. Mahmood, Z.; Shukla, Y. Death receptors: Targets for cancer therapy. *Exp. Cell Res.* **2010**, *316*, 887–899. [CrossRef] [PubMed]
90. Lee, E.W.; Seo, J.; Jeong, M.; Lee, S.; Song, J. The roles of FADD in extrinsic apoptosis and necroptosis. *BMB Rep.* **2012**, *45*, 496–508. [CrossRef] [PubMed]
91. Kim, H.J.; Hawke, N.; Baldwin, A.S. NF-kappaB and IKK as therapeutic targets in cancer. *Cell Death Differ.* **2006**, *13*, 738–747. [CrossRef]
92. Nakajima, S.; Kitamura, M. Bidirectional regulation of NF-κB by reactive oxygen species: A role of unfolded protein response. *Free Radic. Biol. Med.* **2013**, *65*, 162–174. [CrossRef]
93. Napetschnig, J.; Wu, H. Molecul ar basis of NF-κB signaling. *Annu. Rev. Biophys.* **2013**, *42*, 443–468. [CrossRef] [PubMed]

94. Rascio, F.; Spadaccino, F.; Rocchetti, M.T.; Castellano, G.; Stallone, G.; Netti, G.S.; Ranieri, E. The pathogenic role of PI3K/AKT pathway in cancer onset and drug resistance: An updated review. *Cancers* **2021**, *13*, 3949. [CrossRef] [PubMed]
95. Mohammad, R.M.; Muqbil, I.; Lowe, L.; Yedjou, C.; Hsu, H.Y.; Lin, L.T.; Siegelin, M.D.; Fimognari, C.; Kumar, N.B.; Dou, Q.P.; et al. Broad targeting of resistance to apoptosis in cancer. *Semin. Cancer Biol.* **2015**, *35*, 78–103. [CrossRef] [PubMed]
96. Yuan, L.; Cai, Y.; Zhang, L.; Liu, S.; Li, P.; Li, X. Promoting apoptosis, a promising way to treat breast cancer with natural products: A comprehensive review. *Front. Pharmacol.* **2022**, *12*, 801662. [CrossRef]
97. Dar, P.A.; Mir, S.A.; Bhat, J.A.; Hamid, A.; Singh, L.R.; Malik, F.; Dar, T.A. Ananti-cancerous protein fraction from *Withania somnifera* induces ROS dependent mitochondria-mediated apoptosis in human MDA-MB-231 breast cancer cells. *Int. J. Biol. Macromol.* **2019**, *135*, 77–87. [CrossRef] [PubMed]
98. Widodo, N.; Priyandoko, D.; Shah, N.; Wadhwa, R.; Kaul, S.C. Selective killing of cancer cells by Ashwagandha leaf extract and its component Withanone involves ROS signaling. *PLoS ONE* **2010**, *5*, e13536. [CrossRef] [PubMed]
99. Sehrawat, A.; Samanta, S.K.; Hahm, E.R.; St Croix, C.; Watkins, S.; Singh, S.V. Withaferin A-mediated apoptosis in breast cancer cells is associated with alterations in mitochondrial dynamics. *Mitochondrion* **2019**, *47*, 282–293. [CrossRef] [PubMed]
100. Hahm, E.-R.; Singh, S.V. Autophagy fails to alter withaferin A-mediated lethality in human breast cancer cells. *Curr. Cancer Drug Targets* **2013**, *13*, 640–650. [CrossRef]
101. Jamalzadeh, L.; Ghafoori, H.; Aghamaali, M.; Sariri, R. Induction of apoptosis in human breast cancer MCF-7 cells by a semi-synthetic derivative of artemisinin: A caspase-related mechanism. *Iran. J. Biotechnol.* **2017**, *15*, 157–165. [CrossRef]
102. Hahm, E.-R.; Singh, S.V. Withaferin A-induced apoptosis in human breast cancer cells is associated with suppression of inhibitor of apoptosis family protein expression. *Cancer Lett.* **2013**, *334*, 101–108. [CrossRef]
103. Pimentel, J.M.; Zhou, J.Y.; Wu, G.S. The role of TRAIL in apoptosis and immunosurveillance in cancer. *Cancers* **2023**, *15*, 2752. [CrossRef] [PubMed]
104. Ralff, M.D.; El-Deiry, W.S. TRAIL pathway targeting therapeutics. *Expert. Rev. Precis. Med. Drug Dev.* **2018**, *3*, 197–204. [CrossRef]
105. Yuan, X.; Gajan, A.; Chu, Q.; Xiong, H.; Wu, K.; Wu, G.S. Developing TRAIL/TRAIL death receptor-based cancer therapies. *Cancer Metastasis Rev.* **2018**, *37*, 733–748. [CrossRef] [PubMed]
106. Snajdauf, M.; Havlova, K.; Vachtenheim, J., Jr.; Ozaniak, A.; Lischke, R.; Bartunkova, J.; Smrz, D.; Strizova, Z. The TRAIL in the treatment of human cancer: An update on clinical trials. *Front. Mol. Biosci.* **2021**, *8*, 628332. [CrossRef] [PubMed]
107. Kundu, M.; Endo, Y.; Dine, J.L.; Lipkowitz, S. Targeting TRAIL death receptors in triple-negative breast cancers: Challenges and strategies for cancer therap. *Cells* **2022**, *11*, 3717. [CrossRef] [PubMed]
108. Nagalingam, A.; Kuppusamy, P.; Singh, S.V.; Sharma, D.; Saxena, N.K. Mechanistic elucidation of the antitumor properties of withaferin a in breast cancer. *Cancer Res.* **2014**, *74*, 2617–2629. [CrossRef] [PubMed]
109. Zhao, H.; Martin, T.A.; Davies, E.L.; Ruge, F.; Yu, H.; Zhang, Y.; Teng, X.; Jiang, W.G. The clinical implications of RSK1-3 in human breast cancer. *Anticancer Res.* **2016**, *36*, 1267–1274. [CrossRef] [PubMed]
110. Zhang, X.; Mukerji, R.; Samadi, A.K.; Cohen, M.S. Down-regulation of estrogen receptor-alpha and rearranged during transfection tyrosine kinase is associated with withaferin a-induced apoptosis in MCF-7 breast cancer cells. *BMC Compl. Altern. Med.* **2011**, *11*, 84. [CrossRef]
111. Hayden, M.S.; Ghosh, S. Signalling to NF-κB. *Genes Dev.* **2004**, *18*, 2195–2224. [CrossRef]
112. Powers, M.V.; Workman, P. Targeting of multiple signaling pathways by heat shock protein 90 molecular chaperone inhibitors. *Endocr. Relat. Cancer* **2006**, *13*, 125–135. [CrossRef]
113. Wang, H.-C.; Tsai, Y.-L.; Wu, Y.-C.; Chang, F.-R.; Liu, M.-H.; Chen, W.-Y.; Wu, C.-C. Withanolides-induced breast cancer cell death is correlated with their ability to inhibit heat protein 90. *PLoS ONE* **2012**, *27*, 1984–2009. [CrossRef]
114. Bar-Natan, M.; Nelson, E.A.; Xiang, M.; Frank, D.A. STAT signaling in the pathogenesis and treatment of myeloid malignancies. *JAKSTAT* **2012**, *1*, 55–64. [CrossRef] [PubMed]
115. Morris, R.; Kershaw, N.J.; Babon, J.J. The molecular details of cytokine signaling via the JAK/STAT pathway. *Protein Sci.* **2018**, *27*, 1984–2009. [CrossRef] [PubMed]
116. Yu, H.; Pardoll, D.; Jove, R. STATs in cancer inflammation and immunity: A leading role for STAT3. *Nat. Rev. Cancer* **2009**, *9*, 798–809. [CrossRef] [PubMed]
117. Zhang, X.; Blaskovich, M.A.; Forinash, K.D.; Sebti, S.M. Withacnistin inhibits recruitment of STAT3 and STAT5 to growth factor and cytokine receptors and induces regression of breast tumours. *Br. J. Cancer* **2014**, *26*, 894–902. [CrossRef] [PubMed]
118. Ling, X.; Arlinghaus, R.B. Knockdown of STAT3 expression by RNA interference inhibits the induction of breast tumors in immunocompetent mice. *Cancer Res.* **2005**, *65*, 2532–2536. [CrossRef] [PubMed]
119. Halim, C.E.; Deng, S.; Ong, M.S.; Yap, C.T. Involvement of STAT5 in oncogenesis. *Biomedicines* **2020**, *8*, 316. [CrossRef]
120. Igelmann, S.; Neubauer, H.A.; Ferbeyre, G. STAT3 and STAT5 activation in solid cancers. *Cancers* **2019**, *11*, 1428. [CrossRef] [PubMed]
121. Hahm, E.R.; Lee, J.; Singh, S.V. Role of mitogen-activated protein kinases and mcl-1 in apoptosis induction by withaferin a in human breast cancer cells. *Mol. Carcinog.* **2014**, *53*, 907–916. [CrossRef]
122. Yang, S.; Liu, G. Targeting the Ras/Raf/MEK/ERK pathway in hepatocellular carcinoma. *Oncol. Lett.* **2017**, *13*, 1041–1047. [CrossRef]

123. Jiang, M.; Wen, F.; Cao, J.; Li, P.; She, J.; Chu, Z. Genome-wide exploration of the molecular evolution and regulatory network of mitogen-activated protein kinase cascades upon multiple stresses in Brachypodium distachyon. *BMC Genom.* **2015**, *16*, 228. [CrossRef] [PubMed]
124. Ward, A.F.; Braun, B.S.; Shannon, K.M. Targeting oncogenic Ras signaling in hematologic malignancies. *Blood* **2012**, *120*, 3397–3406. [CrossRef] [PubMed]
125. Liu, F.; Yang, X.; Geng, M.; Huang, M. Targeting ERK, an Achilles' Heel of the MAPK pathway, in cancer therapy. *Acta Pharm. Sin. B* **2018**, *8*, 552–562. [CrossRef] [PubMed]
126. Yue, J.; López, J.M. Understanding MAPK signaling pathways in apoptosis. *Int. J. Mol. Sci.* **2020**, *21*, 2346. [CrossRef] [PubMed]
127. Castoria, G.; Migliaccio, A.; Di Domenico, M.; Lombardi, M.; de Falco, A.; Varricchio, L.; Bilancio, A.; Barone, M.V.; Auricchio, F. Role of atypical protein kinase C in estradiol-triggered G1/S progression of MCF-7 cells. *Mol. Cell Biol.* **2004**, *24*, 7643–7653. [CrossRef] [PubMed]
128. Hong, K.; Choi, Y. Role of estrogen and RAS signaling in repeated implantation failure. *BMB Rep.* **2018**, *51*, 225–229. [CrossRef] [PubMed]
129. Acconcia, F.; Totta, P.; Ogawa, S.; Cardillo, I.; Inoue, S.; Leone, S.; Trentalance, A.; Muramatsu, M.; Marino, M. Survival versus apoptotic 17β-estradiol effect: Role of ERα and ERβ activated non-genomic signaling. *J. Cell Physiol.* **2005**, *203*, 193–201. [CrossRef] [PubMed]
130. Björnström, L.; Sjöberg, M. Mechanisms of estrogen receptor signaling: Convergence of genomic and nongenomic actions on target genes. *Mol. Endocrinol.* **2005**, *19*, 833–842. [CrossRef] [PubMed]
131. Cheng, J.; Lee, E.J.; Madison, L.D.; Lazennec, G. Expression of estrogen receptor b in prostate carcinoma cells inhibits invasion and proliferation and triggers apoptosis. *FEBS Lett.* **2004**, *566*, 169–172. [CrossRef]
132. Paruthiyil, S.; Parmar, H.; Kerekatte, V.; Cunha, G.R.; Firestone, G.L.; Leitman, D.C. Estrogen receptor b inhibits human breast cancer cell proliferation and tumor formation by causing a G2 cell cycle arrest. *Cancer Res.* **2004**, *64*, 423–428. [CrossRef]
133. Sayeed, A.; Konduri, S.D.; Liu, W.; Bansal, S.; Li, F.; Das, G.M. Estrogen receptor alpha inhibits p53-mediated transcriptional repression: Implications for the regulation of apoptosis. *Cancer Res.* **2007**, *67*, 7746–7755. [CrossRef] [PubMed]
134. Esseghir, S.; Todd, S.K.; Hunt, T.; Poulsom, R.; Plaza-Menacho, I.; Reis-Filho, J.S.; Isacke, C.M. A role for glial cell derived neurotrophic factor induced expression by inflammatory cytokines and RET/GFR alpha 1 receptor upregulation in breast cancer. *Cancer Res.* **2007**, *67*, 11732–11741. [CrossRef]
135. Janku, F.; McConkeya, D.J.; Hong, D.S.; Kurzrock, R. Autophagy as a target for anticancer therapy. *Nat. Rev. Clin. Oncol.* **2011**, *8*, 528–539. [CrossRef] [PubMed]
136. Muniraj, N.; Siddharth, S.; Nagalingam, A.; Walker, A.; Woo, J.; Gyorffy, B.; Gabrielsona, E.; Saxena, N.K.; Sharma, D. Withaferin A inhibits lysosomal activity to block autophagic flux and induces apoptosis via energetic impairment in breast cancer cells. *Carcinogenesis* **2019**, *40*, 1110–1120. [CrossRef] [PubMed]
137. Ghosh, K.; De, S.; Mukherjee, S.; Das, S.; Ghosh, A.N.; Sengupta, S.B. Withaferin A induced impaired autophagy and unfolded protein response in human breast cancer cell-lines MCF-7 and MDA-MB-231. *Toxicol. Vitr.* **2017**, *44*, 330–338. [CrossRef] [PubMed]
138. Ghosh, K.; De, S.; Das, S.; Mukherjee, S.; Bandyopadhyay, S. Withaferin A induces ROS-mediated paraptosis in human breast cancer cell-lines MCF-7 and MDA-MB-231. *PLoS ONE* **2016**, *11*, e168488. [CrossRef]
139. Biswal, B.M.; Sulaiman, A.M.; Ismail, H.C.; Zakaria, H.; Jalil Abdul, M.I.; Muhammad, K.I. AOS14 Phase II clinical study of combination chemotherapy with herb *Withania somnifera* (ashwagandha) in breast cancer. *Eur. J. Cancer* **2012**, *48*, 8–9. [CrossRef]
140. Biswal, B.M.; Sulaiman, S.A.; Ismail, H.C.; Zakaria, H.; Musa, K.I. Effect of *Withania somnifera* (Ashwagandha) on the development of chemotherapy-induced fatigue and quality of life in breast cancer patients. *Integr. Cancer Ther.* **2013**, *12*, 312–322. [CrossRef] [PubMed]
141. Afewerky, H.K.; Ayodeji, A.E.; Tiamiyu, B.B.; Orege, J.I.; Okeke, E.S.; Oyejobi, A.O.; Bate, P.N.N.; Adeyemi, S.B. Critical review of the *Withania somnifera* (L.) Dunal: Ethnobotany, pharmacological efficacy, and commercialization significance in Africa. *Bull. Natl. Res. Cent.* **2021**, *45*, 176. [CrossRef]
142. Björnsson, H.K.; Björnsson, E.S.; Avula, B.; Khan, I.A.; Jonasson, J.C.; Ghabril, M.; Hayashi, P.H.; Navarro, V. Ashwagandha-induced liver injury: A case series from Iceland and the US Drug-Induced Liver Injury Network. *Liver Int.* **2020**, *40*, 825–829. [CrossRef]
143. Lopresti, A.L.; Smith, S.J. Ashwagandha (*Withania somnifera*) for the treatment and enhancement of mental and physical conditions: A systematic review of human trialsexternal link disclaimer. *J. Herb. Med.* **2021**, *28*, 100434. [CrossRef]
144. Gannon, J.M.; Forrest, P.E.; Roy Chengappa, K.N. Subtle changes in thyroid indices during a placebo-controlled study of an extract of *Withania somnifera* in persons with bipolar disorder. *J. Ayurveda Integr. Med.* **2014**, *5*, 241–245. [CrossRef]
145. Smith, S.J.; Lopresti, A.L.; Teo, S.Y.M.; Fairchild, T.J. Examining the effects of herbs on testosterone concentrations in men: A systematic review. *Adv. Nutr.* **2021**, *12*, 744–765. [CrossRef] [PubMed]
146. Lopresti, A.L.; Drummond, P.D.; Smith, S.J. A randomized, double-blind, placebo-controlled, crossover study examining the hormonal and vitality effects of Ashwagandha (*Withania somnifera*) in aging, overweight males. *Am. J. Mens. Health* **2019**, *13*, 1557988319835985. [CrossRef] [PubMed]
147. Cheah, K.L.; Norhayati, M.N.; Husniati Yaacob, L.; Abdul Rahman, R. Effect of ashwagandha (*Withania somnifera*) extract on sleep: A systematic review and meta-analysis. *PLoS ONE* **2021**, *16*, e0257843. [CrossRef]

148. Verma, N.; Gupta, S.K.; Tiwari, S.; Mishra, A.K. Safety of ashwagandha root extract: A randomized, placebo-controlled, study in healthy volunteers. *Complement. Ther. Med.* **2021**, *57*, 102642. [CrossRef]
149. Choudhary, D.; Bhattacharyya, S.; Bose, S. Efficacy and safety of Ashwagandha (*Withania somnifera* (L.) Dunal) root extract in improving memory and cognitive functions. *J. Diet Suppl.* **2017**, *14*, 599–612. [CrossRef]

current issues in molecular biology

Review

Chemopreventive Agents from Nature: A Review of Apigenin, Rosmarinic Acid, and Thymoquinone

Reem Fawaz Abutayeh [1,*], Maram Altah [2,*], Amani Mehdawi [2], Israa Al-Ataby [1] and Adel Ardakani [3]

1 Faculty of Pharmacy, Applied Science Private University, Amman 11937, Jordan; israa.adnan1985@yahoo.com
2 School of Pharmacy, Al-Qadisiyah College, Amman 11118, Jordan; amanimehdawi@aqc.edu.jo
3 College of Pharmacy, Amman Arab University, Amman 11953, Jordan; a.ardakani@aau.edu.jo
* Correspondence: r_abutayeh@asu.edu.jo (R.F.A.); maram.altah@aqc.edu.jo (M.A.); Tel.: +962-799-567-613 (R.F.A.)

Abstract: Cancer, a major challenge to global health and healthcare systems, requires the study of alternative and supportive treatments due to the limitations of conventional therapies. This review examines the chemopreventive potential of three natural compounds: rosmarinic acid, apigenin, and thymoquinone. Derived from various plants, these compounds have demonstrated promising chemopreventive properties in in vitro, in vivo, and in silico studies. Specifically, they have been shown to inhibit cancer cell growth, induce apoptosis, and modulate key signaling pathways involved in cancer progression. The aim of this review is to provide a comprehensive overview of the current research on these phytochemicals, elucidating their mechanisms of action, therapeutic efficacy, and potential as adjuncts to traditional cancer therapies. This information serves as a valuable resource for researchers and healthcare providers interested in expanding their knowledge within the field of alternative cancer therapies.

Keywords: natural chemoprevention; anti-cancer phytochemicals; natural chemotherapy; apigenin; rosmarinic acid; thymoquinone

1. Introduction

In both industrialized and developing countries, cancer is considered a high-profile disease that damages the body's systems. Conventional treatments such as surgery, chemotherapy, and radiotherapy are commonly employed but often come with severe side effects, potential recurrence, and/or treatment failure. As a result, there is a growing interest in complementary and alternative medicine (CAM) for cancer treatment and prevention. Natural products, including herbal and phytochemical compounds, are the main biology-based practices within CAM, and they have grown to be a multibillion-dollar industry worldwide. Their long history of use supports their adoption in health promotion and disease prevention and treatment [1].

Phytochemicals such as carotenoids, polyphenols, and flavonoids have been studied for their potential in cancer prevention and treatment. These compounds are present in plant-based foods, beverages, supplements, and traditional herbal remedies [1,2]. Scientists have been particularly interested in phytochemicals because they target the biological pathways in mammalian cells that are involved in inflammatory processes and cancer development. These pathways include control of the cell cycle, apoptosis, angiogenesis, and metastasis. Epidemiological studies suggest that regularly ingesting phytochemicals can reduce the incidence of various cancers.

Many phytochemicals, including assorted polyphenols, are rapidly eliminated from the human body. However, they remain promising chemopreventive and/or chemotherapeutic agents due to their ability to target multiple cancer cell mechanisms with minimal toxicity to normal cells. Phytochemicals can be administered alone or in combination with conventional chemotherapeutic agents to explore synergistic or enhanced cytotoxic

effects. Such combination treatments are also investigated for their potential to overcome chemotherapy-induced resistance, reduce adverse effects, and improve the safety profile for normal cells [2].

Cancer chemoprevention involves the use of natural, synthetic, or biological chemical agents to reverse, inhibit, or prevent carcinogenic initiation or the progression of cancer. This approach is considered one of the most effective strategies to reduce the risk of cancer development and recurrence. Bioactive molecules used in chemoprevention can target different stages of carcinogenesis, acting as inhibitors of carcinogen formation, and interfering with the initiation or post-initiation steps to halt or reverse the development of premalignant cells [3–5].

Several interconnected mechanisms of chemoprevention include the modulation of phase I and phase II metabolic enzymes [6], oxidative stress, inflammatory pathways such as the COX-2 pathway, signal transduction, and hormones [7].

In this review, we summarize the mechanisms of three natural phytochemicals—rosmarinic acid, apigenin, and thymoquinone—with different chemical structures and derived from commonly used plants. Although numerous in vivo and in vitro studies support their chemopreventive potential, further research is needed to fully understand their mechanisms of action, to determine the most effective dosages and routes of administration, and to confirm their safety and efficacy in a clinical setting.

Despite their distinct chemical structures and mechanisms of action, these compounds share common bioactivities, such as antioxidant and anti-inflammatory properties, cancer growth inhibition, apoptosis promotion, and the modulation of cell proliferation and survival pathways [5–7].

2. Rosmarinic Acid (RA)

Rosmarinic acid (RA) is a polyphenolic acid found in various herbs and plants, including rosemary, sage, lemon balm, marjoram, thyme, and oregano. The richest sources of RA are members of the Lamiaceae family. RA exhibits antioxidant and anti-inflammatory properties and can inhibit the growth of cancer cells in vitro. It has been shown to suppress the expression of genes involved in cancer cell proliferation and metastasis, as well as inducing apoptosis through the modulation of signaling pathways related to cell survival and death. A summary of RA's chemopreventive properties is shown in Figure 1.

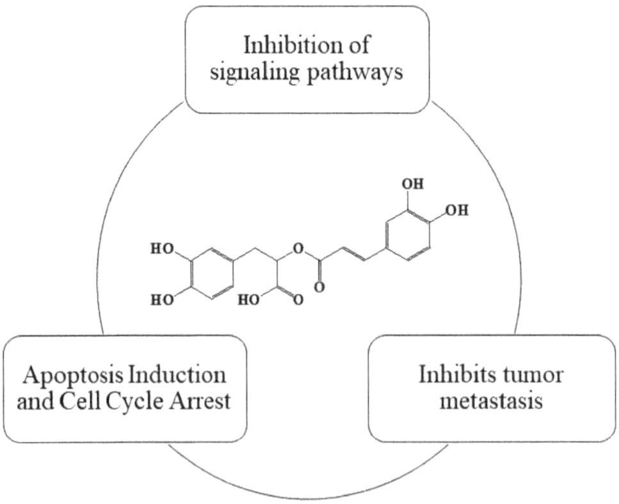

Figure 1. Summary of RA's chemopreventive properties.

2.1. Source and Chemical Structure

RA ($C_{18}H_{16}O_8$), an ester of caffeic acid and 3,4-dihydroxy phenyl lactic acid (Figure 2), is considered one of the most important polyphenolic compounds present in nature [8,9].

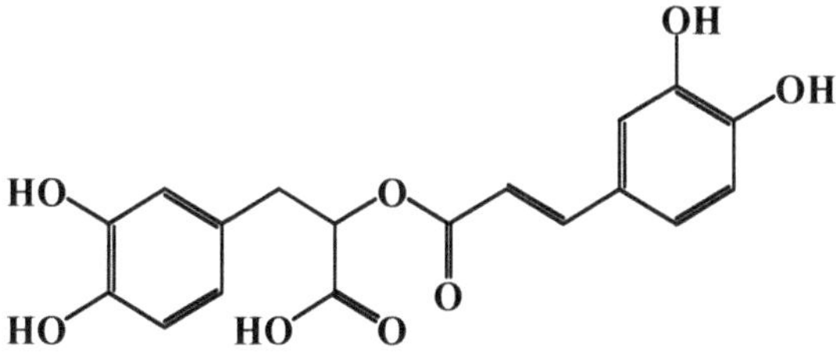

Figure 2. Chemical structure of RA (ChemDraw Ultra 7.0).

Although RA is widespread throughout the plant kingdom, it was first isolated and characterized in 1958 from rosemary (*Rosmarinus officinalis*, Family: Lamiaceae) and named after it. However, rosemary is not considered the primary source or the richest source of RA [9,10]. For example, a high-performance liquid chromatographic analysis of 29 plants belonging to the Labiatae family revealed that Mentha species had the highest RA content, with a considerable concentration ranging from 19.3 to 58.5 mg/g compared to that found in rosemary (7.2 mg/g) [11].

2.2. In Vivo and In Vitro Studies of RA

2.2.1. In Vitro Studies of RA

Given its strong antioxidant properties, RA has been extensively investigated for its chemopreventive potential, and consequently, additional mechanisms of action have been proposed. Yang et al. (2021) reported that RA inhibited tumor metastasis in the human colorectal cancer cell line HT-29, and its effect was mediated primarily by suppressing epithelial–mesenchymal transition [12]. RA also restricted apoptosis and tumor growth in hepatic cancer-induced nude mice in a dose-dependent manner. The inhibitory activity of RA was further illustrated to take place via the PI3K/AKT/mTOR signaling pathway in SMMC-7721 hepatocellular carcinoma cell lines [13]. Moreover, RA demonstrated chemotherapeutic potential in OVCAR-3 ovarian cancer cells, causing cellular shrinkage, apoptosis, and cell migration suppression in a time- and concentration-dependent manner at 10, 40, and 160 µM concentrations after 48 and 72 h [14].

In triple-negative breast cancer cell lines (MDA-MB-231 and MDA-MB-468), RA induced apoptosis and cell cycle arrest by altering the transcription of multiple apoptosis-related genes in both cell lines [15]. RA also inhibited glucose uptake and lactate production in human gastric cancer (MKN45) cell lines in vitro, demonstrating an anti-Warburg effect at concentrations up to 600 µM, and suppressed gastric tumor growth in a mouse xenograft model treated with 2 mg/kg of RA for 14 weeks [16].

2.2.2. In Vivo Studies of RA

Despite its notable cytotoxic effects in vitro, RA extracts have been less extensively studied in vivo in animal cancer models. The available studies (shown in Table 1) have not fully elucidated the mechanisms underlying RA's chemopreventive effects. Furtado et al. (2015) investigated RA's anti-carcinogenic capability and showed that RA, orally administered at doses up to 16 mg/kg/day, successfully reduced the extent and frequency of DNA damage and tumor formation in rats treated with the colon carcinogen 1,2-dimethylhydrazine (DMH) at a dosage of 40 mg/kg [17]. Likewise, when RA was orally administered at a dose of 5 mg/kg for 30 weeks, it prevented tumor formation and induced apoptosis in DMH-induced rats. RA prevented colon cancer by inducing pro-apoptotic protein expression [18]. Additionally, an oral dose of 100 mg/kg/day of RA was administered

to a skin cancer animal model for a week. RA prevented tumor formation and induced apoptosis in Swiss albino mice treated with dimethylbenz(a)anthracene (DMBA) [19].

RA's chemopreventive mechanism of action was further investigated using colorectal cancer animal models. Colorectal cancer was induced in male BALB/c mice and then was treated with a 30 mg/kg/day oral dose of RA for a week, and it was found to suppress tumor progression in mice through the inhibition of TLR4-mediated NF-κB and STAT3 activation. This mechanism was also proven in vitro using the HCT116 colorectal carcinoma cell line, where RA competitively inhibited the TLR4-MD-2 complex [20].

RA enhanced tumor sensitivity to several chemotherapeutic drugs, such as cisplatin and doxorubicin, which are common chemotherapeutic agents capable of inducing multi-drug-resistant (MDR) gene expression. When RA and doxorubicin were given in combination in a breast cancer mouse model, the combination exhibited better pharmacokinetics and anti-cancer efficacy than doxorubicin alone [21]. Also, RA enhanced the apoptotic effect of doxorubicin by activating the mitochondria-mediated signaling pathway in HepG2 and Bel-7402 cell lines [22]. In another study, the efficacy of RA was tested in cisplatin-resistant NSCLC lung cancer cells both in vitro and in xenograft tumors in nude mice. The combination therapy resulted in the significant downregulation of MDR1 mRNA and P-GP expression in vitro and a marked inhibition of NSCLC xenograft tumor growth in nude mice [23]. Similarly, the inhibition of renal cancer cell invasion and migration using cisplatin was augmented when combined with RA [24].

Regarding RA's apparent toxicity in vivo, Xue et al. (2021) reported that the body weight of mice did not show obvious changes during RA treatment. Furthermore, no systemic toxicity was observed in histopathological examination of the major organs, including the heart, liver, spleen, lungs, and kidneys [21].

Table 1. Summary of in vivo studies of rosmarinic acid (RA).

Study Focus	Animal Model	RA Dose and Route of Administration	Findings	Reference
Prevention of colon cancer induced by 1,2-dimethylhydrazine (DMH)	Rats	Oral, up to 16 mg/kg/day	RA significantly reduced DNA damage and tumor formation	[17]
Prevention of colon cancer induced by DMH	Rats	Oral at 5 mg/kg/day for 30 weeks	RA prevented tumor formation and induced apoptosis	[18]
Prevention of skin cancer induced by DMBA	Swiss Albino mice	Oral at 100 mg/kg/day for a week	RA prevented skin cancer and induced apoptosis	[19]
Mechanisms of RA anti-cancer activity in colorectal cancer	Male BALB/c mice	30 mg/kg/day for a week	RA suppressed tumor progression by inhibiting TLR4-mediated NF-κB and STAT3 activation	[20]
Enhancement of doxorubicin's efficacy in breast cancer	Female BALB/C mice	IV 8 mg/kg combined with doxorubicin	Combination showed better pharmacokinetics and anti-cancer efficacy than doxorubicin alone	[21]
Enhancement of cisplatin's efficacy in cisplatin-resistant NSCLC lung cancer	Xenograft in nude female BALB mice	Intraperitoneal, combined with cisplatinvolume of administration of 10 μL/g	Significant inhibition of tumor growth with cisplatin combined with RA when compared to cisplatin alone	[23]

2.3. *In Silico Studies of RA*

The effect of RA on cell lines has been extensively studied, showing its ability to induce apoptosis in cancer cells—a critical mechanism for cancer treatment. Although many modeling studies are found for RA, they mainly address its activity in other fields of pharmacological activities, such as its antiviral, antimicrobial, and anti-diabetic potential activities, among others. Chemoprevention-related in silico studies remain limited. Anwar et al. (2020) studied the activity of RA's anti-cancer effect in relation to microtubule affinity regulating kinase (MARK4) inhibition. RA demonstrated excellent binding affinity to the active site and formed several hydrogen bonds with critical residues, which led to MARK4 inhibition and apoptosis induction [25]. Jelić et al. (2007) studied the modes of RA binding to the Fyn tyrosine kinase and concluded that it binds to the non-ATP binding site of the kinase. The Fyn tyrosine kinase is an Src-family enzyme involved in T-cell receptor signal transduction and was found to be inhibited experimentally by RA. This study combined experimental and computational methods in order to understand the mechanism of RA chemoprevention activity [26].

RA's ability to induce apoptosis and inhibit cancer cell growth by regulating signaling pathways makes it a promising candidate for further development as an anti-cancer drug. However, more studies are needed to fully understand the mechanisms of its anti-cancer effects and to optimize its therapeutic potential. In vitro and in vivo studies of RA used various concentrations of RA and different cancer cell lines or animal models to investigate the underlying mechanisms of RA's chemoprevention effect.

3. Apigenin

Apigenin is a flavonoid that is found in a variety of plants, including parsley, celery, and chamomile. It has been shown to have antioxidant, anti-inflammatory, and anti-cancer properties. In vitro studies have demonstrated that apigenin inhibits the growth of cancer cells, induces cell cycle arrest, and promotes apoptosis. Additionally, apigenin has been shown to modulate signaling pathways involved in cell proliferation and survival and to inhibit angiogenesis and metastasis. A summary of apigenin's chemopreventive properties is shown in Figure 3

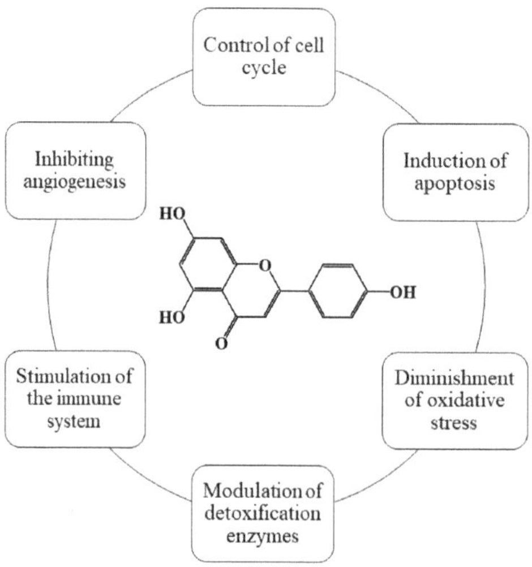

Figure 3. Summary of apigenin's chemopreventive properties.

3.1. *Source and Chemical Structure*

Apigenin (4′, 5, 7-trihydroxyflavone; $C_{15}H_{10}O_5$) is a flavonoid with a molecular weight of 270.24 g/mol. Its chemical structure is shown in Figure 4. Apigenin is mainly found in parsley, which is scientifically named *Petroselinum crispum*, from the family Umbelliferae (also called Apiaceae) [27,28].

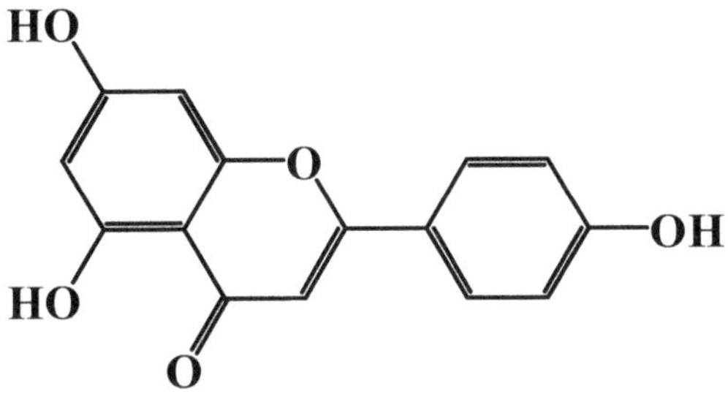

Figure 4. Chemical structure of apigenin (ChemDraw Ultra 7.0).

It is also found in different quantities in a variety of other plants, including celery, basil, chamomile, and many others. Table 2 presents common sources of apigenin along with the approximate quantities found in each.

Table 2. Sources and quantities of apigenin.

Source	Quantity of Apigenin (mg/kg)	Reference
Chinese cabbage	187.0	[29]
Bell pepper	272.0	[29]
Garlic	217.0	[29]
Bilimbi fruit	458.0	[29]
French peas	176.0	[29]
Guava	579.0	[29]
Wolfberry leaves	547.0	[29]
Daun turi	39.5	[29]
Kadok	34.5	[29]
Celery seeds	786.5	[30]
Spinach	620	[30]
Parsley	450.4	[30]
Marjoram	44.0	[30]
Oregano	35.0	[30]
Sage	24.0	[30]
Chamomile	30–50	[30]
Rosemary	5.5	[30]
Pistachio	0.3	[30]

3.2. In Vitro and In Vivo Studies of Apigenin

3.2.1. In Vitro Studies

In vitro studies have been pivotal in illuminating the mechanisms through which apigenin exerts its anti-cancer effects. These studies have demonstrated that apigenin can inhibit the proliferation of various cancer cell lines, including prostate [31–36], breast [37–41], colon [42,43], and lung cancers [44,45]. The mechanisms involved include the modulation of cell cycle regulatory proteins [46,47], the inhibition of angiogenesis [48,49], and the modulation of key signaling pathways, such as the PI3K/AKT/mTOR [50] and PI3K/Akt/FoxO 3a pathways [35,51], which are crucial for cancer cell survival and proliferation.

Apigenin reduces the viability of cancer cells in a dose-dependent manner, where in an MTT assay, apigenin treatment significantly decreased the viability of human breast cancer MCF-7 cells, indicating its potential to selectively target cancerous cells [52]. It exerts its anti-cancer effects through the induction of apoptosis in various cancer cell lines and through multiple pathways. It triggers the activation of caspases, which are essential executors of apoptosis. Studies have demonstrated that it increases the activity of caspase-3 and caspase-9, leading to the cleavage of poly (ADP-ribose) polymerase (PARP), a hallmark of apoptosis. Moreover, it disrupts mitochondrial membrane potential, leading to the release of cytochrome c into the cytosol, which subsequently activates the apoptotic machinery. This mitochondrial pathway is crucial to the intrinsic apoptosis pathway [53].

Furthermore, apigenin alters the expression of the Bcl-2-family proteins, which are key regulators of apoptosis. It downregulates anti-apoptotic proteins like Bcl-2 and Bcl-xL while upregulating pro-apoptotic proteins such as Bax, promoting apoptosis in cancer cells [33].

Apigenin also induces DNA damage in cancer cells, leading to cell cycle arrest and apoptosis. This is evidenced by the increased expression of γ-H2AX, a marker of DNA double-strand breaks, following apigenin treatment [54].

Overall, these in vitro studies underscore the potential of apigenin as a chemopreventive agent by demonstrating its ability to reduce cell viability and induce apoptosis in cancer cells through various molecular mechanisms, including the modulation of signaling pathways, cell proliferation, apoptosis, inflammation, and angiogenesis.

3.2.2. In Vivo Studies

In vivo studies examined the effect of the dietary consumption of apigenin (0.1%) in the prevention of cancer in azoxymethane-induced colon rat models. Apigenin triggered the apoptosis of luminal surface colonocytes, reduced the incidence of aberrant crypt foci, and decreased peritoneal metastasis incidence [55]. Additionally, dietary intake of apigenin (0.2%) for six weeks in nude mice with A549 lung cancer xenografts reduced tumor volume, attributed to the suppression of the HIF-1α–vascular endothelial growth factor pathway [56].

One notable in vivo study used a transgenic mouse prostate adenocarcinoma (TRAMP) model, where TRAMP mice were given 20 and 50 μg/mouse of apigenin orally for 20 weeks. This study revealed that apigenin reduced tumor volumes and distant organ metastasis, attributed to the suppression of the PI3K/Akt/Forkhead box O-signaling pathway [35].

Furthermore, oral administration of apigenin (2.5 mg/kg) in hamsters with DMBA-induced oral cancer for 15 weeks reduced tumor volume and incidence and modulated markers of cell proliferation, apoptosis, inflammation, and angiogenesis [57,58].

Oral administration of apigenin (3 mg/kg) in nude mice bearing human lung cancer xenografts decreased the tumor volume and wet weight, reduced serum IGF-I levels, and induced apoptosis and cell cycle arrest [59]. Additionally, oral administration of apigenin in $Apc^{Min/+}$ mice contributed to a reduction in polyp numbers through the activation of p53 [60].

Topical application of apigenin (5 and 20 μmol) in murine skin tumorigenesis, initiated by DMBA and promoted by TPA in SENCAR mice, resulted in a marked reduction in the incidence and number of papillomas and carcinomas [61].

In UVB-induced skin inflammation in SKH-1 hairless mice, topical application of apigenin (5 μM) prior to UVB exposure reduced UVB-induced ear edema and COX-2 expression, modulated HIF-1α, and suppressed mTOR signaling [62].

As for its toxicity, apigenin was found to have no apparent in vivo toxicity in xenograft tumor models, including regular mice [32], BALB/c mice [54], and athymic nude mice [44]. The safety of apigenin was demonstrated at doses of 30 mg/kg and 10 μg/mouse intraperitoneally for 21 days [44,54], as well as at doses of 20 and 50 μg/mouse/day for up to 56 days [32]. Its non-toxicity was assessed by monitoring body weight changes [32,44], blood cell count differences [54], and liver mass and histological variations [44] compared to control groups, respectively. A summary of apigenin's in vivo studies are shown in Table 3.

Table 3. Summary of in vivo studies of apigenin as a chemopreventive agent.

Study Model	Apigenin Dosage and Administration	Key Findings	Reference
Colon carcinogenesis in rats	Dietary intake of 0.1% apigenin	Triggered apoptosis of luminal surface colonocytes, reduced aberrant crypt foci, decreased peritoneal metastasis	[55]
Lung cancer xenografts in nude mice	Dietary intake of 0.2% apigenin for 6 weeks	Reduced tumor volume, suppressed HIF-1α-VEGF pathway	[56]
Prostate cancer in TRAMP mice	Oral administration of 20 and 50 μg/mice for 20 weeks	Reduced tumor volumes and distant organ metastasis by suppressing PI3K/Akt/FoxO pathway	[35]
DMBA-induced oral carcinogenesis in hamsters	Oral administration of 2.5 mg/kg for 15 weeks	Reduced tumor volume and incidence, modulated cell proliferation, apoptosis, inflammation, and angiogenesis markers	[57]
Lung cancer xenografts in nude mice	Oral administration of 3 mg/kg	Decreased tumor volume and wet weight, reduced serum IGF-I levels, induced apoptosis and cell cycle arrest	[59]
APCMin/+ mice model	Oral administration of apigenin	Reduction in polyp number by activation of p53	[60]
Murine skin tumorigenesis in SENCAR mice	Topical application of 5 and 20 μmol	Marked reduction in the incidence and number of papillomas and carcinomas	[61]
UVB-induced skin inflammation in SKH-1 mice	Topical application of 5 μM prior to UVB exposure	Reduced UVB-induced ear edema and COX-2 expression, modulated HIF-1α, and suppressed mTOR signaling	[62]

3.3. *In Silico Studies of Apigenin*

Apigenin was effectively docked with the cellular tumor antigen p53, caspase-3, and the mucosal addressin cell adhesion molecule 1, exhibiting significant interactions based on their calculated binding energies [63]. Another in silico study using molecular dynamics simulation evaluated apigenin's binding propensity towards class I histone deacetylase (HDAC) isoforms. The study found apigenin to have a high binding affinity for most of the class I HDACs, particularly demonstrating stability in the binding pocket of the HDAC2 isoform, with numerous contacts persisting for more than 30% of the simulation duration [64].

4. Thymoquinone (TQ)

TQ has antioxidant, anti-inflammatory, immunomodulatory, anti-histaminic, anti-microbial, and anti-tumor action, making it a promising natural chemopreventive agent [53–56]. A summary of its chemopreventive properties are shown in Figure 5.

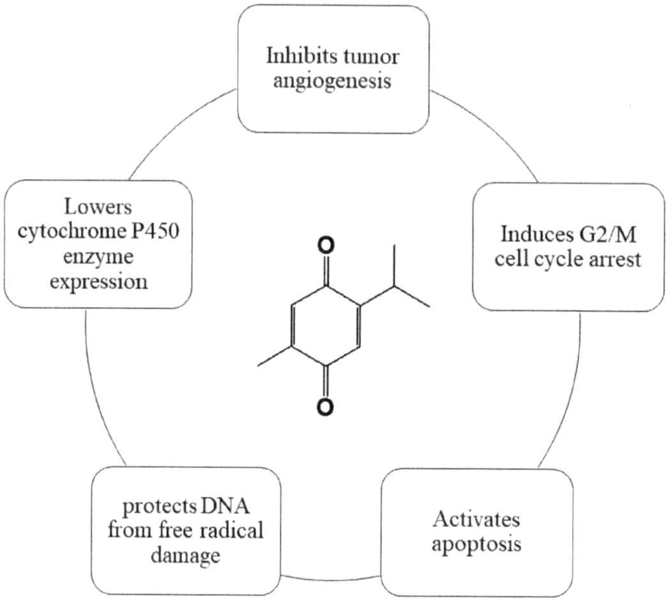

Figure 5. Summary of TQ's chemopreventive properties.

4.1. Source and Chemical Structure

Thymoquinone (TQ) is the main bioactive terpene constituent (Figure 6) found in the volatile oil isolated from *Nigella sativa* (black cumin, black seed), which has been used as a traditional medicine in many countries [52,53]. It can also be found in other plants, as shown in Table 4.

Table 4. Common sources and quantities of TQ.

Source	Quantity of TQ (mg/kg)	Reference
Eupatorium cannabinum L.	8	[51]
Juniperus communis L.	6 free TQ, 15 glycosidically bound TQ	[51]
Monarda didyma L.	3029	[51]
Monarda didyma L.	3425	[51]
Monarda media Willd.	2995	[51]
Monarda menthifolia Graham	1381	[51]
Satureja hortensis L.	217	[51]
Satureja montana L.	1052	[51]
Thymus pulegioides L.	233	[51]
Thymus serpyllum L.	233	[51]
Thymus vulgaris L.	300	[51]
Nigella sativa L.	1881	[51]

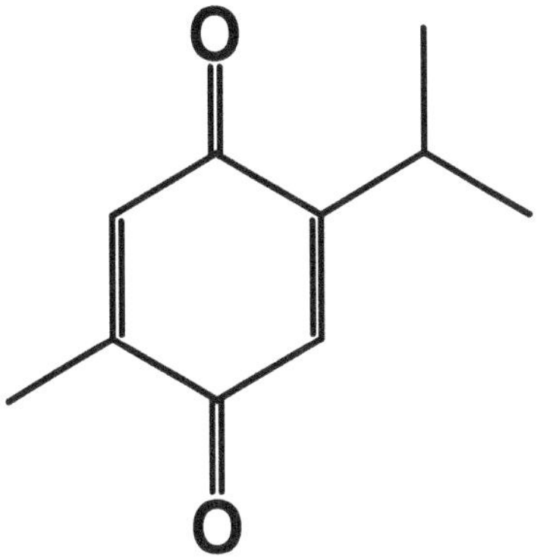

Figure 6. Chemical structure of TQ (ChemDraw Ultra 7.0).

4.2. In Vivo and In Vitro Studies of TQ

4.2.1. In Vitro Studies of TQ

TQ has been shown to inhibit the proliferation of various cancer cell lines, including those from colon and colorectal [65–67], breast [68–70], pancreatic [71], and other types of cancer [72,73]. This inhibition is often mediated through the modulation of cell cycle regulatory proteins. TQ can induce cell cycle arrest at different phases, primarily G1/S and G2/M, by regulating cyclins and cyclin-dependent kinases (CDKs) [74].

In addition, TQ induces apoptosis by activating both intrinsic and extrinsic apoptotic pathways, increasing the expression of pro-apoptotic proteins such as Bax and p53, while decreasing the levels of anti-apoptotic proteins like Bcl-2 [75,76]. TQ also induces the activation of caspases, which are crucial executors of apoptosis [77].

Furthermore, TQ exhibits potent anti-inflammatory effects by inhibiting the expression of pro-inflammatory cytokines such as TNF-α, IL-1β, and IL-6. It also suppresses the NF-κB signaling pathway, which is often upregulated in cancer and associated with inflammation and cell survival [78].

TQ has been shown to induce oxidative stress selectively in cancer cells, leading to cell death. It increases reactive oxygen species (ROS) generation, which can damage cellular components and induce apoptosis. Conversely, TQ enhances the antioxidant defense mechanisms in normal cells, thereby protecting them from oxidative damage [79,80].

Moreover, TQ inhibits key processes involved in cancer metastasis and angiogenesis. It downregulates the expression of matrix metalloproteinases (MMPs), enzymes that degrade the extracellular matrix and facilitate metastasis. Additionally, TQ reduces the expression of vascular endothelial growth factor (VEGF), thereby inhibiting angiogenesis and restricting tumor growth [81,82].

In vitro studies utilizing MCF-7 breast cancer cells have shown that TQ induces cell cycle arrest at the G1 phase and promotes apoptosis through the upregulation of p21 and p27 and the downregulation of cyclin D1 [66]. Likewise, studies on PC-3 prostate cancer cells have demonstrated that TQ induces apoptosis through the mitochondrial pathway and inhibits cell proliferation by suppressing the AKT signaling pathway [79, 82]. In addition, studies with HCT-116 colon cancer cells have found that TQ treatment results in significant inhibition of cell proliferation and the induction of apoptosis via the modulation of the Wnt/β-catenin signaling pathway [79,83]. TQ has also been shown to sensitize pancreatic cancer cells to gemcitabine, a standard chemotherapeutic agent, by enhancing ROS production and downregulating NF-κB signaling, leading to increased apoptosis [84,85].

These in vitro cytotoxicity studies and their findings highlight the potential of TQ as a chemopreventive agent by demonstrating its ability to inhibit cell proliferation, induce apoptosis, exert anti-inflammatory effects, modulate oxidative stress, and inhibit metastasis and angiogenesis.

4.2.2. In Vivo Studies of TQ

Numerous in vivo studies have examined TQ's potential therapeutic effects, particularly in cancer treatment. A summary of in vivo studies of TQ are found in Table 5 These studies have highlighted TQ's ability to inhibit tumor growth, metastasis, and angiogenesis across various cancer models, supporting further exploration of TQ as a therapeutic agent.

Several studies have investigated TQ's effects on different types of cancer in animal models. In a study on Ehrlich acid solid tumors in mice, TQ was administered via intraperitoneal injection at a dose of 10 mg/kg for four weeks (five doses per week). The results showed that TQ reduced oxidative stress, prevented necrosis, and enhanced tissue regeneration [86].

In another study on thioacetamide-induced liver cancer in rats, TQ was given through oral gavage at a dose of 20 mg/kg body weight for 16 weeks. The findings indicated that TQ induced apoptosis by upregulating TRAIL and caspase-3, downregulated Bcl2 and TGF-β1, improved liver function, and reduced hepatocellular carcinoma progression [87].

In a study on mouse epithelial breast cancer cell line (EMT6/P) xenografts in BALB/C mice, the co-administration of TQ with piperine prevented tumor growth by decreasing VEGF expression and increasing serum INF-γ levels, leading to apoptosis [88].

Similarly, in a study on breast cancer cell lines in BALB/C mice, the co-administration of TQ with resveratrol induced apoptosis and decreased VEGF expression [89]. Furthermore, a study on breast cancer in mice, where TQ was administered orally at a dose of 65 mg/kg body weight, revealed that TQ reduced tumor markers, suppressed histopathological changes, and regulated the expression of Brca1, Brca2, P53, and Id-1 mutation [90].

Roepke et al. (2007) conducted a study on osteosarcoma (OS), using human osteosarcoma cell lines MG63 and MNNG/HOS in a xenograft mouse model. TQ was administered in vivo at a dose of 6 mg/kg/day, significantly reducing the expression of NF-κB protein in OS tumors [75].

Another study on human pancreatic ductal adenocarcinoma (PDAC) cells showed that TQ dose-dependently arrested the G2 cell cycle phase and reduced cell growth and viability, increased p53 and p21 expression, and decreased Bcl-2 expression, leading to tumor size reductions [91].

Additionally, Peng et al. (2013) studied SaOS-2 cells (human osteosarcoma) and found that TQ exhibited pro-apoptotic effects in a concentration-dependent manner, reducing cancer cell proliferation through various molecular pathways, including ROS generation and MAPK signaling. TQ also reduced the DNA-binding activity of NF-κB in a dose-dependent manner and significantly attenuated the expression of the NF-κB protein in osteosarcoma tumors [92].

Table 5. Summary of in vivo studies of TQ as a chemopreventive agent.

Cancer Type	Cell Lines	Animal Model	TQ Dosage	Mechanism of TQ Action	Overall Outcome	References
Bladder cancer	T-24 and 253 J cell lines	Xenograft mouse	10 mg/kg/3 days	↑ E-cadherin, ↓ N-cadherin, vimentin, Wnt/β-catenin, MYC, axin-2, MMP7, cyclin D1	Augmentation of gemcitabine anti-cancer activities through the upregulation of apoptosis and autophagy processes	[93]
Breast cancer	MDA-MB-231 and MDA-MB-436	Xenograft mouse	5 mg/kg/day	↑ miR-361, ↓ Rac, RhoA, VEGF-A	Angiogenesis and metastasis suppression and a decrease in tumor weight	[94]
Cervical cancer	SiHa cell lines	-	-	↑ p53, ↓ Bcl-2	Cell cycle arrest at the sub-G1 phase, induction of apoptosis and necrosis	[95]

Table 5. *Cont.*

Cancer Type	Cell Lines	Animal Model	TQ Dosage	Mechanism of TQ Action	Overall Outcome	References
Glioblastoma	S6 cell lines	-	-	↓ ERK, FAK, MMP-2, MMP-9	Reduced cell survival, migration, adhesion, and metastasis processes	[96]
Liver cancer	SNU-7721 and HepG2 cell lines	Xenograft rats	20 mg/kg/day	↑ Bax, caspase-8, ↓ Bcl-2, VEGF	Cell cycle arrest at G2/M phase and induction of apoptosis	[97]
Prostate cancer	DU-145, PC-3	Xenograft mouse	5–30 mg/kg/2 days	↑ E-cadherin, ↓ Slug, TGF-β, Smad-2, Smad-3, vimentin	Reduced cell survival, migration, and invasion	[98]
Prostate cancer	PC-3, LNCaP	Xenograft mouse	10–20 mg/kg/day	↑ p21, p27, caspases; ↓ Bcl-2, Cyclin D1, CDK4	Induction of apoptosis, cell cycle arrest, inhibition of tumor growth	[99]
Gastric cancer	BGC-823, HGC-27, MGC-803, SGC-7901	Xenograft mouse	20 mg/kg/day	↑ Bax, caspase-3, caspase-9, cytochrome c, ↓ Bcl-2	Increased sensitivity to 5-FU, induction of apoptosis, decrease in tumor weight	[100]
Gastric cancer	BGC-823, HGC-27, SGC-7901	Xenograft mouse	10–30 mg/kg/2 days	↑: Bax, caspase-3, caspase-7, caspase-9 ↓: Bcl-2, cyclin D, c-Src, JAK2, STAT3, survivin, VEGF	Inhibition of cell growth and angiogenesis, apoptosis induction, and reduction in tumor weight	[72]
	HGC-27, MGC-803, and SGC-7901	Xenograft mouse	10 mg/kg/2 days	↑: AIF, Bax, caspase-3, caspase-9, cytochrome c, PTEN ↓: Bcl-2, cyclin D1, p-gp	Increased sensitivity to cisplatin, induction of apoptosis, decrease in tumor weight	[101]
Colorectal cancer	HCT 116wt, DLD-1, HT29	-	25 mg/kg/day	↓ ERK1/2, MEK, PAK1	Decreased cell viability, induction of apoptosis and necrosis, decrease in tumor weight	[102]
Colorectal cancer	5FU-resistant HCT116	Xenograft mouse	20 mg/kg/2 days	↑ p21, p53, γH2AX, ↓ CD44, EpCAM, ki67, NF-κB, MEK	Induction of apoptosis, reduced cell invasion and migration, decrease in tumor weight	[103]
	Irinotecan (CPT-11)-resistant LoVo cell lines			↓: IKKα/β, NF-κB, Snail, Twist, vimentin, MMP-2, MMP-9, ERK1/2, PI3K	Increased cell rate, mitochondrial membrane permeability, induction of apoptosis and autophagy	[104]
Pancreatic cancer	PANC-1, BxPC-3	Xenograft mouse	5 mg/kg/day	↑ Bax, caspase-3, p53; ↓ Bcl-2, NF-κB	Induction of apoptosis, suppression of tumor growth	[105]
Lung cancer	A549	-	-	↓: cyclin D1, ERK1/2, MMP-2, MMP-9, PCNA	Decreased rate of cancer cell proliferation, migration, invasion, and metastasis, cell cycle arrest at the G0/G1 phase	[106]
Lung cancer	A549	-	-	↓: Bcl-2	Decreased cell viability and induction of Apoptosis, as well as necrosis Depolymerization of microtubules and disruption of mitotic spindle organization, promotion of apoptosis, and decrease in cell viability	[107,108]

Table 5. *Cont.*

Cancer Type	Cell Lines	Animal Model	TQ Dosage	Mechanism of TQ Action	Overall Outcome	References
Ovarian cancer	ID8_NGL, NCI/ADR, and OVCAR-3	Xenograft mouse	20 mg/kg/2 days	↓: Bcl-2, PCNA	Increased cell death, sensitivity of cancer cells to cisplatin, induced apoptosis	[109]
Ovarian cancer	SK-OV-3 cell lines	-	-	↓: Bcl-2	Induced apoptosis, cell cycle arrest at the S phase, and reduced anti-cancer impact of cisplatin	[110]

↑ upregulate, ↓ downregulate.

4.3. *In Silico Studies of TQ*

A reverse in silico study was applied to TQ against a variety of targets involved in metastasis and apoptosis to search for potential targets involved in cancer therapy. The results found that TQ successfully binds to apoptotic targets such as TRAIL-R, Bcl-2, MDM2, Bak, Bax, and PARP [111]. TQ was docked to the active site of the target PTEN, which is a negative regulator of the PI3K/AKT pathway. TQ illustrated a great binding affinity to PTEN, with the potential to inhibit abnormal cell proliferation via modulating the activity of PTEN [112]. Furthermore, TQ's position as a p53 activator and preventative anti-cancer agent against lung cancer is implicated by the docking data [113].

5. Comparison of RA, Apigenin, and TQ: Chemopreventive Mechanisms and Extraction Methods

In vitro studies have significantly advanced our understanding of the chemopreventive mechanisms of RA, apigenin, and TQ, revealing both common pathways and unique targets affected by each compound, as shown in Table 6. Apigenin inhibits cancer cell proliferation by modulating cell cycle regulatory proteins, inducing cell cycle arrest [47], and promoting apoptosis [37,114]. It affects key signaling pathways such as PI3K/AKT and MAPK, inhibits angiogenesis, and disrupts the mitochondrial membrane, leading to apoptosis [48]. TQ similarly induces cell cycle arrest and apoptosis but also prominently activates both intrinsic and extrinsic apoptotic pathways and modulates oxidative stress by increasing ROS generation selectively in cancer cells. Additionally, TQ has potent anti-inflammatory effects, inhibiting pro-inflammatory cytokines and the NF-κB signaling pathway, and suppresses metastasis and angiogenesis by downregulating MMPs and VEGF [85]. RA also shows potential in cancer prevention through its strong antioxidant properties and modulation of several signaling pathways, including PI3K/AKT/mTOR [12]. It induces apoptosis and cell cycle arrest in various cancer cells, suppresses metastasis, and exhibits anti-Warburg effects by inhibiting glucose uptake and lactate production [16]. Collectively, these compounds target cell proliferation, apoptosis, angiogenesis, and inflammatory pathways but with unique aspects of their mechanisms, such as RA's anti-Warburg effect and TQ's ROS-mediated cytotoxicity. Table 6 illustrates a concise comparison of the chemopreventive mechanisms for RA, apigenin, and TQ.

The interest in the various bioactivities of RA, apigenin, and TQ has led to the development of efficient methods of extraction from their natural sources. For RA, the methods include vibration, maceration with stirring, heat reflux, Soxhlet solvent extraction, and recent innovations like ultrasound-assisted, microwave-assisted, enzyme-assisted, and pressurized-liquid extraction, with the solvent choice playing a crucial role in yield optimization [115]. Apigenin extraction benefits from advanced techniques such as dynamic maceration and the use of ionic liquid analogs, specifically deep eutectic solvents (DESs), which offer efficient and environmentally friendly alternatives [116]. TQ extraction involves hydrodistillation (HD) using a Clevenger-type apparatus, dry steam distillation (SD), steam distillation of crude oils obtained by solvent extraction (SE-SD), and supercritical fluid extraction (SFE-SD), with CO2 as the preferred solvent due to its cost-effectiveness and safety [117]. These varied methods reflect ongoing efforts to optimize the extraction processes for these valuable phytochemicals.

Table 6. Comparison of mechanisms and molecular targets of apigenin, RA, and TQ.

Compound	Key Mechanisms	Specific Targets	References
Apigenin	Inhibits proliferation, induces apoptosis, modulates cell cycle	Cell cycle regulatory proteins, PI3K/AKT, MAPK, caspases, Bcl-2 family, mitochondrial membrane potential	[33,53]
Rosmarinic Acid (RA)	Induces apoptosis, inhibits metastasis, affects glucose metabolism (anti-Warburg effect) [13,16]	PI3K/AKT/mTOR, epithelial–mesenchymal transition, apoptosis-related genes, glucose uptake, and lactate production [13,16]	[13,16]
Thymoquinone (TQ)	Induces cell cycle arrest and apoptosis, modulates oxidative stress, anti-inflammatory, inhibits metastasis and angiogenesis	Cyclins, CDKs, p53, Bcl-2, Bax, NF-κB, ROS, MMPs, VEGF	[69,75,77,78,89]

6. Clinical Studies

Among the three natural compounds—rosmarinic acid (RA), apigenin, and thymoquinone (TQ)—there are no adequate clinical studies supporting their use as chemopreventive agents, despite promising data from in vivo and in vitro studies [115–120].

One clinical study involving apigenin, titled "Dietary Bioflavonoid Supplementation for the Prevention of Neoplasia Recurrence" (ClinicalTrials.gov Identifier: NCT00609310), aimed to evaluate the efficacy of bioflavonoid supplementation in reducing the recurrence of colorectal neoplasia. Conducted by Technische Universität Dresden, this phase 2 interventional study involved 382 participants aged 50 to 75 years who had recently undergone surgical resection for stage 2 or 3 colorectal cancer. It was designed as a double-blind, randomized, placebo-controlled trial, with the participants divided into two groups. The experimental group received a daily dietary supplement containing a mixture of bioflavonoids, specifically 20 mg of apigenin and 20 mg of epigallocatechin gallate (EGCG) from chamomile and green tea extracts, along with vitamins and folic acid. The primary objective was to determine whether this supplementation could decrease the rate of neoplasia recurrence over a three-year period. The secondary outcomes included overall survival, recurrence-free survival, and serum levels of the bioflavonoids. Despite its promising design, the study's recruitment status was listed as suspended as of the last update in February 2012, with the reasons for suspension unspecified.

TQ was investigated for its long-term safety in healthy human subjects at a dosage of 200 mg/day for 90 days. Hematological and biochemical parameters, including kidney and liver function tests and lipid profiles, were examined alongside anthropometric measurements to monitor safety. The study participants did not exhibit any side effects, indicating that TQ was well tolerated over the studied period [119].

A recent clinical study involving TQ, titled "Clinical and Immunohistochemical Evaluation of Chemopreventive Effect of Thymoquinone on Oral Potentially Malignant Lesions" (ClinicalTrials.gov Identifier: NCT03208790), investigated the potential of TQ, derived from Nigella sativa, as a chemopreventive agent for oral potentially malignant lesions (OPMLs). Conducted by Cairo University, this randomized, controlled, parallel-group trial involved 48 participants aged 18 to 75 years with histologically and clinically confirmed OPMLs. The participants were divided into three groups: Group A received Nigella sativa buccal tablets containing 10 mg of TQ; Group B received Nigella sativa buccal tablets containing 5 mg of TQ; Group C received placebo buccal tablets. The primary goal was to assess the clinical response by measuring the dimensions of the lesions at baseline and after three months of treatment. The secondary outcomes included immunohistochemical evaluations for markers of cell proliferation (Ki-67) and apoptosis (caspase-3). While specific results from the study are not detailed in the available summaries, the trial aimed to determine whether TQ could reduce lesion size and affect molecular markers indicative of malignant transformation. The study concluded in March 2020, but detailed results have not been posted publicly. This study represents a significant step in exploring natural compounds like TQ for cancer chemoprevention, specifically in OPMLs, although further detailed results are necessary to confirm its efficacy and potential for clinical use. According to the database, the study completed phase 2, with the last update posted on 20 April 2021 [121–123].

7. Conclusions

In this review, we highlight the chemopreventive potential of rosmarinic acid (RA), apigenin, and thymoquinone (TQ). These compounds, derived from widely used plants, exhibit diverse chemical structures and functions, including their ability to act as antioxidants, cell signaling modulators, and inhibitors of cell proliferation. Extensive in vitro, in vivo, and in silico studies provide a robust foundation for their chemopreventive properties. However, transitioning these agents into clinical use necessitates further clinical, toxicological, and pharmacokinetic studies to confirm their safety and efficacy in humans. Addressing pharmacokinetics and bioavailability challenges through advanced formulations, drug delivery systems, and chemical optimization is essential. Computational methods such as computer-aided drug design (CADD) and molecular dynamics simulations can significantly reduce the research costs and expedite the development of more potent and more selective chemopreventive derivatives.

Continuous investigation into these natural products could lead to complementary or alternative cancer treatments with fewer adverse effects than conventional therapies. Thus, future research should focus on the following: (1) conducting well-designed clinical trials to establish effective dosages, formulations, and delivery methods; (2) investigating the anti-metastatic potential and synergistic effects of RA, apigenin, and TQ in combination with other chemotherapeutic agents; and (3) long-term safety and toxicology studies to assess the potential adverse effects of their chronic use.

By addressing these research objectives, the potential of chemopreventive agents like RA, apigenin, and TQ in cancer treatment can be fully realized, leading to improved patient outcomes and innovative therapeutic options.

Author Contributions: Conceptualization: R.F.A. and M.A.; Methodology: R.F.A. and M.A.; Investigation: M.A., A.M. and I.A.-A.; Original Draft Preparation: M.A., A.M., I.A.-A., R.F.A.; Review and Editing:. R.F.A., M.A. and A.A.; Visualization: M.A.; Supervision: R.F.A. and A.A.; Project Administration: M.A. and R.F.A. All authors have read and agreed to the published version of the manuscript.

Funding: This research received no funding.

Conflicts of Interest: The authors declare no conflict of interest.

References

1. Akhtar, M.S.; Swamy, M.K. *Anticancer Plants: Mechanisms and Molecular Interactions*; Springer Science and Business Media LLC: Dordrecht, The Netherlands, 2018; Volume 4. [CrossRef]
2. Russo, M.; Spagnuolo, C.; Tedesco, I.; Russo, G.L. Phytochemicals in Cancer Prevention and Therapy: Truth or Dare? *Toxins* **2010**, *2*, 517–551. [CrossRef] [PubMed]
3. Benetou, V.; Lagiou, A.; Lagiou, P. Chemoprevention of Cancer: Current Evidence and Future Prospects. *F1000Research* **2015**, *4*, 916. [CrossRef] [PubMed]
4. Ranjan, A.; Ramachandran, S.; Gupta, N.; Kaushik, I.; Wright, S.; Srivastava, S.; Das, H.; Srivastava, S.; Prasad, S.; Srivastava, S.K. Role of Phytochemicals in Cancer Prevention. *Int. J. Mol. Sci.* **2019**, *20*, 4981. [CrossRef] [PubMed]
5. Dmitrovsky, E.; Sporn, M.B. Chemoprevention, Pharmacology of. In *Encyclopedia of Cancer*, 2nd ed.; Bertino, J.R., Ed.; Academic Press: Cambridge, MA, USA, 2002; pp. 449–455. [CrossRef]

6. Hodges, R.E.; Minich, D.M. Modulation of Metabolic Detoxification Pathways Using Foods and Food-Derived Components: A Scientific Review with Clinical Application. *J. Nutr. Metab.* **2015**, *2015*, 760689. [CrossRef] [PubMed]
7. Abel, E.L.; DiGiovanni, J. Environmental Carcinogenesis. In *The Molecular Basis of Cancer*, 4th ed.; Mendelsohn, J., Gray, J.W., Howley, P.M., Israel, M.A., Eds.; Elsevier Inc.: Amsterdam, The Netherlands, 2014; pp. 103–128. [CrossRef]
8. Alagawany, M.; Abd El-Hack, M.E.; Farag, M.R.; Gopi, M.; Karthik, K.; Malik, Y.S.; Dhama, K. Rosmarinic Acid: Modes of Action, Medicinal Values and Health Benefits. *Anim. Health Res. Rev.* **2017**, *18*, 167–176. [CrossRef] [PubMed]
9. Wang, H.; Provan, G.J.; Helliwell, K. Determination of Rosmarinic Acid and Caffeic Acid in Aromatic Herbs by HPLC. *Food Chem.* **2004**, *87*, 307–311. [CrossRef]
10. Petersen, M. Rosmarinic Acid: New Aspects. *Phytochem. Rev.* **2013**, *12*, 207–227. [CrossRef]
11. Shekarchi, M.; Hajimehdipoor, H.; Saeidnia, S.; Gohari, A.R.; Hamedani, M.P. Comparative Study of Rosmarinic Acid Content in Some Plants of Labiatae Family. *Pharmacogn. Mag.* **2012**, *8*, 37–41. [CrossRef] [PubMed]
12. Yang, K.; Shen, Z.; Zou, Y.; Gao, K. Rosmarinic Acid Inhibits Migration, Invasion, and p38/AP-1 Signaling via miR-1225-5p in Colorectal Cancer Cells. *J. Recept. Signal Transduct. Res.* **2021**, *41*, 284–293. [CrossRef]
13. Wang, L.; Yang, H.; Wang, C.; Shi, X.; Li, K. Rosmarinic Acid Inhibits Proliferation and Invasion of Hepatocellular Carcinoma Cells SMMC 7721 via PI3K/AKT/mTOR Signal Pathway. *Biomed. Pharmacother.* **2019**, *120*, 109443. [CrossRef]
14. Zhang, Y.; Hu, M.; Liu, L.; Cheng, X.L.; Cai, J.; Zhou, J.; Wang, T. Cytotoxic Effects of Rosmarinic Acid in OVCAR-3 Ovarian Cancer Cells Are Mediated via Induction of Apoptosis, Suppression of Cell Migration and Modulation of lncRNA MALAT-1 Expression. *J. BUON* **2018**, *23*, 763–768. [PubMed]
15. Messeha, S.S.; Zarmouh, N.O.; Asiri, A.; Soliman, K.F.A. Rosmarinic Acid-Induced Apoptosis and Cell Cycle Arrest in Triple-Negative Breast Cancer Cells. *Eur. J. Pharmacol.* **2020**, *885*, 173419. [CrossRef] [PubMed]
16. Han, S.; Yang, S.; Cai, Z.; Pan, D.; Li, Z.; Huang, Z.; Zhang, P.; Zhu, H.; Lei, L.; Wang, W. Anti-Warburg Effect of Rosmarinic Acid via miR-155 in Gastric Cancer Cells. *Drug Des. Devel. Ther.* **2015**, *9*, 2695–2703. [CrossRef] [PubMed]
17. Furtado, R.A.; Oliveira, B.R.; Silva, L.R.; Cleto, S.S.; Munari, C.C.; Cunha, W.R.; Tavares, D.C. Chemopreventive Effects of Rosmarinic Acid on Rat Colon Carcinogenesis. *Eur. J. Cancer Prev.* **2015**, *24*, 106–112. [CrossRef] [PubMed]
18. Venkatachalam, K.; Gunasekaran, S.; Namasivayam, N. Biochemical and Molecular Mechanisms Underlying the Chemopreventive Efficacy of Rosmarinic Acid in a Rat Colon Cancer. *Eur. J. Pharmacol.* **2016**, *791*, 37–50. [CrossRef] [PubMed]
19. Sharmila, R.; Manoharan, S. Anti-Tumor Activity of Rosmarinic Acid in 7,12-Dimethylbenz(a)Anthracene (DMBA) Induced Skin Carcinogenesis in Swiss Albino Mice. *Indian. J. Exp. Biol.* **2012**, *50*, 187–194. [PubMed]
20. Jin, B.R.; Chung, K.S.; Hwang, S.; Hwang, S.N.; Rhee, K.J.; Lee, M.; An, H.J. Rosmarinic Acid Represses Colitis-Associated Colon Cancer: A Pivotal Involvement of the TLR4-Mediated NF-κB-STAT3 Axis. *Neoplasia* **2021**, *23*, 561–573. [CrossRef]
21. Xue, X.; Ricci, M.; Qu, H.; Lindstrom, A.; Zhang, D.; Wu, H.; Lin, T.Y.; Li, Y. Iron-Crosslinked Rososome with Robust Stability and High Drug Loading for Synergistic Cancer Therapy. *J. Control. Release* **2021**, *329*, 794–804. [CrossRef]
22. Huang, Y.; Cai, Y.; Huang, R.; Zheng, X. Rosmarinic Acid Combined with Adriamycin Induces Apoptosis by Triggering Mitochondria-Mediated Signaling Pathway in HepG2 and Bel-7402 Cells. *Med. Sci. Monit.* **2018**, *24*, 7898–7908. [CrossRef]
23. Liao, X.Z.; Gao, Y.; Sun, L.L.; Liu, J.H.; Chen, H.R.; Yu, L.; Chen, Z.Z.; Chen, W.H.; Lin, L.Z. Rosmarinic Acid Reverses Non-Small Cell Lung Cancer Cisplatin Resistance by Activating the MAPK Signaling Pathway. *Phytother. Res.* **2020**, *34*, 1142–1153. [CrossRef]
24. Chou, S.T.; Ho, B.Y.; Tai, Y.T.; Huang, C.J.; Chao, W.W. Bidirect Effects from Cisplatin Combined with Rosmarinic Acid (RA) or Hot Water Extracts of Glechoma hederacea (HWG) on Renal Cancer Cells. *Chin. Med.* **2020**, *15*, 77. [CrossRef] [PubMed]
25. Anwar, S.; Shamsi, A.; Shahbaaz, M.; Queen, A.; Khan, P.; Hasan, G.M.; Islam, A.; Alajmi, M.F.; Hussain, A.; Ahmad, F.; et al. Rosmarinic Acid Exhibits Cytotoxic Effects via MARK4 Inhibition. *Sci. Rep.* **2020**, *10*, 10300. [CrossRef]
26. Jelić, D.; Mildner, B.; Koštrun, S.; Nujić, K.; Verbanac, D.; Čulić, O.; Antolović, R.; Brandt, W. Homology Modeling of Human Fyn Kinase Structure: Discovery of Rosmarinic Acid as a New Fyn Kinase Inhibitor and in Silico Study of Its Possible Binding Modes. *J. Med. Chem.* **2007**, *50*, 1090–1100. [CrossRef] [PubMed]
27. Ali, F.; Rahul; Naz, F.; Jyoti, S.; Siddique, Y.H. Health Functionality of Apigenin: A Review. *Int. J. Food Prop.* **2017**, *20*, 1197–1238. [CrossRef]
28. Mozafarian, V. *Flora of Iran*; Forest & Ranglands Research Institute Press: Tehran, Iran, 2007; Volume 1, p. 54.
29. Miean, K.H.; Mohamed, S. Flavonoid (Myricetin, Quercetin, Kaempferol, Luteolin, and Apigenin) Content of Edible Tropical Plants. *J. Agric. Food Chem.* **2001**, *49*, 3106–3112. [CrossRef] [PubMed]
30. Cannataro, R.; Fazio, A.; La Torre, C.; Caroleo, M.C.; Cione, E. Polyphenols in the Mediterranean Diet: From Dietary Sources to MicroRNA Modulation. *Antioxidants* **2021**, *10*, 328. [CrossRef] [PubMed]
31. Gupta, S.; Afaq, F.; Mukhtar, H. Selective Growth-Inhibitory, Cell-Cycle Deregulatory and Apoptotic Response of Apigenin in Normal Versus Human Prostate Carcinoma Cells. *Biochem. Biophys. Res. Commun.* **2001**, *287*, 914–920. [CrossRef] [PubMed]
32. Shukla, S.; Fu, P.; Gupta, S. Apigenin Induces Apoptosis by Targeting Inhibitor of Apoptosis Proteins and Ku70-Bax Interaction in Prostate Cancer. *Apoptosis* **2014**, *19*, 883–894. [CrossRef] [PubMed]
33. Gupta, S.; Afaq, F.; Mukhtar, H. Involvement of Nuclear Factor-Kappa B, Bax, and Bcl-2 in Induction of Cell Cycle Arrest and Apoptosis by Apigenin in Human Prostate Carcinoma Cells. *Oncogene* **2002**, *21*, 3727–3738. [CrossRef]
34. Erdogan, S.; Doganlar, O.; Doganlar, Z.B.; Serttas, R.; Turkekul, K.; Dibirdik, I.; Bilir, A. The Flavonoid Apigenin Reduces Prostate Cancer CD44(+) Stem Cell Survival and Migration Through PI3K/Akt/NF-κB Signaling. *Life Sci.* **2016**, *162*, 77–86. [CrossRef]

35. Shukla, S.; Bhaskaran, N.; Babcook, M.A.; Fu, P.; MacLennan, G.T.; Gupta, S. Apigenin Inhibits Prostate Cancer Progression in TRAMP Mice via Targeting PI3K/Akt/FoxO Pathway. *Carcinogenesis* **2014**, *35*, 452–460. [CrossRef] [PubMed]
36. Mirzoeva, S.; Franzen, C.A.; Pelling, J.C. Apigenin Inhibits TGF-β-Induced VEGF Expression in Human Prostate Carcinoma Cells via a Smad2/3- and Src-Dependent Mechanism. *Mol. Carcinog.* **2014**, *53*, 598–609. [CrossRef] [PubMed]
37. Seo, H.; Ku Mo, J.; Choi, H.; Woo, J.; Jang, B.; Go, H.; Ko, S. Apigenin Induces Caspase-Dependent Apoptosis by Inhibiting Signal Transducer and Activator of Transcription 3 Signaling in HER2-Overexpressing SKBR3 Breast Cancer Cells. *Mol. Med. Rep.* **2015**, *12*, 2977–2984. [CrossRef] [PubMed]
38. Tseng, T.-H.; Chien, M.-H.; Lin, W.-L.; Wen, Y.-C.; Chow, J.-M.; Chen, C.-K.; Lee, W.-J. Inhibition of MDA-MB-231 Breast Cancer Cell Proliferation and Tumor Growth by Apigenin Through Induction of G2/M Arrest and Histone H3 Acetylation-Mediated p21(WAF1/CIP1) Expression. *Environ. Toxicol.* **2017**, *32*, 434–444. [CrossRef] [PubMed]
39. Cao, X.; Liu, B.; Cao, W.; Zhang, W.; Zhang, F.; Zhao, H.; Meng, R.; Zhang, L.; Niu, R.; Hao, X.; et al. Autophagy Inhibition Enhances Apigenin-Induced Apoptosis in Human Breast Cancer Cells. *Chin. J. Cancer Res.* **2013**, *25*, 212–222. [CrossRef]
40. Seo, H.-S.; Ku, J.M.; Choi, H.-S.; Woo, J.-K.; Jang, B.-H.; Shin, Y.C.; Ko, S.-G. Induction of Caspase-Dependent Apoptosis by Apigenin by Inhibiting STAT3 Signaling in HER2-Overexpressing MDA-MB-453 Breast Cancer Cells. *Anticancer. Res.* **2014**, *34*, 2869–2882.
41. Seo, H.-S.; Jo, J.K.; Ku, J.M.; Choi, H.-S.; Choi, Y.K.; Woo, J.-K.; Ko, S.-G. Induction of Caspase-Dependent Extrinsic Apoptosis by Apigenin Through Inhibition of Signal Transducer and Activator of Transcription 3 (STAT3) Signalling in HER2-Overexpressing BT-474 Breast Cancer Cells. *Biosci. Rep.* **2015**, *35*, e00276. [CrossRef] [PubMed]
42. Shao, H.; Jing, K.; Mahmoud, E.; Huang, H.; Fang, X.; Yu, C. Apigenin Sensitizes Colon Cancer Cells to Antitumor Activity of ABT-263. *Mol. Cancer Ther.* **2013**, *12*, 2640–2650. [CrossRef] [PubMed]
43. Lee, Y.; Sung, B.; Kang, Y.J.; Kim, D.H.; Jang, J.-Y.; Hwang, S.Y.; Kim, N.D. Apigenin-Induced Apoptosis is Enhanced by Inhibition of Autophagy Formation in HCT116 Human Colon Cancer Cells. *Int. J. Oncol.* **2014**, *44*, 1599–1606. [CrossRef]
44. Chen, M.; Wang, X.; Zha, D.; Cai, F.; Zhang, W.; He, Y.; Hua, Z.-C. Apigenin Potentiates TRAIL Therapy of Non-Small Cell Lung Cancer via Upregulating DR4/DR5 Expression in a p53-Dependent Manner. *Sci. Rep.* **2016**, *6*, 35468. [CrossRef]
45. Zhou, Z.; Tang, M.; Liu, Y.; Zhang, Z.; Lu, R.; Lu, J. Apigenin Inhibits Cell Proliferation, Migration, and Invasion by Targeting Akt in the A549 Human Lung Cancer Cell Line. *Anti-Cancer Drugs* **2017**, *28*, 446–456. [CrossRef] [PubMed]
46. Shukla, S.; Gupta, S. Apigenin: A Promising Molecule for Cancer Prevention. *Pharm. Res.* **2010**, *27*, 962–978. [CrossRef] [PubMed]
47. Yin, F.; Giuliano, A.E.; Van Herle, A.J. Signal Transduction Pathways Involved in Apigenin-Induced Apoptosis and Cell-Cycle Arrest in Human Breast Cancer Cells. *Nutr. Cancer* **2001**, *39*, 114–126.
48. Fang, J.; Xia, C.; Cao, Z.; Zheng, J.Z.; Reed, E.; Jiang, B.H. Apigenin Inhibits VEGF and HIF-1 Expression via PI3K/AKT/p70S6K1 and HDM2/p53 Pathways. *FASEB J.* **2005**, *19*, 342–353. [CrossRef]
49. Zhang, Q.Y.; Wang, F.X.; Jia, K.K.; Kong, L.D. Natural Product Apigenin Inhibits Angiogenesis: Implication in Its Anti-Inflammatory and Anti-Oxidative Therapeutic Effects. *Cell. Mol. Biol.* **2017**, *63*, 14–21.
50. Tong, X.; Pelling, J.C. Targeting the PI3K/Akt/mTOR Axis by Apigenin for Cancer Prevention. *Anti-Cancer Agents Med. Chem.* **2013**, *13*, 971–978. [CrossRef] [PubMed]
51. Táborský, J.; Kunt, M.; Klouček, P.; Lachman, J.; Zelený, V.; Kokoška, L. Identification of potential sources of thymoquinone and related compounds in asteraceae, cupressaceae, lamiaceae, and ranunculaceae families. *Open Chem.* **2012**, *10*, 1899–1906. [CrossRef]
52. Long, X.; Fan, M.; Bigsby, R.M.; Nephew, K.P. Apigenin Inhibits Antiestrogen-Resistant Breast Cancer Cell Growth through Estrogen Receptor-α-Dependent and Estrogen Receptor-α-Independent Mechanisms. *Mol. Cancer Ther.* **2008**, *7*, 2096–2108. [CrossRef]
53. Wang, I.K.; Lin-Shiau, S.Y.; Lin, J.K. Induction of Apoptosis by Apigenin and Related Flavonoids through Cytochrome c Release and Activation of Caspase-9 and Caspase-3 in Leukemia HL-60 Cells. *Eur. J. Cancer* **1999**, *35*, 1517–1525. [CrossRef] [PubMed]
54. Meng, S.; Zhu, Y.; Li, J.F.; Wang, X.; Liang, Z.; Li, S.Q.; Xu, X.; Chen, H.; Liu, B.; Zheng, X.Y.; et al. Apigenin Inhibits Renal Cell Carcinoma Cell Proliferation. *Oncotarget* **2017**, *8*, 19834–19842. [CrossRef]
55. Leonardi, T.; Vanamala, J.; Taddeo, S.S.; Davidson, L.A.; Murphy, M.E.; Patil, B.S. Apigenin and Naringenin Suppress Colon Carcinogenesis through the Aberrant Crypt Stage in Azoxymethane-Treated Rats. *Exp. Biol. Med.* **2010**, *235*, 710–717. [CrossRef]
56. King, J.C.; Lu, Q.Y.; Li, G.; Moro, A.; Takahashi, H.; Chen, M. Evidence for Activation of Mutated p53 by Apigenin in Human Pancreatic Cancer. *Biochim. Biophys. Acta* **2012**, *1823*, 593–604. [CrossRef]
57. Silvan, S.; Manoharan, S. Apigenin Prevents Deregulation in the Expression Pattern of Cell-Proliferative, Apoptotic, Inflammatory, and Angiogenic Markers During 7,12-Dimethylbenz[a]anthracene-Induced Hamster Buccal Pouch Carcinogenesis. *Arch. Oral. Biol.* **2013**, *58*, 94–101. [CrossRef] [PubMed]
58. Silvan, S.; Manoharan, S.; Baskaran, N.; Anusuya, C.; Karthikeyan, S.; Prabhakar, M.M. Chemo-Preventive Potential of Apigenin in 7,12-Dimethylbenz[a]anthracene-Induced Experimental Oral Carcinogenesis. *Eur. J. Pharmacol.* **2011**, *670*, 571–577. [CrossRef]
59. Liu, L.Z.; Fang, J.; Zhou, Q.; Hu, X.; Shi, X.; Jiang, B.H. Apigenin Inhibits Expression of Vascular Endothelial Growth Factor and Angiogenesis in Human Lung Cancer Cells: Implication of Chemoprevention of Lung Cancer. *Mol. Pharmacol.* **2005**, *68*, 635–643. [CrossRef] [PubMed]
60. Zhong, Y.; Krisanapun, C.; Lee, S.H.; Nualsanit, T.; Sams, C.; Peungvicha, P. Molecular Targets of Apigenin in Colorectal Cancer Cells: Involvement of p21, NAG-1 and p53. *Eur. J. Cancer* **2010**, *46*, 3365–3374. [CrossRef]

61. Wei, H.; Tye, L.; Bresnick, E.; Birt, D.F. Inhibitory Effect of Apigenin, a Plant Flavonoid, on Epidermal Ornithine Decarboxylase and Skin Tumor Promotion in Mice. *Cancer Res.* **1990**, *50*, 499–502. [PubMed]
62. Bridgeman, B.B.; Wang, P.; Ye, B.; Pelling, J.C.; Volpert, O.V.; Tong, X. Inhibition of mTOR by Apigenin in UVB-Irradiated Keratinocytes: A New Implication of Skin Cancer Prevention. *Cell. Signal.* **2016**, *28*, 460–468. [CrossRef]
63. Kasilingam, T.; Elengoe, A. In Silico Molecular Modeling and Docking of Apigenin Against the Lung Cancer Cell Proteins. *Asian J. Pharm. Clin. Res.* **2018**, *11*, 246–252. [CrossRef]
64. Ganai, S.A.; Farooq, Z.; Banday, S.; Altaf, M. In Silico Approaches for Investigating the Binding Propensity of Apigenin and Luteolin Against Class I HDAC Isoforms. *Future Med. Chem.* **2018**, *10*, 1925–1945. [CrossRef]
65. Wirries, A.; Breyer, S.; Quint, K.; Schobert, R.; Ocker, M. Thymoquinone Hydrazone Derivatives Cause Cell Cycle Arrest in p53-Competent Colorectal Cancer Cells. *Exp. Ther. Med.* **2010**, *1*, 369–375. [CrossRef] [PubMed]
66. Gali-Muhtasib, H.; Kuester, D.; Mawrin, C.; Bajbouj, K.; Diestel, A.; Ocker, M.; Schneider-Stock, R. Thymoquinone Triggers Inactivation of the Stress Response Pathway Sensor CHEK1 and Contributes to Apoptosis in Colorectal Cancer Cells. *Cancer Res.* **2008**, *68*, 5609–5618. [CrossRef] [PubMed]
67. Kundu, J.; Choi, B.Y.; Jeong, C.-H.; Kundu, J.K.; Chun, K.-S. Thymoquinone Induces Apoptosis in Human Colon Cancer HCT116 Cells Through Inactivation of STAT3 by Blocking JAK2- and Src-Mediated Phosphorylation of EGF Receptor Tyrosine Kinase. *Oncol. Rep.* **2014**, *32*, 821–828. [CrossRef] [PubMed]
68. Motaghed, M.; Al-Hassan, F.M.; Hamid, S.S. Cellular responses with thymoquinone treatment in human breast cancer cell line MCF-7. *Pharmacogn. Res.* **2013**, *5*, 200–206. [CrossRef]
69. Woo, C.C.; Hsu, A.; Kumar, A.P.; Sethi, G.; Tan, K.H. Thymoquinone inhibits tumor growth and induces apoptosis in a breast cancer xenograft mouse model: The role of p38 MAPK and ROS. *PLoS ONE* **2013**, *8*, e75356. [CrossRef] [PubMed]
70. Arafa, E.-S.A.; Zhu, Q.; Shah, Z.I.; Wani, G.; Barakat, B.M.; Racoma, I.; Wani, A.A. Thymoquinone up-regulates PTEN expression and induces apoptosis in doxorubicin-resistant human breast cancer cells. *Mutat. Res.* **2011**, *706*, 28–35. [CrossRef] [PubMed]
71. Chehl, N.; Chipitsyna, G.; Gong, Q.; Yeo, C.J.; Arafat, H.A. Anti-inflammatory effects of the Nigella sativa seed extract, thymoquinone, in pancreatic cancer cells. *HPB* **2009**, *11*, 373–381. [CrossRef] [PubMed]
72. Zhu, W.-Q.; Wang, J.; Guo, X.-F.; Liu, Z.; Dong, W.-G. Thymoquinone inhibits proliferation in gastric cancer via the STAT3 pathway in vivo and in vitro. *World J. Gastroenterol.* **2016**, *22*, 4149–4159. [CrossRef]
73. Ahmad, I.; Muneer, K.M.; Tamimi, I.A.; Chang, M.E.; Ata, M.O.; Yusuf, N. Thymoquinone suppresses metastasis of melanoma cells by inhibition of NLRP3 inflammasome. *Toxicol. Appl. Pharmacol.* **2013**, *270*, 70–76. [CrossRef]
74. Woo, C.C.; Kumar, A.P.; Sethi, G.; Tan, K.H. Thymoquinone: Potential cure for inflammatory disorders and cancer. *Biochem. Pharmacol.* **2012**, *83*, 443–451. [CrossRef]
75. Roepke, M.; Diestel, A.; Bajbouj, K.; Walluscheck, D.; Schonfeld, P.; Roessner, A.; Gali-Muhtasib, H. Lack of p53 augments thymoquinone-induced apoptosis and caspase activation in doxorubicin-resistant liver cancer cells. *Oncogene* **2007**, *26*, 3493–3503.
76. Gali-Muhtasib, H.; Diab-Assaf, M.; Boltze, C.; Al-Hmaira, J.; Hartig, R.; Roessner, A.; Schneider-Stock, R. Thymoquinone extracted from black seed triggers apoptotic cell death in human colorectal cancer cells via a p53-dependent mechanism. *Int. J. Oncol.* **2004**, *25*, 857–866.
77. El-Mahdy, M.A.; Zhu, Q.; Wang, Q.E.; Wani, G.; Wani, A.A. Thymoquinone induces apoptosis through activation of caspase-3 and caspase-8 and mitochondrial events in p53-null myeloblastic leukemia HL-60 cells. *Int. J. Cancer* **2005**, *117*, 409–417. [CrossRef]
78. Sethi, G.; Ahn, K.S.; Aggarwal, B.B. Targeting nuclear factor-κB activation pathway by thymoquinone: Role in suppression of antiapoptotic gene products and enhancement of apoptosis. *Mol. Cancer Res.* **2008**, *6*, 1059–1070. [CrossRef]
79. Kaseb, A.O.; Chinnakannu, K.; Chen, D.; Sivanandam, A.; Tejwani, S.; Menon, M.; Dou, Q.P. Androgen receptor and E2F-1 targeted thymoquinone therapy for hormone-refractory prostate cancer. *Cancer Res.* **2007**, *67*, 7782–7788. [CrossRef] [PubMed]
80. Nagi, M.N.; Al-Shabanah, O.A. The potential role of thymoquinone (TQ) in the treatment of the oxidative stress in STZ diabetic rats. *Res. Commun. Mol. Pathol. Pharmacol.* **1999**, *104*, 211–224.
81. Yi, T.; Cho, S.G.; Yi, Z.; Pang, X.; Rodriguez, M.; Wang, Y.; Liu, M. Thymoquinone inhibits tumor angiogenesis and tumor growth through suppressing AKT and extracellular signal-regulated kinase signaling pathways. *Mol. Cancer Ther.* **2008**, *7*, 1789–1796. [CrossRef]
82. Mu, L.; Fang, Q.; Chen, X. Thymoquinone induces apoptosis in PC-3 prostate cancer cells through mitochondrial-dependent apoptosis pathway. *Nat. Prod. Commun.* **2014**, *9*, 325–328.
83. Gali-Muhtasib, H.; Roessner, A.; Schneider-Stock, R. Thymoquinone: A promising anti-cancer drug from natural sources. *Int. J. Biochem. Cell Biol.* **2006**, *38*, 1249–1253. [CrossRef] [PubMed]
84. Banerjee, S.; Padhye, S.; Azmi, A.; Wang, Z.; Philip, P.A.; Kucuk, O.; Sarkar, F.H.; Mohammad, R.M. Review on molecular and therapeutic potential of thymoquinone in cancer. *Nutr. Cancer* **2010**, *62*, 938–946. [CrossRef]
85. Ravindran, J.; Nair, H.B.; Aggarwal, B.B. Thymoquinone inhibits NF-κB signaling in human multiple myeloma cells and suppresses osteoclastogenesis. *Clin. Cancer Res.* **2009**, *15*, 273–282.
86. Meral, I.; Pala, M.; Akbas, F.; Ustunova, S.; Yildiz, C.; Demirel, M. Effects of thymoquinone on liver miRNAs and oxidative stress in Ehrlich acid mouse solid tumor model. *Biotech. Histochem.* **2018**, *93*, 301–308. [CrossRef] [PubMed]
87. Helmy, S.A.; El-Mesery, M.; El-Karef, A.; Eissa, L.A.; El Gayar, A.M. Thymoquinone upregulates TRAIL/TRAILR2 expression and attenuates hepatocellular carcinoma in vivo model. *Life Sci.* **2019**, *233*, 116673. [CrossRef] [PubMed]

88. Shabani, H.; Karami, M.H.; Kolour, J.; Sayyahi, Z.; Parvin, M.A.; Soghala, S.; Baghini, S.S.; Mardasi, M.; Chopani, A.; Moulavi, P.; et al. Anticancer activity of thymoquinone against breast cancer cells: Mechanisms of action and delivery approaches. *Biomed. Pharmacother.* **2023**, *165*, 114972. [CrossRef] [PubMed]
89. Talib, W.H. Regressions of breast carcinoma syngraft following treatment with piperine in combination with thymoquinone. *Sci. Pharm.* **2017**, *85*, 27. [CrossRef] [PubMed]
90. Dehghani, H.; Hashemi, M.; Entezari, M.; Mohsenifar, A. The comparison of anticancer activity of thymoquinone and nanothymoquinone on human breast adenocarcinoma. *Iran. J. Pharm. Res.* **2015**, *14*, 539. [PubMed]
91. Relles, D.; Chipitsyna, G.I.; Gong, Q.; Yeo, C.J.; Arafat, H.A. Thymoquinone promotes pancreatic cancer cell death and reduction of tumor size through combined inhibition of histone deacetylation and induction of histone acetylation. *Adv. Prev. Med.* **2016**, *2016*, 1407840. [CrossRef] [PubMed]
92. Peng, L.; Liu, A.; Shen, Y.; Xu, H.Z.; Yang, S.Z.; Ying, X.Z.; Liao, W.; Liu, H.X.; Lin, Z.Q.; Chen, Q.Y.; et al. Antitumor and anti-angiogenesis effects of thymoquinone on osteosarcoma through the NF-κB pathway. *Oncol. Rep.* **2013**, *29*, 571–578. [CrossRef] [PubMed]
93. Zhang, M.; Du, H.; Huang, Z.; Zhang, P.; Yue, Y.; Wang, W.; Liu, W.; Zeng, J.; Ma, J.; Chen, G.; et al. Thymoquinone induces apoptosis in bladder cancer cell via endoplasmic reticulum stress-dependent mitochondrial pathway. *Chem. Biol. Interact.* **2018**, *292*, 65–75. [CrossRef]
94. Sutton, K.M.; Greenshields, A.L.; Hoskin, D.W. Thymoquinone, a bioactive component of black caraway seeds, causes G1 phase cell cycle arrest and apoptosis in triple-negative breast cancer cells with mutant p53. *Nutr. Cancer.* **2014**, *66*, 408–418. [CrossRef] [PubMed]
95. Ng, W.K.; Yazan, L.S.; Ismail, M. Thymoquinone from Nigella sativa was more potent than cisplatin in eliminating of SiHa cells via apoptosis with down-regulation of Bcl-2 protein. *Toxicol. Vitro.* **2011**, *25*, 1392–1398. [CrossRef] [PubMed]
96. Krylova, N.G.; Drobysh, M.S.; Semenkova, G.N.; Kulahava, T.A.; Pinchuk, S.V.; Shadyro, O.I. Cytotoxic and antiproliferative efects of thymoquinone on rat C6 glioma cells depend on oxidative stress. *Mol. Cell Biochem.* **2019**, *462*, 195–206. [CrossRef]
97. ElKhoely, A.; Hafez, H.F.; Ashmawy, A.M.; Badary, O.; Abdelaziz, A.; Mostafa, A.; Shouman, S.A. Chemopreventive and therapeutic potentials of thymoquinone in HepG2 cells: Mechanistic perspectives. *J. Nat. Med.* **2015**, *69*, 313–323. [CrossRef]
98. Kou, B.; Liu, W.; Zhao, W.; Duan, P.; Yang, Y.; Yi, Q.; Guo, F.; Li, J.; Zhou, J.; Kou, Q. Thymoquinone inhibits epithelial–mesenchymal transition in prostate cancer cells by negatively regulating the TGF-β/Smad2/3 signaling pathway. *Oncol. Rep.* **2017**, *38*, 3592–3598. [CrossRef] [PubMed]
99. Alshyarba, M.; Otifi, H.; Al Fayi, M.; A Dera, A.; Rajagopalan, P. Thymoquinone inhibits IL-7-induced tumor progression and metastatic invasion in prostate cancer cells by attenuating matrix metalloproteinase activity and Akt/NF-κB signaling. *Biotechnol. Appl. Biochem.* **2021**, *68*, 1403–1411. [CrossRef] [PubMed]
100. Lei, X.; Lv, X.; Liu, M.; Yang, Z.; Ji, M.; Guo, X.; Dong, W. Thymoquinone inhibits growth and augments 5-fuorouracil-induced apoptosis in gastric cancer cells both in vitro and in vivo. *Biochem. Biophys. Res. Commun.* **2012**, *417*, 864–868. [CrossRef]
101. Ma, J.; Hu, X.; Li, J.; Wu, D.; Lan, Q.; Wang, Q.; Tian, S.; Dong, W. Enhancing conventional chemotherapy drug cisplatin-induced antitumor efects on human gastric cancer cells both in vitro and in vivo by thymoquinone targeting PTEN gene. *Oncotarget* **2017**, *8*, 85926. [CrossRef] [PubMed]
102. El-Baba, C.; Mahadevan, V.; Fahlbusch, F.B.; Rau, T.T.; Gali-Muhtasib, H.; Schneider-Stock, R. Thymoquinone-induced conformational changes of PAK1 interrupt prosurvival MEK–ERK signaling in colorectal cancer. *Mol. Cancer.* **2014**, *13*, 201. [CrossRef]
103. Chen, M.C.; Lee, N.H.; Hsu, H.H.; Ho, T.J.; Tu, C.C.; Chen, R.J.; Lin, Y.M.; Viswanadha, V.P.; Kuo, W.W.; Huang, C.Y. Inhibition of NF-κB and metastasis in irinotecan (CPT-11)-resistant LoVo colon cancer cells by thymoquinone via JNK and p38. *Environ. Toxicol.* **2017**, *32*, 669–678. [CrossRef]
104. Chen, M.-C.; Lee, N.-H.; Hsu, H.-H.; Ho, T.-J.; Tu, C.-C.; Hsieh, D.J.-Y.; Lin, Y.-M.; Chen, L.-M.; Kuo, W.-W.; Huang, C.-Y. Thymoquinone induces caspase-independent, autophagic cell death in CPT-11-resistant lovo colon cancer via mitochondrial dysfunction and activation of JNK and p38. *J. Agric. Food Chem.* **2015**, *63*, 1540. [CrossRef]
105. Mu, G.G.; Zhang, L.L.; Li, H.Y.; Liao, Y.; Yu, H.G. Thymoquinone pretreatment overcomes the insensitivity and potentiates the antitumor efect of gemcitabine through abrogation of Notch1, PI3K/Akt/mTOR regulated signaling pathways in pancreatic cancer. *Digest Dis. Sci.* **2015**, *60*, 1067–1080. [CrossRef] [PubMed]
106. Patel, S.S.; Acharya, A.; Ray, R.S.; Agrawal, R.; Raghuwanshi, R.; Jain, P. Cellular and molecular mechanisms of curcumin in prevention and treatment of disease. *Crit. Rev. Food Sci. Nutr.* **2020**, *60*, 887–939. [CrossRef] [PubMed]
107. Samarghandian, S.; Azimi-Nezhad, M.; Farkhondeh, T. Thymoquinone-induced antitumor and apoptosis in human lung adenocarcinoma cells. *J. Cell Physiol.* **2019**, *234*, 10421–10431. [CrossRef] [PubMed]
108. Acharya, B.R.; Chatterjee, A.; Ganguli, A.; Bhattacharya, S.; Chakrabarti, G. Thymoquinone inhibits microtubule polymerization by tubulin binding and causes mitotic arrest following apoptosis in A549 cells. *Biochimie* **2014**, *97*, 78–91. [CrossRef] [PubMed]
109. Wilson, A.J.; Saskowski, J.; Barham, W.; Yull, F.; Khabele, D. Thymoquinone enhances cisplatin-response through direct tumor efects in a syngeneic mouse model of ovarian cancer. *J. Ovarian Res.* **2015**, *8*, 46. [CrossRef] [PubMed]
110. Liu, X.; Dong, J.; Cai, W.; Pan, Y.; Li, R.; Li, B. The efect of thymoquinone on apoptosis of SK-OV-3 ovarian cancer cell by regulation of Bcl-2 and Bax. *Int. J. Gynecol. Cancer.* **2017**, *27*, 1596–1601. [CrossRef] [PubMed]

111. Sundaravadivelu, S.; Raj, S.K.; Kumar, B.S.; Arumugamand, P.; Ragunathan, P.P. Reverse Screening Bioinformatics Approach to Identify Potential Anti Breast Cancer Targets Using Thymoquinone from Neutraceuticals Black Cumin Oil. *Anti-Cancer Agents Med. Chem.* **2019**, *19*, 599–609. [CrossRef] [PubMed]
112. Nithya, G.; Ilakkia, A.; Sakthisekaran, D. In silico docking studies on the anti-cancer effect of thymoquinone on interaction with phosphatase and tensin homolog located on chromosome 10q23: A regulator of PI3K/AKT pathway. *Asian J. Pharm. Clin. Res.* **2015**, *8*, 192–195.
113. Durga, B.; Julius, A. In-Silico Docking studies of thymoquinone as potential anti-cancer drug target on Lung Cancer Cells. *Eur. J. Mol. Clin. Med.* **2020**, *7*, 1706–1716.
114. Choi, E.J.; Kim, G.H. Apigenin induces apoptosis through a mitochondria/caspase-pathway in human breast cancer MDA-MB-453 cells. *J. Clin. Biochem. Nutr.* **2009**, *44*, 260–265. [CrossRef]
115. Guan, H.; Luo, W.; Bao, B.; Cao, Y.; Cheng, F.; Yu, S.; Fan, Q.; Zhang, L.; Wu, Q.; Shan, M. A Comprehensive Review of Rosmarinic Acid: From Phytochemistry to Pharmacology and Its New Insight. *Molecules* **2022**, *27*, 3292. [CrossRef] [PubMed]
116. Salehi, B.; Venditti, A.; Sharifi-Rad, M.; Kręgiel, D.; Sharifi-Rad, J.; Durazzo, A.; Lucarini, M.; Santini, A.; Souto, E.B.; Novellino, E.; et al. The Therapeutic Potential of Apigenin. *Int. J. Mol. Sci.* **2019**, *20*, 1305. [CrossRef]
117. Talib, W.H.; Alsalahat, I.; Daoud, S.; Abutayeh, R.F.; Mahmod, A.I. Plant-Derived Natural Products in Cancer Research: Extraction, Mechanism of Action, and Drug Formulation. *Molecules* **2020**, *25*, 5319. [CrossRef] [PubMed]
118. Rahmani, A.H.; Alsahli, M.A.; Almatroudi, A.; Almogbel, M.A.; Khan, A.A.; Anwar, S.; Almatroodi, S.A. The Potential Role of Apigenin in Cancer Prevention and Treatment. *Molecules* **2022**, *27*, 6051. [CrossRef] [PubMed]
119. Thomas, J.V.; Mohan, M.E.; Prabhakaran, P.; Maliakel, B.; Krishnakumar, I.M. A phase I clinical trial to evaluate the safety of thymoquinone-rich black cumin oil (BlaQmax®) on healthy subjects: Randomized, double-blinded, placebo-controlled prospective study. *Toxicol. Rep.* **2022**, *9*, 999–1007. [CrossRef]
120. Tavakkoli, A.; Mahdian, V.; Razavi, B.M.; Hosseinzadeh, H. Review on Clinical Trials of Black Seed (Nigella sativa) and Its Active Constituent, Thymoquinone. *J. Pharmacopunct.* **2017**, *20*, 179–193. [CrossRef]
121. Clinical and Immunohisochemical Evaluation of Chemopreventive Effect of Thymoquinone on Oral Potenti. Available online: https://ctv.veeva.com/study/clinical-and-immunohisochemical-evaluation-of-chemopreventive-effect-of-thymoquinone-on-oral-potenti (accessed on 16 May 2024).
122. ClinicalTrials.gov Identifier: NCT03208790. Available online: https://classic.clinicaltrials.gov/ct2/show/NCT03208790 (accessed on 16 May 2024).
123. ClinicalTrials.gov Study: NCT03208790. Available online: https://clinicaltrials.gov/study/NCT03208790?intr=Thymoquinone&cond=Cancer&limit=100&page=1&rank=1 (accessed on 16 May 2024).

MDPI AG
Grosspeteranlage 5
4052 Basel
Switzerland
Tel.: +41 61 683 77 34

Current Issues in Molecular Biology Editorial Office
E-mail: cimb@mdpi.com
www.mdpi.com/journal/cimb

www.ingramcontent.com/pod-product-compliance
Lightning Source LLC
Chambersburg PA
CBHW061501210926
51850CB00008B/1781